D0911289

Oxf
Mu
Nursing

DATE DUE

Oxford Handbooks in Nursing

Oxford Handbook of Midwifery
Janet Medforth, Susan Battersby, Maggie Evans, Beverley Marsh, and Angela Walker

Oxford Handbook of Mental Health Nursing
Edited by Patrick Callaghan and Helen Waldock

Oxford Handbook of Children's and Young People's Nursing
Edited by Edward Alan Glasper, Gillian McEwing, and Jim Richardson

Oxford Handbook of Nurse Prescribing
Sue Beckwith and Penny Franklin

Oxford Handbook of Cancer Nursing
Edited by Mike Tadman and Dave Roberts

Oxford Handbook of Cardiac Nursing
Edited by Kate Johnson and Karen Rawlings-Anderson

Oxford Handbook of Primary Care Nursing
Edited by Vari Drennan and Claire Goodman

Oxford Handbook of Gastrointestinal Nursing
Edited by Christine Norton, Julia Williams, Claire Taylor, Annmarie Nunwa, and Kathy Whayman

Oxford Handbook of Respiratory Nursing
Terry Robinson and Jane Scullion

Oxford Handbook of Nursing Older People
Beverley Tabernacle, Marie Barnes, and Annette Jinks

Oxford Handbook of Clinical Skills in Adult Nursing
Jacqueline Randle, Frank Coffey, and Martyn Bradbury

Oxford Handbook of Emergency Nursing
Robert Crouch, Alan Charters, Mary Dawood, and Paula O'Gara

Oxford Handbook of Dental Nursing
K Seymour, DYD Samarawickrama, EC Boon, RL Parr

Oxford Handbook of Diabetes Nursing
Lorraine Avery, Sue Beckwith, Janet Sumner

Oxford Handbook of Musculoskeletal Nursing
Susan Oliver

Oxford Handbook of Women's Health Nursing
Ali Kubba, Sunanda Gupta, and Debra Holloway

Oxford Handbook of Perioperative Practice
Suzanne Hughes and Andy Mardell

Oxford Handbook of Critical Care Nursing
Sheila Adam and Sue Osborne

Oxford Handbook of Neuroscience Nursing
Sue Woodward, Cath Waterhouse

Oxford Handbook of General & Adult Nursing
Ann Close and George Castledine

Oxford Handbook of
Musculoskeletal Nursing

Edited by

Susan M. Oliver

Nurse Consultant Rheumatology FRCN, MSc RN
Chair of the Royal College of Nursing Rheumatology Forum
Chief Nurse Adviser for the National Rheumatoid Arthritis
Society, Barnstaple, UK

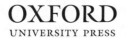

OXFORD
UNIVERSITY PRESS

OXFORD
UNIVERSITY PRESS

Great Clarendon Street, Oxford OX2 6DP

Oxford University Press is a department of the University of Oxford.
It furthers the University's objective of excellence in research, scholarship,
and education by publishing worldwide in

Oxford New York

Auckland Cape Town Dar es Salaam Hong Kong Karachi
Kuala Lumpur Madrid Melbourne Mexico City Nairobi
New Delhi Shanghai Taipei Toronto

With offices in

Argentina Austria Brazil Chile Czech Republic France Greece
Guatemala Hungary Italy Japan Poland Portugal Singapore
South Korea Switzerland Thailand Turkey Ukraine Vietnam

Oxford is a registered trade mark of Oxford University Press
in the UK and in certain other countries

Published in the United States
by Oxford University Press Inc., New York

© Oxford University Press, 2009

The moral rights of the author have been asserted
Database right Oxford University Press (maker)

First published 2009

British Library Cataloguing in Publication Data
Data available

Library of Congress Cataloging-in-Publication Data
Oxford handbook of musculoskeletal nursing / edited by Susan Oliver.
   p. ; cm.
  Includes index.
  ISBN 978-0-19-923833-0 (alk. paper)
  1. Musculoskeletal system--Diseases--Nursing--Handbooks, manuals,
etc. I. Oliver, Susan M.
  [DNLM: 1. Musculoskeletal Diseases--nursing--Handbooks. WY 49 O98
2009]
  RC925.5.O94 2009
  616.7'0231--dc22

                                                    2009009505

Typeset by Cepha Imaging Private Ltd., Bangalore, India
Printed in China
on acid-free paper through
Asia Pacific Offset

ISBN 978–0–19–923833–0

10 9 8 7 6 5 4 3 2 1

Foreword

Musculoskeletal conditions affect millions of people, adults and children in the UK today. Individuals who live with these conditions need a range of high-quality support and treatment; from simple advice on how to remain well and independent to complex, highly specialized advice and care. Musculoskeletal conditions can be self-limiting or cause longer-term disability. It is vital that we achieve better outcomes for people through an actively managed patient pathway delivered by knowledgeable health and social care professionals.

Nurses and nursing have a crucial role to play in the management of all musculoskeletal conditions and a highly skilled and educated nursing workforce will be able to make a significant difference to those living with the disease. Nurses are not just involved in hands-on nursing care, they are crucial members of the multidisciplinary team required to manage these conditions: they assess, prescribe, treat, address psychological and social support issues, and signpost to other specialists so that individuals and their carers enjoy a good quality of life with impairments from the disease process minimized wherever possible. Nurses are also a catalyst for ensuring service development and innovation in musculoskeletal care.

The profile of musculoskeletal problems has been raised considerably over the last 2 years with the publication of the Musculoskeletal Services Framework (DH, 2006). Our ageing population will further increase the demand for treatment of age-related musculoskeletal conditions like rheumatoid and osteoarthritis so it is vital that good quality educational resources are available for the workforce. This handbook will thus be an excellent resource for the education of nurses at all levels of training both pre- and post-registration and I am delighted to recommend this text to you.

Dr Peter Carter OBE, PhD, MBA, MCIPD
Chief Executive and General Secretary
Royal College of Nursing

A doctor's perspective

Nurses and practitioners are continuing to extend and develop their roles, with the focus on improving patient outcomes. The content and scope of this handbook provides a very welcome addition to the field of musculoskeletal nursing and complements and builds on similar handbooks that were previously developed for doctors. A 'must have' for all rheumatology units and all nurses involved in the care of patients with arthritis.

David G. I. Scott
Consultant Rheumatologist,
Honorary Professor of Rheumatology
Clinical Director Comprehensive
Local Research Network for
Norfolk and Suffolk
Patient Involvement Officer
Royal College of Physicians
Department of Rheumatology
Norfolk and Norwich
University Hospital

A patient's perspective

The National Rheumatoid Arthritis Society (NRAS) very much welcome publication of the *Oxford Handbook of Musculoskeletal Nursing* which will be a valuable reference tool for all nurses involved in the care of patients with rheumatoid arthritis (as well as other conditions). Specialist nurses play a pivotal role within the multidisciplinary team and are valued highly by patients who usually see the nurse specialist as the team member who provides emotional and educational support as well as ongoing medical care. In a changing NHS, where patient safety and governance issues are more important than ever, this Handbook will be essential for all nurses, and indeed other practitioners, involved in musculoskeletal medicine. Susan Oliver, as our Chief Nurse Adviser for NRAS, has recognized the need to raise the knowledge and expertise of nurses and practitioners in all care settings who provide care to those with a musculoskeletal condition. We warmly welcome this publication.

Ailsa Bosworth
Chief Executive
National Rheumatoid Arthritis Society
Joint Chair, Rheumatology Futures
Group Project

Preface

The book sets out to be a definitive quick reference resource for nurses but also highlights the significant improvements in management of many musculoskeletal conditions (MSCs) in the last 10 years. It is a useful stepping stone and quick resource for the newly qualified nurse who wishes to enhance their knowledge of MSCs but also supports nurses working in a range of care settings who have identified the significant number of patients who come through their department with a MSC but present for the management of other conditions.

A strong focus in developing the content for this book has been that of providing an evidence-base for nurses who wish to innovate or extend their role delivering high-quality care in a range of settings. The content includes walk-in clinics, nurse consultation, physical examination, joint injections, and treatment issues for the nurse prescriber to consider. A patient-centred and holistic approach is outlined to support conditions such as osteoarthritis, vasculitis, scleroderma, rheumatoid arthritis, gout, and back pain as well as discussing how to assess changes in health status using validated tools. Sexual issues, social and psychological needs, and symptom control are addressed with the majority of chapters including a 'frequently asked question' section.

In the last 10 years the evidence-base for MSC has increased significantly. In particular there is now a greater understanding of many musculoskeletal disease pathologies, safety and efficacy of differing treatment modalities, the social and psychological needs of the patient, and, ultimately, the long-term outcomes that can be improved as a result of multi-professional care. There is also a greater awareness of how we work to empower patients to make informed decisions.

The term 'musculoskeletal' covers a wide spectrum of conditions. Some of these may be considered mild and self-limiting but others have a long-term and significant impact upon the individual's quality of life and ability to function. To practitioners working in specialist fields 'musculoskeletal care' straddles traditional specialist fields of practice: that of rheumatology, rehabilitation, sports medicine, and orthopaedics. The future of health relies upon the patient understanding their treatment options and how to access the information or care that they require. The recognition of this approach has led to a stronger focus on services that refer to musculoskeletal services and it is for this reason the term MSCs has been used for this handbook.

Nurses in all care settings should find this handbook a useful resource as people with a MSC present in the community, attend clinics, present for hospital treatments, or are admitted with more than one comorbidity. If we are to provide high-quality care and optimize patient outcomes we need to know when to seek specialist support or have the knowledge and ability to do so.

This handbook focuses on the MSCs that nurses will see frequently and, importantly, highlights where their enhanced knowledge can provide a valuable contribution to improving patient care.

Acknowledgements

I would like to thank all the contributors for their support and excellent work. I would also like to acknowledge the Royal College of Nursing, the Rheumatology Forum Committee, and members of the forum of whom some have contributed to this book, but in all cases strive to improve the care of those with musculoskeletal conditions. The reviewers of this book have provided a valuable contribution and I would like to thank them all including the student nurses, specialist nurses, and medics. A special thanks must go to the team at OUP especially Jamie Hartmann-Boyce. Lastly a very special acknowledgement must go to husband Mike and my family who have had to endure this book writing process.

Susan Oliver
2009

The skeleton used in figures 2.1, 2.3, 4.1, 4.8, 4.10, and 4.12 is reproduced from Castledine and Close, *Oxford Handbook of Adult Nursing*, 2009, with permission from Oxford University Press.

Acknowledgements

Contents

Detailed contents

Contributors

Julian Barratt	London South Bank University and Melbourne Grove Medical Practice, London
Sue Brown	Royal National Hospital for Rheumatic Diseases NHS Foundation Trust, Bath
Maggie Carr	Ashford and St Peters Hospitals NHS Trust, Chertsey
Patricia Cornell	Poole Foundation Trust, Poole
Maureen Cox	Nuffield Orthopaedic Centre, Oxford
Kate Gadsby	Derby Hospitals NHS Trust, Derby
Alison Hammond	Centre for Rehabilitation & Human Performance Research, University of Salford, Manchester
Benny Harston	Hoveton & Wroxham Medical Centre, Norwich
Sheena Hennell	Department of Health, Merseyside
Diane Home	West Middlesex University Hospital NHS Trust, Isleworth
Dawn Homer	University Hospital Birmingham NHS Trust, Selly Oak Hospital, Birmingham
Mike Hurley	King's College London
Liz Hutchinson	Nottingham University Hospitals NHS Trust, Nottingham
Gill Jackson	Leeds Teaching Hospitals NHS Trust, Leeds
Garth Logan	Lisburn Health Centre, Lisburn
Janice Mooney	School of Nursing & Midwifery, University of East Anglia, Norwich
Michael H Oliver	Northern Devon Healthcare Trust, Barnstaple
Susan Quilliam	Cambridge
Sarah Ryan	Haywood Hospital, Stoke on Trent
David Scott	Norfolk & Norwich University Hospital, Norwich
Helen Strike	Bristol Royal Hospital for Children, Bristol
Anne Sutcliffe	Newcastle upon Tyne
Rachel Vincent	Centre for Rheumatology, Royal Free Hospital, London
Ann Wild	Worcestershire Acute Hospitals NHS Trust, Worcestershire
Helen Wilson	Centre for Rheumatology, Royal Free Hospital, London

Symbols and abbreviations

📖	cross reference
⚠	warning
☞	controversial topic
▶	important
▶▶	don't dawdle
↑	increase/d
↓	decrease/d
♂	male
♀	female
🖰	website
1°	primary
2°	secondary
<	less than
>	greater than
∴	therefore
~	approximately
ACA	anti-centromere antibody
ACJ	acromioclavicular joint
ACL	anterior cruciate ligament
ACS	acute compartment syndrome
ADL	activities of daily living
AHI	Arthritis Helplessness Index
ALP	alkaline phosphatase
ANA	anti-nuclear antibody
ANCA	anti-neutrophil cytoplasmic antibody
ANF	anti-nuclear factor
anti-CCP	anti-cyclic citrullinated peptide antibodies
APS	anti-phospholipid syndrome
APTT	activated partial thromboplastin time
ARC	Arthritis Research Campaign
ARMA	Arthritis and Musculoskeletal Alliance
AS	ankylosing spondylitis
ASES	Arthritis Self-Efficacy Scale
AST	aspartate transaminase
AT	assistive technology
AZA	azathioprine
BASDAI	Bath Ankylosing Spondylitis Disease Activity Index

BASFI	Bath Ankylosing Spondylitis Functional Index
BAS-G	Bath Ankylosing Spondylitis Global
BASMI	Bath Ankylosing Spondylitis Measurement Index
BCG	Bacillus Calmette-Guérin
BMD	bone mineral density
BMI	body mass index
BNF	British National Formulary
BSSA	British Sjögren's Syndrome Association
BVAS	Birmingham Vasculitis Activity Score
C&S	culture & sensitivity
CAM	complementary/alterative medicine
c-ANCA	anti-neutrophil cytoplasmic antibody with cytoplasmic staining
CD	cluster differentiation
CHAQ	Childhood Health Assessment Questionnaire
CMCJ	carpometacarpal joint
CMP	clinical management plan
CNS	central nervous system
COMA	Committee on Medical Aspects of Food and Nutrition
cP	centipoise
CPD	calcium pyrophosphate deposition
CPPC	calcium pyrophosphate crystals
CRP	C-reactive protein
CRPS	chronic regional pain syndrome
CSF	cerebrospinal fluid
CSM	Committee on Safety of Medicines
CSS	Churg–Strauss syndrome
CT	computerized tomography
CTD	connective tissue disease
CTPA	computerized tomography pulmonary angiogram
CTS	carpal tunnel syndrome
CV	cardiovascular
DAS	Disease Assessment Score
DIP	distal interphalangeal
dL	decilitre/s
DLF	Disabled Living Foundation
DMARD	disease-modifying anti-rheumatic drugs
dRVVT	dilute Russell's viper venom time
DVT	deep vein thrombosis
DXA	dual energy x-ray absorptiometry
EA	enteropathic arthritis

ECG	electrocardiogram
ECHO	echocardiogram
EMEA	European Medicines Agency
EMS	early morning stiffness
ENA	extractable nuclear antigen
ENT	ear, nose, and throat
EPP	expert patient programme
ESR	erythrocyte sedimentation
FBC	full blood count
g	gram/s
GCA	giant cell arteritis
GGT	gamma glutamyl transpeptidase
GHS	General Household Survey
GI	gastrointestinal
GP	general practitioner
GPwSI	general practitioner with a special interest
H@H	Hospital at home
HA	hyaluronic acid
Hb	haemoglobin
HCP	healthcare professionals
HCQ	hydroxychloroquine
HCT	haematocrit
HLA	human leucocyte antigen
HRCT	high-resolution computed tomography
HRQOL	health-related quality of life
HRT	hormone replacement therapy
HTO	high tibial osteotomy of the knee
IA	intra-articular
ICP	integrated care pathway
IEP	Individual Education Plan
IJD	inflammatory joint disease
IL	interleukin
ILAR	International League of Associations for Rheumatology
ILD	interstitial lung disease
IM	intramuscular
IS	isotope scanning
ITP	idiopathic thrombocytopenic purpura
IV	intravenous
IVF	in vitro fertilization
JCA	juvenile chronic arthritis
JIA	juvenile idiopathic arthritis

JRA	juvenile rheumatoid arthritis
JSN	joint space narrowing
KCT	kaolin clotting time
L	litre
LASS	Local Authority Social Services
LCL	lateral collateral ligament
LFT	liver function test
LTC	long term condition
mcg	microgram/s
MCL	medial collateral ligament
MCP	metacarpophalangeal
MCV	mean corpuscular volume
mesna	2-mercaptoethane sulfonate
MI	myocardial infarction
min	minute/s
mL	millilitre
MMF	mycophenolate mofetil
MORE	Multiple Outcomes of Raloxifene Evaluation
MPA	microscopic polyangiitis
MPN	microscopic polyangiitis nodosa
MPO	myleoperoxidase
MRI	magnetic resonance imaging
MRSA	methicillin-resistant *Staphylococcus aureus*
MSC	musculoskeletal conditions
MSM	monosodium urate monohydrate
MSU	midstream specimen of urine
MTD	multidisciplinary team
MTP	metatarsophalangeal
NHL	non-Hodgkin's lymphoma
NHS	National Health Service
NK	natural killer
NOS	National Osteoporosis Society
NPSA	National Patient Safety Agency
NRAS	National Rheumatoid Arthritis Society
NSAID	non-steroidal anti-inflammatory drug
OA	osteoarthritis
OT	occupational therapist
PAN	polyarteritis nodosa
PCA	patient controlled analgesia
PE	pulmonary embolism
PFT	pulmonary function test

PMR	polymyalgia rheumatica
PPD	purified protein derivative
PPI	proton pump inhibitor
PRMP	Pharmion Risk Management Programme
prn	when necessary (pro re nata)
PROM	patient-reported outcome measure
Psa	psoriatic arthritis
PSA	prostate specific antigen
PSV	primary systemic vasculitis
PT	physiotherapist
PTH	parathryroid hormone
PUVA	psoralen plus ultraviolet A light
PUVB	psoralen plus ultraviolet B light
PV	plasma viscosity
RA	rheumatoid arthritis
RAI	Rheumatoid Attitude Index
RASE	Rheumatoid Arthritis Self-Efficacy scale
RBC	red blood cell
RCP	Royal College of Physicians
ReA	reactive arthritis
REMS	regional examination of the musculoskeletal system
RNS	rheumatology nurse specialist
ROAM	range of active movement
ROM	range of motion
RSI	repetitive strain injury
SaO2	oxygen saturation of arterial blood
SARA	sexually-acquired reactive arthritis
SAS	sulfasalazine
SC	subcutaneous
SD	standard deviation
SE	self-efficacy
sec	second/s
SEN	Special Educational Need
SENCO	Special Educational Needs Coordinator
SGOT	serum glutamic oxaloacetic transaminase
SGPT	serum glutamic pyruvic transaminase
SIGN	Scottish Intercollegiate Guidelines
SLA	Service Level Agreement
SLE	systemic lupus erythematosus
SLR	straight leg raising
SNRI	serotonin and noradrenaline reuptake inhibitor

SOB	shortness of breath
SPC	Summary of Product Characteristics
Ssc	systemic sclerosis
SSRI	serotonin-specific reuptake inhibitor
SUA	serum uric acid
TB	tuberculosis
TCA	tricyclic anti-depressant
TEA	total elbow arthroplasty
THR	total hip arthroplasty/replacement
TKR	total knee arthroplasty/replacement
TNFa	tumour necrosis factor alpha
TPMT	thiopurine methyl transferase
TPR	temperature, pulse, respiration
TSA	total shoulder arthroplasty
URTI	upper respiratory tract infection
US	ultrasound
UTI	urinary tract infection
VAS	Visual Analogue Scale
VDI	Vasculitis Damage Index
WBC	white blood cell
WG	Wegener's granulomatosis
WHO	World Health Organization

Introduction

Musculoskeletal conditions

There are >200 musculoskeletal conditions (MSCs) that affect all age groups from the very young to the elderly. MSCs are common and are generally referred to by the public as 'arthritis'—a term referring to disorders of the muscles, joints, bones, or connective tissues (Figs. 1.1, 1.2).

MSCs are also the major cause of morbidity throughout Europe, substantially affecting health and quality of life and causing significant costs to health and society.

Key facts about MSCs:
- Pain is the predominant feature and the main reason for seeking medical advice.
- Currently, individuals experiencing musculoskeletal symptoms constitute up to 30% of general practitioner (GP) consultations.
- In England and Wales, MSC are reported as the 2nd largest group (22%) receiving incapacity benefit.
- Some MSCs can be mild and self-limiting; others can involve ongoing treatment with cytotoxic therapies and significant reductions in life expectancy or affect long-term functional ability.
- Affect all ages but become increasingly common with ageing.
- One-quarter of adults in Europe are affected by longstanding musculoskeletal problems.
- Represent a major cause of physical disability.
- Numbers are set to rise with ↑ elderly and obese population.
- Evidence suggests that soft tissue and back disorders represent the most common types of patient self-reported pain and limited activity in the young and middle aged.

The major MSC that present a significant burden are outlined (Table 1.1).

The UK General Household Survey (GHS) has highlighted the significant unmet needs of individuals with joint pain as high level of self-reported joint pain are noted yet there continues to be the mistaken belief that 'nothing can be done' and thus many individuals fail to seek medical advice. There will be an ↑ need for specialist expertise in managing the MSCs where the prevalence ↑ with age (e.g. osteoarthritis (OA), gout, and osteoporosis). Nurses and allied healthcare professionals play an essential role providing:
- Key information and support to patients.
- Enhancing self-management principles to enable individuals to manage their symptoms effectively.
- Expertise must recognize conditions that require proactive management to optimize patient outcomes and improve functional ability and life expectancy.

There is a public health need to increase awareness of factors that can improve a 'bone healthy lifestyle' in the general population improving general health and fitness, reducing obesity and risks of trauma.

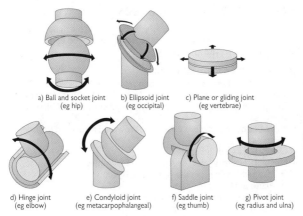

a) Ball and socket joint
(eg hip)

b) Ellipsoid joint
(eg occipital)

c) Plane or gliding joint
(eg vertebrae)

d) Hinge joint
(eg elbow)

e) Condyloid joint
(eg metacarpophalangeal)

f) Saddle joint
(eg thumb)

g) Pivot joint
(eg radius and ulna)

Fig. 1.1 Types of joints. Reproduced with permission of Clinical Skills Ltd.

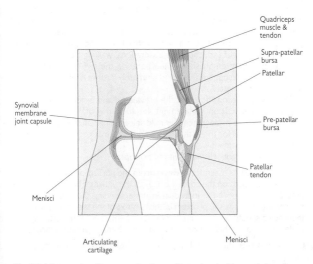

Quadriceps
muscle &
tendon

Supra-patellar
bursa

Patellar

Synovial
membrane
joint capsule

Pre-patellar
bursa

Patellar
tendon

Menisci

Articulating
cartilage

Menisci

Fig. 1.2 Joint capsule with surrounding tissues. Reproduced with permission of Clinical Skills Ltd. 📖 For a frontal view of the knee see Fig. 2.2, Normal joint and OA changes in the knee, p.9.

Classifying joint diseases

The way differing MSCs present, which group of tissues and structures are affected, and the persistence of the symptoms all add up to the complexity of diagnosis and management

Joint diseases can be classified as:

- Inflammatory diseases: e.g. rheumatoid arthritis (RA), ankylosing spondylitis (AS), psoriatic arthritis (PsA), juvenile idiopathic arthritis (JIA).
- Connective diseases: e.g. systemic lupus erythematosus (SLE), systemic sclerosis.
- Metabolic bone disorders: e.g. osteoporosis and associated fragility fractures.
- OA and related disorders.
- Non-inflammatory joint pain/soft tissue syndromes:
  - Mild self-limiting conditions (e.g. tennis elbow).
  - Acute or chronic.
  - Mono (single joint) or poly (many joint).
- Back pain or spinal conditions.
- Major trauma to joints and surrounding tissues (requiring surgical or medical management).
- Sports or occupational injuries e.g. trauma, sports injuries, mechanical disorders, occupational, or changes as a result of destructive joint diseases.

There are a variety of ways of classifying MSCs and referral pathways to diagnosis and treatment are usually based upon early decisions about those potentially requiring surgery (orthopaedic) or medical management (rheumatology). These referral pathways and management approaches have not always served patients well; for example, a patient may ultimately require knee replacement but may be wish initially to consider a conservative route of weight reduction and adaptations, walking aids, etc. There is now an increasing emphasis on incorporating the two disciplines more closely to improve patient flows and ultimately pathways of care using the term 'musculoskeletal'.

There is also recognition that the prevalence and incidence of MSCs is set to rise. The focus on management should be that of:
- Rapid proactive management for mild self-limiting conditions.
- Prompt referral for those that have conditions that require specialist advice and treatment.
- Encourage patient self-management principles.

A clear diagnosis is essential; however, from the nursing perspective clarity needs also to focus on the consequences to the patient. This should include how best to support the individual in understanding their condition and how best to manage the problem in the context of the individual's daily life. Individuals should be supported to enable them to be active participants in decisions about their treatment including self-management principles.

📖 Also see Education, social, and psychological issues, pp. 320–22.

Table 1.1 Musculoskeletal conditions

Inflammatory	Most common is RA. Others include JIA, diffuse connective tissue disorders, crystal related arthropathies, infectious arthritis, PsA
Metabolic bone diseases	Osteoporosis, Paget's disease, metabolic, endocrine, and other systemic arthropathies
OA	Idiopathic but also associated with aging. Secondary forms of OA and related conditions
Osteoporosis	Associated with fractures
Back pain and spinal disorders	Low back pain and diseases of the spine, trauma, mechanical injury, inflammation, infection, and tumors
Major musculoskeletal injuries including severe limb trauma	Resulting in permanent disability including fractures, blood vessels, and nerve injuries
Occupational musculoskeletal injuries	Work-related injuries: repetition, direct pressure, high force, vibration or prolonged constraint on posture
Sports injuries	Physical activity or sports-related injuries

Website resources

Patient information websites

- Arthritis Research Campaign for leaflets or website access:
  ⌁ www.arc.org.uk
- Abilitynet information on computing and disability:
  ⌁ www.disabilitynet.org.uk
- Benefit enquiries: ⌁ www.dwp.gov.uk
- BMJ Best Treatments: ⌁ www.besttreatments.bmj.com
- Citizen's advice bureau: ⌁ www.adviceguide.org.uk
- Community Legal Service Direct for guidance on work related issues:
  ⌁ www.clsdirect.org.uk
- Department of Health: ⌁ www.dh.gov.uk/
- Disabled Living Foundation advice on equipment and aids/advice:
  ⌁ www.dlf.org.uk/
- Family Planning Association: ⌁ www.fpa.org.uk
- Patient UK. Information on all conditions: ⌁ www.patient.co.uk
- Sexual health policy team: ⌁ www.playingsafely.co.uk
- The Arthritis and Musculoskeletal Alliance (ARMA) link for over 30 support groups and guidance on Standards of Care for those with MSC: ⌁ www.arma.uk.net
- The National Institute of Health and Clinical Excellence:
  ⌁ www.nice.org.uk
- The Royal British Legion Legionline. Financial social and emotion support to former service people and their dependents:
  ⌁ www.britishlegion.org.uk
- The Queen Elizabeth's Foundation Mobility Centre. Advice on assessment and driving instruction: ⌁ www.qefd.org.uk
- Volunteering in the community: ⌁ www.reach-online.org.uk

Patient organizations

- Ankylosing Spondylitis: www.nass.co.uk
- Antiphospholipid syndrome: www.hughes-syndrome.org.
- Back Care: www.backcare.org.uk
- British Sjogren's Syndrome Society: www.bssa.uk.net
- Carers UK: www.carersuk.org
- Fibromyalgia Association UK: www.fibromyalgia-associationuk.org
- Lupus UK: www.lupusuk.com
- Prodigy: www.patient.co.uk/pils
- Patient experiences of conditions: www.healthtalkonline.org
- Raynauds and Scleroderma Society: www.raynauds.org.uk
- National Rheumatoid Arthritis Society: www.rheumatoid.org.uk
- Scleroderma Society: www.sclerodermasociety.co.uk
- The British Pain Society: www.britishpainsociety.org.uk
- The Myositis Support Group: www.myositis.org.uk
- The National Osteoporosis Society: www.nos.org.uk

Employment information

- ACAS: www.acas.org.uk
- Age positive: www.agepositive.gov.uk
- College of Occupational Therapists: www.cot.org.uk
- Commission for Equality and Human Rights: www.cehr.org.uk
- Employment tribunals: www.employmenttribunals.gov.uk
- Ergonomics Society: www.ergonomics.org.uk
- New deal 50 plus: www.jobcentreplus.gov.uk

Assessment tools

- EuroQuol: www.euroqol.org
- Short Form 36 and Sickness Impact Profile: http://www.outcomes-trust.org/instruments.htm#SIP.
- Fatigue Tool (FACIT): http://www.facit.org
- Low Back Pain Tool. The Chartered Society of Physiotherapy (LBP tools): www.csp.org.uk

Osteoarthritis

Overview

Introduction

OA is a common MSC that is characterized by changes to the structure of a joint and the joints affected. OA can develop in any joint and is most commonly referred to as a syndrome of joint pain and changes in functional ability impacting upon the individual's quality of life. Joint changes are slowly progressive and will result in changes to synovial joints affecting changes to subchondral bone, loss of articular cartilage, formation of osteophytes, and thickening of the joint capsule (Fig. 2.1). This can result in mal-alignment of normal joint anatomy.

Higher numbers of ♀ populations have severe OA. Generalized and nodal OA is more common in post-menopause ♀ but can occur in those in their 40s.

Estimates of OA prevalence vary depending upon how OA is defined (clinically or radiographically) but there are ~8.5 million people in the UK with OA. Figures for those affected with OA are set to rise due to:
* ↑ growing elderly and chronic disease populations.
* ↑ obesity.
* ↓ physical activity.

It is unusual to see OA changes in those <40 years of age and the prevalence of OA does increase with age. ~half of adults aged >50 years will have radiographic evidence of OA, yet not all will be symptomatic. For example, 25% of individuals x-rayed demonstrate evidence of knee OA but only 13% are symptomatic. The prevalence of symptomatic radiographic knee OA in the UK for those >55 years is estimated to be ~10%. Symptomatic OA is the most common joint disorder in the elderly. See Box 2.1 for causes of OA.

Box 2.1 Causes of OA can be attributed to:

* 1° idiopathic.
* 2° to:
  * Local mechanical causes—post trauma, sports injury (e.g. rugby player).
  * Metabolic or systemic predisposition (e.g. familial OA).
  * 2° to pre-existing joint disease (e.g. RA or gout).
  * Haemachromatosis.
  * Hypermobility.

Further reading

Hakim A, Clunie G, Haq I (eds) (2006). *Oxford Handbook of Rheumatology*, 2nd edn. Oxford University Press, Oxford.

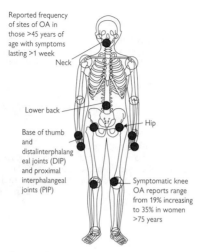

Reported frequency of sites of OA in those >45 years of age with symptoms lasting >1 week

Neck

Lower back

Base of thumb and distalinterphalangeal joints (DIP) and proximal interphalangeal joints (PIP)

Hip

Symptomatic knee OA reports range from 19% increasing to 35% in women >75 years

Fig. 2.1 Joints affected in OA.

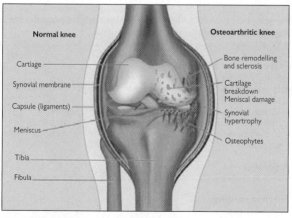

Normal knee

Cartilage

Synovial membrane

Capsule (ligaments)

Meniscus

Tibia

Fibula

Osteoarthritic knee

Bone remodelling and sclerosis

Cartilage breakdown Meniscal damage

Synovial hypertrophy

Osteophytes

Fig. 2.2 Normal joint and OA changes in the knee. Reproduced with permission from *Practice Nursing* (2008).

Clinical features and investigations

OA is a heterogeneous group of conditions sharing common features (such as anatomical changes) yet functional impairment, pain, and stiffness vary significantly and do not necessarily correlate with radiological damage.

The features of OA can be categorized as:
• Nodal generalized OA (tends to affect small joints).
• Erosive OA (uncommon): episodes of inflammation and erosive changes on x-ray.
• Large-joint OA.

In OA the most common joints affected are:
• Distal and proximal joints of the fingers and thumb (Fig. 2.3):
  • Changes at base of thumb (carpometacarpal, (CMC)).
  • PIP joints (Bouchard's nodes can sometimes be palpated).
  • DIP joints (Heberden's nodes can sometimes be palpated).
• The weight-bearing lower limbs:
  • Hip and knee.
  • Feet (commonly hallux valgus (bunion)).
• Spine (facet joints).

Signs and symptoms
• See Boxes 2.1, 2.2, and Fig. 2.1.

Diagnosis and investigations

OA is chiefly a clinical diagnosis requiring a thorough musculoskeletal examination, history taking, and patient reported symptoms (📖 see Assessing the pain, p.292). The presence of joint pain for most days of the previous month is used in many diagnostic criteria.[1]

Where diagnosis is in doubt, or in complex cases, further investigations may include:
• Radiological or MRI investigations.
• Synovial fluid analysis e.g. to exclude gout.
• Evidence of mechanical problems e.g. true 'locking of joint' or loose bodies—may require referral.
• Blood tests for evidence of inflammatory markers—erythrocyte sedimentation rate (ESR), C-reactive protein (CRP)—or urate.
• 2° OA as a result of other conditions e.g. haemachromatosis or Wilson disease.

Reference
1. Arden N, Cooper C (eds) (2006). *Osteoarthritis Handbook*. Taylor and Francis, London.

Further reading
NICE (2007). *Guidance on Osteoarthritis*. NICE, London.

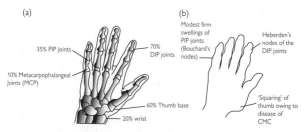

Fig. 2.3 The osteoarthritic hand. a) Joint involvement. b) Fingers and thumb affected by OA. Reproduced with kind permission from *Practice Nursing*.

Box 2.2 Signs on examination

- Mild cool effusions—non-inflammatory.
- Restricted, painful ROMs.
- Crepitus on movement.
- Stiffness of joint on movement —'gelling'.
- Tenderness on palpation around joint margin of affected joint.
- Changes at joint margins e.g. 'squaring' of OA base of thumb or presence of bony changes/thickening of joint on palpation.

Box 2.3 Symptoms of OA

The key symptom related to OA is that of joint pain usually in association with:

- Activity and relieved when the joint is rested—particularly in early phases of OA.
- In lower limbs, joint pain may be exacerbated by weight bearing.
- Pain is often accompanied by stiffness (lasting <30min) after periods of prolonged rest or inactivity. Often referred to as 'gelling'.

In addition, individuals may:

- Complain of 'crepitus' (grating sound) on movement.
- Report changes in functional ability—↓ in range of motion (ROM) and ↓ joint stability.

Hip and knee

Weight-bearing joints affected by OA commonly result in significant disability. Hip and knee OA show variable outcomes and rates of progression. Hip OA tends to show the worst overall outcome of the major sites affected by OA.

Diagnostic features for peripheral joint OA

- Persistent joint pain worse with activity.
- Age ≥45 years.
- Morning stiffness lasting no more than 30minutes—'gelling'.
- Absence of raised inflammatory markers—ESR, CRP, plasma viscosity (PV).

In addition the most common problems related to hip and knee OA include:

- Pain on walking/using stairs/prolonged standing.
- Getting in and out of buses or cars/getting up from low chairs/toilets.
- Adjusting footwear.

Hip OA

Radiological evidence suggests that >210,000 people have moderate-to-severe OA of the hips in the UK. Symptomatic radiographic hip OA reports vary between 5–9%. The course of the disease varies with some cases showing rapid deterioration and requiring prompt surgery to those with mild symptoms and slower progression (Box 2.4).

Knee OA

The prevalence of knee pain (lasting >1 week in the past month) is high in adults >45 years (19%) and in ♀ >75 years (35%). In the UK, >0.5.million people have x-ray evidence of moderate-to-severe OA of the knee.

The knee is complex with two joints (tibiofemoral and patellofemoral sharing a joint cavity) but three compartments (medial and lateral tibiofemoral and patellofemoral). Obesity is an important contributing factor in OA of the knee. The subtle changes in load bearing of the joint may be as a result of underlying disorders of the anatomy. If there are varus or valgus deformities the load distribution of the joint will be altered and will result in different stresses to the joint (see Fig. 2.4).

The most common presentation for symptomatic knee OA is combined tibiofemoral and patellofemoral changes including irregularly distributed loss of cartilage, sclerosis of subchondral bone, and osteophytes. The predisposing factors for 2° knee OA fall into two groups:

- Young ♂ with isolated knee OA—usually due to previous trauma or surgical interventions e.g. meniscectomy.
- Middle aged (predominantly ♀) with generalized OA.

Obesity is strongly associated with OA of the knee; see Box 2.4. The core management principles for OA are outlined in Advice and general management issues 🔲 p.22.

Box 2.4 Signs, symptoms, and investigations for hip and knee OA

Signs and symptoms for hip OA

- Pain and stiffness of hip particularly on activity (walking)—reports of pain in buttock, groin, front of thigh, or in the knee (20%).
- Changes in gait (antalgic gait)—Trendelenburg sign (tipping of pelvis before walking).
- Loss of internal rotation ↑ pain.
- Crepitus may be audible.
- Joint swelling cannot be detected on examination.
- X-ray are not indicated routinely but if done must be standing anterior–posterior view.

Specific investigations for hip OA

X-ray to:

- Examine degree of damage.
- Confirm diagnosis or identify contributing factors e.g. susceptibility following trauma, avascular necrosis.

Signs and symptoms for knee OA

- Pain and stiffness on mobilizing or weight bearing.
- Crepitus maybe audible.
- Joint changes may be palpable around the joint margin—osteophytes.
- Later stages may show signs of muscle wasting and valgus or varus deformity.
- Pain on climbing stairs or sensation of 'giving way'.
- Effusions may be present with 2° inflammatory process—aspirate from an OA joint with mild or no inflammation is viscous with low cell count, unlike inflammatory fluid which has a high cell count and is non-viscous.

Specific investigations for knee OA

- Crepitus or bony swelling may be present on joint margins

Further reading

Jordan KM, Arden NK, Doherty M, *et al.* (2003). EULAR recommendations 2003: an evidence based approach to the management of knee osteoarthritis: *Annals of the Rheumatic Diseases*, **62**, 1145–55.

NICE (2008). *Osteoarthritis.* NICE, London.

Zhang W, Doherty M, Arden N, *et al.* (2005). EULAR evidence based recommendations for the management of hip osteoarthritis. *Annals of Rheumatic Diseases*, **64**, 669–81.

Treatment of hip and knee OA

Treatment for hip and knee OA should be considered in the context of:
- A tailored assessment of risk factors relating to knee or hip OA:
  - Knee: obesity, adverse mechanical factors, physical activity.
  - Hip: as for hip plus dysplasia.
- General risk factors: age, co-morbidities, poly-pharmacy.
- Level of pain intensity and resulting functional disability.
- Location and degree of structural damage.
- Signs of inflammation e.g. joint effusion in knee pain.
- Patient needs and expectations.

Options to consider in the management of hip and knee OA

- Educating the patient in the condition and how to self-manage. Consider referral for self-management courses (􀤓 See Self-management, pp.324, 326).
- Walking aids (sticks) and use of insoles (wedged insoles for knee).
- Exercises e.g. aerobic, quadriceps, and muscle strengthening.
- Weigh reduction if obese or overweight.
- Analgesia:
  - First choice paracetamol for long-term pain relief but as part of a comprehensive treatment package (regular dosing regimen to maximum indicated doses). Refer to *BNF*.[1]
  - Consider topical NSAIDs or capsaicin (knee).
  - Additional pain relief may be required. This treatment option must be based upon a patient-centred risk assessment and contraindications/cautions and patient choice. Consider:
    —NSAIDs may be indicated for short-term pain relief. Prescribe at lowest effective dose for shortest duration. Refer to *BNF*.[2]
    —Compound analgesia or opiates may be indicated for some patients.
- Self-management aids (thermotherapy, walking aids, footwear, pacing, and muscle strengthening exercises) (􀤓 see Self-management, pp.324, 326).
  - If patient is taking glucosamine sulfate at a dose of 1250–1500mg once a day advise them to review benefit in pain relief at 3 months; if pain relief benefits not achieved advise stopping. Note: the strongest evidence has been based upon a daily dose of 1500mg; however, the BNF refers to licensed indication at 1250mg/day.
- Intra-articular (IA) steroid injection for treatment if a 2° inflammatory component present:
  - Knee—particularly if signs of effusion
  - Hip—injections should be guided by US or x-ray
- Joint replacement surgery for those who have symptomatic and radiographic evidence and where pain, stiffness, and reduced function impact on quality of life and fail to respond adequately to non-surgical treatments.
- Knee: a knee brace may reduce pain and improve function.
- Hip: osteotomy and joint-preserving surgical interventions should be considered in young adults who are symptomatic—particularly if presence of dysplasia or varus/valgus deformity.
- Hip: manual therapies (stretching of shortened muscles).

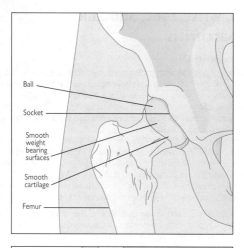

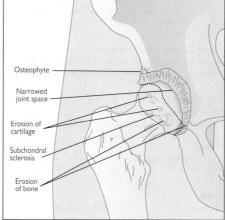

Fig. 2.4 OA of the hip. Reproduced with permission of Clinical Skills Ltd.

References

1. Joint Formulary Committee (2008). *British National Formulary*, 56th edn, section 4.7, Analgesics. British Medical Association and Royal Pharmaceutical Society of Great Britain, London.

2. Joint Formulary Committee (2008). *British National Formulary*, 56th edn, section 10, Musculoskeletal and joint diseases. British Medical Association and Royal Pharmaceutical Society of Great Britain, London.

Hand, wrist, foot, and ankle osteoarthritis

Hand and wrist OA

Symptomatic hand OA with radiographic evidence suggests is <3% of the population in the UK. Statistics show reported hand pain ranges from 12% in adults >45 years to 30% in adults >50 years. Many people fail to seek medical advice yet the impact and associated disability are significant, affecting many activities related to dexterity and hand function (📖 2° Functional issues, pp.304, 306).

Prevalence of hand OA is higher in ♀ and ↑ with age, yet has a good prognosis. Hand OA is associated with knee OA and obesity. Hallmarks of OA include nodes which may be initially painful (active) but usually settle with bony overgrowth (osteophytes) (📖 see Fig. 2.3, p.11).
- Heberden's nodes—DIP swelling on superior-lateral margins of joint.
- Bouchard's nodes—PIP swelling on superior-lateral margins of joint.

Poorly localized pain and tenderness around the wrist may be related to thumb OA. Crepitus may be present. In severe disease, deformities and 'squaring off of the base of thumb' can be seen. The loss of movement and joint deformity in the thumb and digits required particularly for pinch grip may create functional problems due to loss of manual dexterity. Loss of movement in the wrist and functional changes are similar to those outlined for the hand.

Hand and wrist OA core treatment issues
- Refer to core management advice on all OA treatments.
- Core treatment should be provided to those presenting with symptomatic OA of hand or foot.

Treatment should be individualized and considered in the context of:
- Patient anxieties, needs, and expectations.
- Level of pain, impact on functioning, and quality of life.
- Type of OA – nodal, erosive, traumatic.
- Localization.
- Severity of structural damage.
- Additional risk factors – age, work-related issues, comorbidities.
- See Boxes 2.5 and 2.6.

Foot and ankle OA
Ankle involvement is uncommon (related to previous injury e.g. previous fracture site); however, the forefoot is the main site for OA of the 1st metatarsophalangeal (MTP) joint. Hallux valgus (bunion) is extremely common in ♀ (Fig. 2.5). Relationship to generalized OA is unclear. The bunion is related to the use of modern footwear and is painful on walking or localized pressure.

📖 Also see Treatment options, p.24.

Box 2.5 Hand- and wrist-specific treatment issues

- Education and advice on avoiding mechanical aggravating factors.
- Topical NSAID or capsaicin cream.
- Joint protection—based upon expert opinion and limited research evidence:
  - Referral to occupational therapist for joint protection and assistive devices e.g. tap turners.
  - A wrist component to splints for base of thumb will improve efficacy.
- Local heat or cold applications (as an adjunct to treatments) encourage self-management strategies and can be safely used.
- Surgery may be beneficial for severe base of thumb if refractory to conventional treatment.

Box 2.6 Foot-specific treatment issues

- Advice on the use of insoles, and footwear with shock absorbing properties —limited evidence but cost effective.
- Topical NSAID or capsaicin cream.
- Referral for footwear advice may be appropriate depending upon functional issues and severity.
- Hallux valgus and hallux rigidus—surgery may be appropriate to correct deformities.

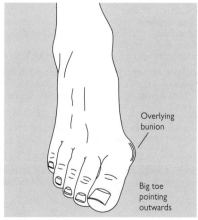

Example of bunion (hallux valgus) OA of foot.
ARC leaflet on OA.

Fig. 2.5 OA foot bunion (hallux valgus). Reproduced with kind permission from the Arthritis Research Campaign (ARC).

Neck and spine

Joints of the spinal column may show many of the changes evident in peripheral joints. If symptoms are not due to serious pathology, pain in spinal joint can be managed in the same way as peripheral joint pain.

Prevalence of spinal (back and neck) pain

- Back and neck pain are very common, about 60–80% of people will get spinal pain at some time in their life.
- Often starts for no apparent reason, or after everyday activities e.g. gardening, poor sitting or sleep postures, working environment.
- Recovery (or lack of) is unpredictable.
- <5% of people with spinal pain have a diagnosable condition, such as irritation of a nerve root (radicular pain) or spinal stenosis.
- Very few (<1%) have a serious medical problem.

Natural course of spinal pain

- Most spinal pain resolves within 6–8 weeks.
- Most people have long-term episodic periods of relatively little or no pain interspersed with acute 'flares' of pain.
- 15–20% develop chronic, disabling pain.

Examination and investigations

- Rarely establish a clear-cut cause of the pain.
- This often results in multiple, inconsistent, false diagnoses, inappropriate advice, anxiety, and undermining confidence in management and reinforcing unhelpful health beliefs.

Management

Reducing the likelihood of acute spinal pain becoming chronic and disabling is a key aim of management.

- Be honest about the limitations of investigations and diagnosis.
- Avoid confusing pseudo-diagnoses.
- Reassure people this does not mean they cannot be helped.

Individuals with one or more 'yellow flags' should be closely monitored and referred (ideally to a multidisciplinary, back assessment clinic) if their symptoms have not significantly eased within 6 weeks of presentation.

Yellow flags

The main reasons for developing chronic, disabling pain are the presence of psychological and social 'yellow flags'. (Box 2.7)

Red flags

People who present with a 'red flag' (Box 2.8) should be closely assessed and, if necessary, referred for investigation to eliminate serious pathology.

Box 2.7 'Yellow flags' for the risk for developing chronic pain and disability

- Belief that pain and activity are harmful.
- 'Sickness behaviours'—extended rest, fear-avoidance.
- Low or negative moods, social withdrawal.
- Treatment that does not fit best practice—extended bed rest, opiate use.
- Problems with insurance claims and accident compensation.
- History of back pain, time-off, other claims.
- Problems at work, poor job satisfaction.
- Heavy work, unsociable hours.
- Overprotective family or lack of support.

Box 2.8 'Red flags'—if present consider referring for investigation

- Age <20 or >55 years.
- Systemically unwell.
- Weight loss.
- Persistent night pain (lying more than sitting)—indicator to consider malignancy.
- Cancer, steroids, HIV or other significant past history.
- Widespread neurology (>one nerve root) or progressive motor weakness in the legs or gait disturbance.
- Cauda equina syndrome—indicators might include radicular pain, sensory loss, difficulty with micturition, faecal incontinence, saddle anesthesia.
- Thoracic pain.
- Violent trauma: e.g. fall from a height or road traffic accident.
- Constant, progressive, non-mechanical pain—capsular pattern.
- Persisting, severe restriction of lumbar flexion or structural deformity.
- Inflammatory disorders (e.g. AS)—pain worse at night, often accompanied by EMS.

Management of osteoarthritis spinal pain

Encouraging people to stay active is of the utmost importance. Consider:

- Advice to rest completely or take more than a few days off work increases the chance of long-term disability.
- People might take things easier for a day or two, but even during this time they must be encouraged to be gently active.
- Challenge fear-avoidance beliefs and behaviours that lead to muscle weakness, joint damage and pain, reduced activity, disability, and dependency.
- Advise about changing lifestyle to include participation in regular exercise and physical activity.
- Teaching 'rest–activity cycling' (interspersing bouts of exercise and activity with short rests).
- Suggest ways people can protect their back in the work/home environment provides control and avoids exacerbating their pain.
  - Apply heat (place a hot-water bottle wrapped in a towel on back for 5–10min, or take a hot bath) before or after exercise or unavoidable activities that increase pain (gardening, work).
  - Empathetetically explore psychological and social factors (e.g. relationships, work problems) that might contribute to problem.

Advice and general management issues

Overview

OA is a heterogeneous condition. Radiological evidence of OA may be evident yet the individual may be symptom free. OA presents a significant health burden with prevalence set to rise. It is essential for practitioners in all care settings to provide, at the minimum, core information and support to those presenting with symptomatic OA. Pain is the predominant feature and is usually the driver for seeking a medical consultation.

Presentation in the clinical setting can vary significantly, from individuals presenting with OA base of thumb, with an insidious onset of pain and minor functional difficulties right through to others presenting with severe and rapidly progressing joint pain that causes significant loss of function as a result of OA to the hip. There are a number of factors that need to be considered in the management of those with symptomatic OA. Management should be tailored according to:

- Disease presentation, severity, and treatment options.
- Impact of pain, stiffness, and functional changes to the individual.
- Psychological, social (including age, cultural background), and work-related issues.
- Prior understanding and knowledge of the condition and how to self-manage.
- Additional co-morbidities and the vulnerable—consider in treatment plan.

Evidence base behind treatment recommendations are usually based on studies and efficacy of one or two specific joint sites (often the knee joint); ∴ advice and evidence needs to be considered in the context of the specific joints (e.g. weight loss may not be appropriate for OA hand, although evidence suggests OA hand is linked to obesity). Expert opinion and systematic reviews of research evidence identify 'core' aspects of management that should be offered to every person presenting with signs of symptoms of OA.

Core treatment and patient-centred assessment

Decisions about core treatment and additional treatment needs must be considered following a thorough history taking and clinical examination, which should include a holistic assessment to identify the individuals' specific anxieties, needs, and expectations in the context of their condition (Table 2.1). The benefits of a patient-centred approach include:

- The informed patient can consider their pathway of care applying self-management principles with the potential to enhance self-efficacy.
- Improvement in patient outcomes and reduction in resource inefficiencies (↓ referrals and investigations).
- Positive health-seeking behaviours will enable individuals to seek information on their condition, treatment options, and how to access services.

Supporting these principles, verbal information must be reinforced by providing written information. Equally, individuals should be offered a review of educational needs as well as a review of treatment benefits.

Table 2.1 Holistic assessment of OA

Assessment	Consider	Effects on the individual	Consider
Disease	• Joint involved and severity of symptoms	• Joint abnormalities • ↓ muscle strength • ↓ functional ability	• Confirmation of diagnosis • Symptom control/functional ability
Pain	• Pain score • Distribution and description of pain experienced • Duration of pain	• ↓ quality of life • Fatigue, disturbed sleep • Difficulties in work and activities of daily living (ADL)	• Family responsibilities • ADL • Work-related factors
Knowledge/expectations; attitudes and beliefs	• Knowledge of condition • Patient expectations • Health beliefs and behaviours • Coping styles/self-efficacy • Cultural factors	• Ability to undertake positive health-seeking behaviours • Fear and anxieties about limitations • Beliefs about medications	• Educational needs • Concordance • Prior experiences in relation to health and illness • Relationship/support by significant family/friends • Cultural and religious beliefs
Psychological	• Anxiety and depression • Coping styles • Self-image • Perceptions of chronic disease status	• Negative mood, fatigue • Negative coping styles • Poor self-esteem	• Tailored information giving • Support groups • Information sharing and education • Management of comorbidities
Social	• Level of social need • Social support available—significant other	• Financial burden • Social isolation • Loss of independence	• Carer needs and abilities • Maintaining independence and functional ability • Community, voluntary or social services support

Treatment options

There are pharmacological and non-pharmacological treatment options available for OA. A combination of these treatment modalities should be offered to individuals presenting with symptoms, in the context of the joints affected and tailored to specific needs following a full holistic, patient-centred assessment (Fig. 2.6) (📖 also see Nursing issues pp.300, 346, and patient-centred care, pp.314). The level of treatment required and support necessary will vary according to:

- Disease severity and functional loss.
- Impact on the individual's quality of life and ADL.
- Other compounding factors for example co-morbidities.

Core treatments—pharmacological

- Paracetamol (prescribed up to 4g per day) should be regularly taken over 24 hours when pain relief is required. For those failing to achieve pain relief on paracetamol, check dose and frequency of administration (may be sub-optimal).
- Topical NSAIDs (knee and hand) or topical capsaicin cream.
- Where topical NSAIDs and paracetamol are ineffective consider:
  - An NSAID or cyclooxygenase (COX)-2 inhibitor (📖 see NSAID and COX-2, p.412)

  or
  - Addition of an opiate (rarely indicated in OA) after a thorough risk–benefit assessment of the patient has been made (caution in the elderly).

Core treatments—non-pharmacological

Individuals with symptomatic OA should be offered the following core advice and treatments:

- Information and education about the condition and how to self-manage symptoms including non-pharmacological advice and information on complementary therapies.
- Exercise advice—irrespective of age, comorbidity, pain, or severity of condition. Exercises should include:
  - Local muscle strengthening exercises above and below the affected joint, e.g. quadriceps for the knee.
  - General aerobic fitness.
- Consider referral to a self-management programme (e.g. expert patient programme (EPP)) if appropriate.

Review of treatment

For those whose symptoms fail to be managed using core treatments a prompt re-assessment should consider additional treatment options available to the patient.

A review of the individual's holistic assessment should also consider building on information and education about the condition with the aim of enhancing self-efficacy. Building the individual's ability to understand and manage their condition is not a 'one-stop shop' but an ongoing programme of information giving, tailored to their specific needs.

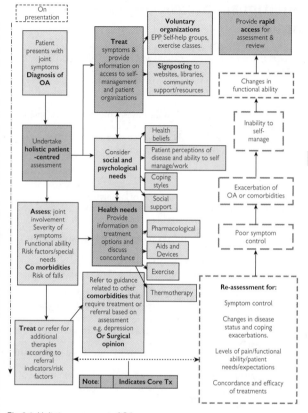

Fig. 2.6 Holistic management of OA

Additional pharmacological treatment options

◆ The use of NSAIDs (traditional and the newer generation of COX-2 inhibitors) may be required for those who have pain unresponsive to core treatments.

The use of these therapies must be considered carefully in the context of:
- The individual's specific gastrointestinal, renal, and cardiovascular risk factors.
- NSAIDs should be prescribed at the lowest possible effective dose for the shortest duration (e.g. to ease the pain during an exacerbation of symptoms). See Box 2.9 for NSAID prescribing advice.

In severe disease, NSAIDs may be required in addition to paracetamol or opiates.

IA joint injections
- For flare of joints—particularly if signs of inflammation (warm, effusion)—consider corticosteroid injections.
- ◆ Hyaluronic acid (HA)—limited evidence in knee OA.

Non-pharmacological options as an adjunct to treatment
- Exercise.
- Weight loss if obese (weight-bearing joints).
- Use of aids and devices/walking aids/insoles—braces may be beneficial in the presence of varus deformity (knee)
- Complementary and alternative therapies for pain relief:
  - ◆ Glucosamine sulfate (1250–1500mg daily for a period of 3 months) may be beneficial for pain relief.
  - ◆ Other compounds that are available include chondroitin sulfate (500mg bd).
  - Fish oil supplements (omega 3 fatty acids) have shown some benefit for pain relief.
- Use of cold packs or hot packs for topical symptom relief.
- Acupuncture may provide pain relief in the short term.

Physiotherapy treatments
- Stretching exercises (hip).
- Land based exercises (knee)—individual or class-based programmes.

Surgical interventions
- For those whose symptoms impact significantly on their quality of life and fail to be adequately controlled using non-surgical management, referral should be considered for joint replacement surgery.
- ◆ If a clear history of mechanical 'locking' arthroscopy or debridement may be required:
  - Arthroscopic lavage and debridement is not considered necessary for the treatment of general symptoms related to OA.
- Osteotomy and joint-preserving procedures should be considered for young adults in the presence of dysplasia or valgus/varus deformity.

Box 2.9 NSAIDs

Note: Consider NSAIDs and COX-2 as a continuum of drugs within one class with differing side-effect profiles (called NSAIDs). Refer to BNF.[1]

All patients:
- Consider prior treatments prescribed and side effects/benefits.
- Review renal function (U&E and electrolytes).
- Prescriptions for NSAIDs should be at the lowest effective dose for shortest duration. NICE recommend the co-prescription of a proton pump inhibitor (PPI) (including COX-2 inhibitors)[2] (📖 see NSAID and COX-2, p.412).
- Review efficacy, health status, and treatment plan.
- Identify risk factors related to changes in treatment e.g. risk of falls with opiates.

Assessment for NSAIDs
Risk factor:
- Age <65 years.
- No gastrointestinal risk factors.
- No cardiovascular risk factors.
- No age-related or renal risk factors.
Prescribing plan: standard NSAID with PPI at lowest possible dose for shortest duration.

Risk factor:
- All age groups.
- Gastrointestinal risk factors and no cardiovascular risks.
Prescribing plan: All NSAIDs are now recommended to be pre-scribed with a PPI (select appropriate therapy with a good GI profile +PPI).[2]

Risk factor: cardiovascular risk—on low-dose aspirin
Prescribing plan: select other analgesia prior to NSAIDs (e.g. opiates).

Risk factor: renal insufficiency or frail elderly.
Prescribing plan: consider compound analgesics (e.g. co-codamol 8/500) or opiates (e.g. tramadol hydrochloride) or other pain-relieving strate-gies where appropriate. (e.g. joint injections). *Caution:* opiates—lower doses in the elderly (opioid side effects).

References

1. Joint Formulary Committee (2008). *British National Formulary*, 56th edn, section 10, Musculoskeletal and joint diseases. British Medical Association and Royal Pharmaceutical Society of Great Britain, London.

2. NICE (2008). *Osteoarthritis: the Care and Management of Osteoarthritis in Adults*. NICE, London.

When to refer

OA is not one clearly defined disease but represents joint failure to a specific site, or sites, accompanied by the symptoms of pain, stiffness, and limited functional ability. In most cases of OA the deterioration is slow with gradual limitation as a result of the symptoms experienced. ~80% of all hip and knee replacements are attributed to OA. Symptoms may be constant or, more commonly, relapsing and remitting.

The first step in the pathway of care must include patient education about the condition and treatments available, encouraging the patient's ability to self-manage using a range of options that might include pharmacological and non-pharmacological pain-relieving strategies. The patient's reported symptoms, joint (or joints) involved, and length of time between relapsing and remitting symptoms will help inform the practitioner of treatment benefits.

In many cases, surgery may never be required although additional treatment options may be needed from time to time. For others, particularly those with load-bearing joints such as the knees or hips, the condition can rapidly deteriorate with the accompanying changes in functional ability. It is therefore important to recognize when to refer patients who do not gain benefit from early treatment. Specific scoring systems have been developed to aid clinicians identify those who need to receive prompt surgery (📖 see Chapter 7, Orthopaedic surgery, p.340).

Joint replacement surgery is expensive, although generally an effective intervention with improved postoperative outcomes.

Features that should prompt the nurse to consider referral for a medical/surgical opinion include:
- Joint pain that wakes the patient at night.
- Moderate-to-severe pain that is not effectively treated by pharmacological or non-pharmacological options.
- Moderate-to-severe functional impairment.
- Joint pain that places a significant burden on the patient e.g. work limitations or loss of independence—inability to undertake ADL effectively.
- Doubts about the diagnosis of OA or changes in symptoms, joints affected.
- Patients who may require psychological assessment, e.g. :
  - Inability to alter perceptions of pain despite treatment with a range of pharmacological options.
  - Patients who demonstrates anxiety, depression, or persistently rates pain as maximum score.

Integrated care pathways (ICPs) are often used to aid management and have particular value in surgical interventions such as total hip or knee replacements.

Factors that need to be considered prior to referral for a surgical intervention will include:
- Has the patient been offered other treatment options (pharmacological and non-pharmacological) without sufficient sustained benefit?
- General health and ability to undergo an anaesthetic.

- The patient's wish to undergo surgery.
- Absence of infections—particularly in or around surrounding tissues.
- The potential success of the proposed surgical intervention, e.g.:
  - Hip and knee replacement surgery will be negatively affected if patient is obese or is unable to actively rehabilitate postoperatively.
  - Patient expectations and ability to rehabilitate needs to be considered.

Equity of access for surgical interventions

Evidence has demonstrated that socially deprived groups, and some ethnic groups or minority groups (e.g. visual impairment) may be less likely to receive total hip or knee replacements.

Lack of access may be related to:

- Lower expectations of treatment access.
- Anxiety in seeking a medical opinion.
- Experiencing difficulty in articulating their needs to healthcare professionals.
- Have other health/comorbidity/risk factors that result in reduced referral for surgical opinion.

Frequently asked questions

I never really know what to do when someone comes into my clinic and start talking about their joint pain. I worry it might be something serious like septic arthritis

Joint pain can cover a multitude of problems including acute conditions such as septic arthritis. The first thing to do is to take a good clinical history and examine the joint(s) affected and compare it against the unaffected joint. Patients with septic arthritis usually have severe pain and will not want you to touch the joint; they may have rapid and dramatic onset of pain, with a tender swollen joint that is warm/hot to touch—however, there are cases that don't always fit this criteria so if the patient presents with the above symptoms, until you have developed your knowledge of joint diseases, ensure your provisional diagnosis is confirmed by the GP/physician. If OA is confirmed make sure you educate the patient about their condition and start the process of self-management.

What is the first thing I should think about when someone presents with newly diagnosed OA?

Undertake a patient-centred consultation (including an assessment of pain). You will then know how much of an issue the joint pain is to the patient and what they understand about their problems. Make sure you start the process promptly when giving information and, based upon the symptoms and joints affected, offer a number of practical tips (e.g. wearing sensible shoes) as well as non-pharmacological options (pacing) and pharmacological support based upon what the patient has already tried. Check the dosages and frequency of self-medications.

It seems to me there still isn't enough evidence to support many of the complementary therapies patients take for their OA—shouldn't I advise them not to take them?

Most patient wish to explore the option of taking complementary therapies and this may enhance their own perception of self-efficacy. You may be asked your opinion of treatment options—the most important thing to say is that although the evidence may not be sufficient for us to recommend such treatments, if they are going to take them they need to ensure they evaluate them carefully in relation to cost and benefits achieved. Importantly, you must encourage an open and transparent relationship so that they will report what therapies they are taking.

How can we help patients with their pain when the risks of NSAIDs and COX-2 therapies now means they can only have these prescribed in the short term and lowest effective dose?

Pain relief is a basic human right and we must ensure patients do get effective treatment. However, we often fail to encourage patients to take their simple analgesia (at maximum prescribed dose on a regular dosing regimen) so we should apply these principles together with an objective assessment of pain (for instance, using a visual analogue scale). Paracetamol can be an effective treatment for many provided it is prescribed at maximum doses and taken at regular intervals to maintain therapeutic levels. NSAIDs and COX-2 do have an important place in the treatment plan, but they must be used with adjunct therapies that will help to moderate the symptoms and reduce reliance on NSAIDs and COX-2s. Remember, topical NSAIDs/capsaicin cream may be of value particularly for small joints. However, the ultimate point must be to ensure that patients who need additional pain relief have an opportunity to make a fully informed decision about their treatment options based upon their individual risk factors.

Which patients should I refer to a self-management programme?

In reality all patients should have access to the same level of care, including self-management. However, it is helpful if you understand a little bit about the patient and their prior knowledge of the condition before asking them whether they would like to participate in a self-management programme. Key points to consider are:
- Able and willingness to attend a self-management course.
- Prior knowledge of the condition and treatment.
- Other comorbidities/conditions/medications.
- Level of social support or other voluntary support accessed.
- Their health beliefs/behaviours.
- Prior history of concordance with treatments/attendance of programmes.
- The individual's ability and wish to socialize/interact within a group setting.

These points are not discriminatory but are of value in considering:
- Which individuals might gain the most benefit from the course.
- When the option would be most positively received by the patient.

Osteoporosis

Overview

Definition

The World Health Organization (WHO, 2001) has defined osteoporosis as 'a progressive systemic skeletal disease characterized by low bone mass and micro-architectural deterioration of bone tissue, with a consequent increase in bone fragility and susceptibility to fracture'.

Clinical features

- Osteoporosis is largely asymptomatic until fractures occur.
- Hip and spine fractures are linked to ↑ mortality and all fractures may lead to disability and reduced quality of life.

Is osteoporosis an important problem?

In the UK, osteoporosis results in >200,000 fractures per year with the commonest ones occurring at the forearm, vertebral body, or femoral neck. Fractures at the spine and forearm are associated with significant morbidity but the most serious consequences arise in patients sustaining hip fracture, with a significant ↑ in mortality of 15–20%, particularly in elderly people.

- Health and social expenditure on the treatment of osteoporotic fractures in the female population was £1.5–1.8 billion in UK in 2000.
- With an ageing population and ↑ in fracture incidence, it is estimated that this may increase to £2.1 billion by 2010.

What happens during bone growth?

Bone mass and bone loss

- Bone is a dynamic tissue that undergoes constant remodelling throughout life; being metabolically active it is continually formed and resorbed by bone cells known as osteoblasts and osteoclasts. This remodelling allows the skeleton to:
  - ↑ in size during growth.
  - Respond to the physical stresses.
  - Repair structural damage due to fatigue or fracture.
- Up to 90% of an individual's bone mass is deposited during skeletal growth. This is followed by a phase of consolidation lasting for up to 15 years. Bone loss starts between the ages of 35–40 years in both sexes, with an acceleration of bone loss in ♀ in the decade following the menopause.

What are the important factors influencing bone mass and bone loss?

Heredity

Genetic factors account for as much as 80% of the variance in peak bone mass and also influence the rates of bone loss.

Activity
Activity is vital as the associated weight bearing and muscular activity stimulates bone formation and ↑ bone mass. Immobilization may result in rapid bone loss and a decline in activity with advancing age is likely to cause further bone loss.

Nutrition
- *Dietary calcium* intake is essential to ensure attainment of peak bone mass. The role of calcium and its effect on bone loss remains controversial but skeletal losses in older life may be accelerated by low calcium diets and evidence suggests that low calcium intakes in childhood and adolescence are associated with an ↑ risk of osteoporosis in later life.
- Prolonged *vitamin D* deficiency in childhood delays puberty and is likely to ↓ bone mass in relation to height attained. With advancing age, vitamin D absorption is reduced due to impaired percutaneous absorption and impaired metabolism. Low vitamin D levels cause ↑ parathryroid hormone (PTH) levels which can lead to ↑ bone loss in the frail older person.
- *Dietary intake* of protein, sodium, fluoride, caffeine, magnesium, vitamin K, and alcohol may also influence bone mass and bone loss, but their importance remains uncertain.

Body weight
Low body weight, associated with amenorrhea and eating disorders may result in ↓ bone mass. Bone loss is more rapid in postmenopausal ♀ with low body weight as there is insufficient fat tissue to convert androgens to oestrogens.

Hormonal
Gonadal hormones are probably the most important determinants of skeletal mass in ♀. Delayed menarche and persisting amenorrhoea may account for an impaired bone mass. Loss of ovarian function at the menopause leads to ↑ bone loss. There is an association between hypogonadism, low body mass, and ↑ bone loss in ♂.

2° causes
Bone mass and bone loss are influenced by a large number of 2° causes, including:
- Medications, particularly oral glucocorticoids.
- Malabsorption disorders e.g. coeliac disease.
- Renal disease.
- Cancer.

Diagnosis

Osteoporosis may go undetected as usually people are asymptomatic. However, an index of suspicion for osteoporosis should be considered in patients who have been admitted to hospital with a low impact fracture, particularly in sites such as the wrist, forearm, or neck of femur, or who have identified risk factors such as:

- Genetic predisposition, particularly parental history of hip fracture <75 years.
- Persistent amenorrhoea (>6 months) or early menopause.
- Malabsorption disorders, e.g. coeliac disease.
- Endocrine disorders, e.g. parathyroid disease.
- Low body mass index (BMI < 19).
- Prolonged use of glucocorticoids (over 3 months).
- Other factors including lifestyle issues e.g. poor dietary calcium intake, smoking, immobility, and high alcohol consumption levels.

Osteoporosis can be detected using:

- Dual energy x-ray absorptiometry (DXA) is the most widely used method of measuring BMD.
- X-rays will detect fractures and may suggest osteoporosis but are too insensitive to measure BMD.

What is a DXA scan?

- A scan that uses minimal doses of radiation and is a quick, non-invasive procedure.
- Provides measurements of BMD at spine and hip and may also perform total body and forearm measurements.
- Confirms the diagnosis of osteoporosis and allows the most appropriate targeting of treatment.

BMD measurements are expressed in standard deviation (SD) units. They are then compared to a reference range of young healthy adults with average bone density. The difference between this average and the reported BMD is then given as a T-score (Box 3.1). A Z-score is also calculated, this compares the reported BMD with an age-matched range.

Box 3.1 T-scores

- Between 0 and −1SD: normal.
- Between −1 and −2.5SD: osteopenia.
- Below −2.5SD: osteoporosis.

Will blood tests diagnose osteoporosis?
- Biochemical tests will not diagnose osteoporosis.
- Biochemical tests may help to identify 2° causes of bone loss, e.g. untreated thyroid disease.
- Specific serum and urine markers can measure bone turnover and may be useful in indicating rapid bone loss and also response to treatment.

Osteoporosis in premenopausal women and men

Osteoporosis in premenopausal ♀ may be as a result of low peak bone mass, ↑ bone loss, or a combination of the two. It may be attributable to an underlying cause but may also be idiopathic.

Common causes

- Menstrual factors include persisting amenorrhoea (>6 months) due to simple oestrogen deficiency or hypothalamic hypogonadism (related to either anorexia nervosa or exercise-induced amenorrhoea).
- The use of Depo-Provera®, particularly when commenced before skeletal maturity, may be associated with low BMD. May be reversible on cessation and restoration of normal menses.
- Underlying 2° causes include:
  - Inflammatory diseases e.g. RA.
  - Endocrine disorders e.g. thyrotoxicosis.
  - Conditions associated with malabsorption, e.g. coeliac disease.
- Glucocorticoid therapy is the most significant cause of drug-induced osteoporosis.
- Lifestyle factors such as:
  - Prolonged immobility—a potent cause of bone loss.
  - Dietary calcium intake in childhood and adolescence may also impact on peak bone mass.
  - Limited data on the relevance of smoking or alcohol intake in premenopausal ♀.

Management

- Investigation for an underlying cause (about 50% of cases may be 2°). If a cause is identified this should be treated appropriately.
- Patient education to increase understanding of osteoporosis and ways to optimize bone health. Reassure that absolute fracture risk is probably low. Occupational assessment and advice may be required.
- Calcium and vitamin D supplements may be required if dietary intake is poor.
- Bisphosphonates are the only licensed therapies for glucocorticoid-induced osteoporosis in premenopausal ♀. Treatment must be made on an individual basis only if the benefit is felt to outweigh the potential risk, e.g. if the patient is at an unacceptably high current risk of fracture.
- ⚠ Bisphosphonates should be avoided during pregnancy and lactation. Patient must be counselled on effective contraception to avoid pregnancy whilst taking treatment.
- Hormone replacement therapy (HRT) may be the optimal approach in hypogonadism.
- The use of teriparatide and strontium ranelate has not been evaluated in premenopausal ♀.
- Raloxifene should not be given to premenopausal ♀ as may increase bone loss.

Osteoporosis in men

Up to 20% of symptomatic vertebral fractures, 25% of forearm fractures, and 30% hip fractures occur in ♂. The lifetime risk for a 50-year-old white ♂ in the UK has been estimated to 2% for the forearm, 2% for the vertebra, and 3% for the hip.

♂ with low trauma fractures tend to have lower BMD, smaller skeletal size, and more disruption of trabecular architecture than ♂ control subjects of the same age.

Causes

Major causes with strong evidence:
- Hypogonadism.
- Alcoholism.
- Oral glucocorticoids.
- Following organ transplant.

Other factors:
- Low BMI.
- Smoking.
- Physical inactivity.
- Poor dietary calcium intake.
- Impaired vitamin D production.
- 2° hyperparathyroidism.
- Malabsorption syndromes.

Management

- Use of DXA to confirm osteoporosis.
- Reference ranges for BMD measurements in ♂ are derived from a smaller sample size than ♀; there is a similar inverse relationship between BMD and fracture risk.
- Investigations to exclude 2° causes. In addition to routine biochemical investigations, testosterone and gonadotrophins should be checked and prostate specific antigen (PSA) should be measured in those with vertebral fractures, to exclude possible malignancy.
- Advice on lifestyle measures to ↓ bone loss, including a balanced diet rich in calcium, weight-bearing exercise, smoking cessation, and moderation of alcohol intake.
- Bisphosphonates are the treatment of choice for most ♂, although alendronate is the only one licensed for idiopathic osteoporosis in ♂.
- Teriparatide is licensed for male osteoporosis but is recommended only when there is severe osteoporosis or intolerance of bisphosphonates.
- Testosterone treatment has shown beneficial effects in study populations but due to potential side effects and cardiovascular risk factor profiles it is has not to date been used widely.

Osteoporotic vertebral and hip fractures

Vertebral fracture

Vertebral fractures commonly present in the lower thoracic or upper lumbar spine and can occur spontaneously or as a result of minimal trauma such as coughing.

The major features may include:

- *Acute back pain:* at the specific site of fracture and may also be referred around the body in a symmetrical fashion and can mimic chest or abdominal discomfort. Pain may be accompanied by paravertebral spasm and can persist for several weeks; during this time back movements—particularly flexion—may be limited.
- *Chronic back pain:* residual pain persists in a proportion of patients requiring long-term management with analgesia, exercises, and various psychological support mechanisms.
- *Kyphosis and height loss* which may subsequently result in ↓ lung and abdominal volumes and skeletal disproportion.
- *Quality of life measures* have indicated a substantial reduction in quality of life following vertebral fracture, comparable with other major diseases. These include a decline in both physical and mental functions with several studies suggesting ↑ anxiety, depression, and impaired mobility.

Hip fracture

- Common complications in the peri- and postoperative phase include cardiac and thromboembolic events, pneumonia, sepsis, urinary tract infections, the development of pressure sores, dehydration, and confusion.
- Longer term there may be loss of function and independence.
- ~40% of patients are unable to walk independently 1 year after hip fracture and 60–80% may become limited in ADL.
- In the first year after hip fracture, ~27% of patients will require nursing home care and 30% will require additional home support.
- Hip fractures are also associated with ↑ mortality with most deaths occurring in the first days and months following the fracture.

Avoiding hip fractures

>95% of hip fractures occur in association with a fall and the highest risk of fracture is observed in those people who have osteoporosis and are also at the highest risk of falling.

How should falls be addressed?

- 30% of people >65 years fall each year and >50% of those living in long-term care fall every year, some repeatedly.
- Recurrent falls are associated with ↑ mortality, ↑ rate of hospitalization, curtailment of daily activities, ↑ fear of falling, and loss of confidence.

Although estimates vary, ~25% of falls result in serious injury with 1 fall in 40 resulting in a fracture. Among older people, falling accounts for 95% of hip fractures.

- >400 potential risk factors for falling have been identified. The most important of these include those related to the environment, gait/balance disorders or weakness, dizziness and vertigo, use of assistive devices, impaired ADL, chronic diseases, and polypharmacy.

Randomized controlled trials of falls prevention strategies have focused on both multifactorial and unifactorial approaches. It is likely that there a number of approaches that should be applied to reduce the risks related to falls and osteoporotic fracture.

NICE guidelines[1] considered the use of multifactorial falls risk assessment; it does not recommend low intensity or untargeted group exercises and unifactorial cognitive/ behavioural interventions (Box 3.2).

Box 3.2 Multifactorial risk assessment and interventions

Multifactorial risk assessment
- Falls history.
- Gait, balance, muscle weakness.
- Osteoporosis risk.
- Perceived functional ability.
- Vision.
- Cognition.
- Urinary continence.
- Home hazards.
- Cardiovascular examination.
- Medication.

Multifactorial interventions
- Strength and balance training.
- Vision assessment.
- Modification of medication.
- Identify future risk.
- Participation in falls-prevention programme.
- Prevention programmes.

Reference

1. Nice (2004). *The assessment and prevention of falls in older people. Clinical Guideline 21.* NICE, London.

Prevention of osteoporosis: lifestyle factors

- Nutritional factors are important to maintain skeletal integrity.
- Tobacco consumption may adversely affect bone density.
- Strongest evidence on beneficial effect of exercise on bone density is during childhood and adolescence. Exercise in later life may improve muscle tone, balance, and ↓ risks related to falls and related fractures.

📖 Osteoporotic vertebral and hip fractures. p.40.

What is important in the diet?

- Calcium intake is important during skeletal growth and peak bone mass development and higher intakes may also be effective in reducing bone loss in late postmenopausal ♀.
- Dairy products are the major sources of calcium and ideally dietary calcium intake should be maintained throughout life to help maintain skeletal integrity (see Table 3.1).

Table 3.1 Calcium requirements: reference nutrition intake (RNI).

Age	Daily intake (mg)
<1	525
1–3	350
4–6	450
7–10	550
11–18	1000(♂); 800(♀)
>19	700

- Vitamin D_3 is necessary for optimal absorption of calcium.
- Exposure to sunlight and subsequent cutaneous production of vitamin D_3 is the major source of this vitamin with only about 10% being derived from the diet.
- Vitamin D deficiency is common in various groups:
  - Frail elderly people with poor nutrition and limited exposure to sunlight. In this group vitamin D deficiency may lead to impaired muscle strength which can ↑ the risk of falls.
  - ↑ skin pigmentation and ↓ sunlight exposure (due to strict dress codes) exposes infants, young children, and pregnant ♀ of Asian, African, and Afro-Caribbean origin to the risk of developing vitamin D deficiency.
  - Strict vegans and individuals with malabsorption syndromes or those who have undergone extensive gastric surgery may be at risk.
- Anti-convulsant therapy may lead to vitamin D deficiency syndrome.
- Low body weight. Bone loss is more rapid in post-menopausal ♀ with low body weight. Eating disorders leading to amenorrhea in young ♀ may also affect bone density. Fruit and vegetables rich in dietary alkali may also benefit bone health.
- Vitamins A, B, C, and K may contribute to bone health but many of the data on these individual nutrients are based on small studies only.

- Carbonated drinks or beverages containing caffeine may be detrimental to bone health but findings are not universal.
- Phytoestrogens are widely distributed within the plant kingdom and have oestrogen-like properties. High intakes of isoflavones and the lignans, which are found in soy products and grains, cereals, and linseed may help to improve bone density although evidence is limited.

Does tobacco and alcohol affect bone density?

Smoking

- Smoking may affect several mechanisms that ↑ fracture risk.
- Current and past smoking may adversely affect BMD. ♀ smokers have earlier menopause and ↑ rate of bone loss after menopause, suggesting that smoking may enhance oestrogen catabolism.
- Smokers are also thinner and ∴ have lower BMI, losing the protective effect of adipose tissue and impairing peripheral oestrogen metabolism.
- Current smoking is associated with a significantly ↑ risk of any kind of fracture in both ♂ and ♀ with the risk slowly ↓ on cessation of smoking.
- Bone loss is reported to be ↑ in ♂ smokers than in ♀ smokers perhaps due to ♂'s higher exposure to cigarette smoking.

Alcohol

- Heavy alcohol consumption is associated with a ↓ in bone density and ↑ fracture risk.
- A probable direct effect of ethanol on osteoblasts but in addition relative malnutrition, lack of exercise, and impaired vitamin D metabolism will ↑ the likelihood of osteoporosis and fractures.

Exercise

- Physical activity—particularly weight bearing exercise—provides the mechanical stimuli or 'loading' important for the maintenance and improvement of bone health as well as enhancing gait, balance, co-ordination, proprioception, reaction time, and muscle strength in elderly people.
- Repetitive (e.g. jumping) or resistance exercise (e.g. weight training) can produce the necessary loading to provide mechanical stimuli.
- Activity needs to be within safe limits but must be more than just customary attempts if it is to produce improvements, e.g. extra walking, at a normal pace, >10min daily has failed to ↑ BMD at vulnerable sites for fracture.
- Exercise benefits to bone are doubled if activity is commenced before or at puberty (for example in gymnastics, tennis, and jumping).
- In adulthood, exercise appears to largely preserve bone but does not add new bone. In the immediate postmenopausal years it is unlikely that exercise will balance the effect of oestrogen deficiency.
- Exercise can reduce the risk of falls in the elderly.
- It is unclear how long benefits of young adulthood exercise will be sustained in advancing years. Evidence supports benefit of earlier sports activities producing lasting benefits until the late 60s but only if activity at a lower level is sustained.

Providing education and support

Where can education have an impact?

- Knowledge and ability to explain issues related to osteoporosis and prevention.
- Guiding on the results of DXA scans and effect on lifestyle and treatment.
- Providing advice on treatment options leading to adherence.

Outline the evidence on the role of diet and exercise

At a population-based level the role and importance of dietary calcium intake and exercise are the major preventive options that have been addressed across various age groups.

- ♀ adolescents have heard about osteoporosis and may have some limited knowledge about dietary calcium intake and exercise but have little concept about types of calcium-rich foods and the specific types of weight-bearing activity required for skeletal preservation. ♀ of this age believe they are unlikely to develop osteoporosis and that it is less serious than heart disease and breast cancer. Health information is commonly sought from brochures, magazines, and the media, suggesting a preference for this source rather than from a healthcare professional.
- In evaluating the impact of osteoporosis knowledge and preventive behaviour in older ♀, there is greater recognition of the condition and a trend towards ↑ dietary calcium intake and weight-bearing activity following education-based programmes.

DXA scans

It has been suggested that information on and explanation of DXA results may influence health-related behaviours with respect to relevant lifestyle changes and also adherence to treatments.

- Several studies have shown that those who understand their DXA results—particularly when they are low—are more likely to be prescribed medication and are more likely to continue treatment on a long-term basis.
- In contrast, those who were either uncertain of their DXA results or thought it did not show osteoporosis were less likely to continue treatment.

Adherence with treatment

Despite studies showing that osteoporosis treatments are generally well tolerated and associated with significant efficacy benefits, adherence to therapies on a long-term basis remains inconsistent.

Factors affecting adherence include:

- Understanding of disease.
- Severity of symptoms.
- Complexity and duration of treatment regimens.
- Immediacy of beneficial effects.
- Perceived or actual side effects.
- Use of concomitant medications

- *The adherence gap: why osteoporosis patients don't continue with treatment.* is a European survey that has highlighted reasons why patients fail to continue with bisphosphonate therapy.[1]
- ♀ report side effects and inconvenience of medication as the most common reasons for discontinuing therapy.
- Physicians attribute non-adherence to lack of patient understanding only.
- 27% of ♀ felt their risk of fracture was the same whether or not they took treatment; 20% were unaware of treatment benefits; and a further 17% did not believe their treatment had any benefit at all.
- This survey suggests that although advice is given it is not always interpreted in the correct manner. Factors that may explain this include a lack of communication skills of both doctor and patient, use of inappropriate terminology, inadequate emphasis on, and repetition of, key features, and diminished motivation.

Education

In a clinical setting most patient education should ideally take place on an individualized basis, with the emphasis on verbal communication.

Patient information leaflets and booklets from various sources including the National Osteoporosis Society (NOS) and pharmaceutical companies provide written information on osteoporosis. Most of these are reasonably composed and have undergone some form of scientific ratification but there have been few attempts to analyse their educational value and effect on relevant behavioural change.

The role of the National Osteoporosis Society

The NOS[2] is a major national charity whose membership comprises people with osteoporosis, their families and carers, and clinical and research professionals. Its activities include:
- Providing information via a comprehensive range of leaflets, newsletters, public meetings, and a helpline staffed by nurse specialists.
- Fundraising activities.
- Media communications.
- Political lobbying.
- Organizing an international conference every 18 months, funding research projects, and supporting studentships.
- Supporting >100 public groups across the UK, assisted by almost 1000 volunteers.

References

1. IPSOS UK (2005). *The adherence gap: why osteoporosis patients don't continue with treatment.* International Osteoporosis Foundation.

2. National Osteoporosis Society: ⌨ www.nos.org.uk Tel: 08451303076 or 01761 471771. Helpline 08454500230 or 01761472721.

Treatment for osteoporosis

What drugs are commonly used?

There are a number of agents that have been shown to prevent bone loss and reduce fracture incidence in postmenopausal ♀ and ↑ evidence to suggest that some of these have similar effects in ♂ (also see Boxes 3.3, 3.4).

- Bisphosphonates; alendronate, etidronate, risedronate (all given orally); ibandronate, given orally and intravenously. Zoledronic acid is an annual infusion.
- HRT.
- Raloxifene.
- Strontium ranelate.
- Teriparatide.

The bisphosphonates, HRT, and raloxifene slow down bone resorption whilst strontium has both an anti-resorptive effect and stimulates bone formation. Teriparatide is an anabolic agent that stimulates bone formation and leads to large ↑ in bone mass

---

Box 3.3 1° Prevention of osteoporotic fragility fractures in postmenopausal ♀

- ♀ aged 70+ who have ≥1 clinical risk factors for # or medical conditions suggestive of low BMD. In ♀ aged 75+ DXA may not be required:
  - Treat with alendronate.
- ♀ aged<70 with medical conditions suggestive of low BMD and at least 1 clinical factor suggestive of ↑ fracture risk and a T-score <–2.5SD:
  - Treat with alendronate.

Box 3.4 2° Prevention of osteoporotic fragility fractures in postmenopausal ♀

- ♀ with fragility fracture + T-score <–2.5 SD.
- In ♀ 75+, DXA may not be necessary if it is clinically inappropriate or unfeasible.
- Treat with alendronate.
- Other options may be considered if alendronate is not tolerated.

▶Calcium + vitamin D recommended in all cases unless clinicians are confident that ♀ have an adequate dietary calcium intake and are vitamin D replete.

Issues related to treatment

Although anti-fracture efficacy is proven, use of therapy in the clinical setting is not always straightforward for varied reasons. Adherence to osteoporosis therapies is generally poor. 77% of patients taking a once-daily bisphosphonate stop treatment within a year with almost two-thirds of patients taking a once-weekly preparation also failing to adhere to treatment. Non-adherence has significant repercussions to prognosis with evidence showing greater fracture reduction in those who adhere to therapy compared to those who do not.

Treatment is long-term; therapies do not provide symptomatic improvement and side effects may present. These include:

- Bisphosphonates may cause upper gastrointestinal symptoms and the dosing instructions may be difficult to follow.
- Strontium is taken as granules dissolved in water, recommended at bedtime. It may be associated with diarrhoea, nausea, and headache, particularly in the first few months. Early trials suggested a possible unexplained small ↑ in the risk of venous thromboembolism.
- Raloxifene, which is taken as a once daily dose, may exacerbate vasomotor symptoms in some ♀ and is also associated with ↑ risk of thromboembolic disease.
- The risk benefit balance of HRT is complex but long-term use, particularly past the age of 60 years, is no longer recommended for the prevention of bone loss.
- Teriparatide requires daily injections for 18 months and it is also an extremely expensive therapy.

Duration of treatment

- Optimal duration of therapy has not been established. For many of the interventions, resumption of bone loss has been shown in the first couple of years after withdrawal of therapy, although it is not certain whether this occurs at the normal rate for age-related bone loss or is accelerated.
- There are slight concerns about long-term suppression of bone turnover with the more potent bisphosphonates and little is known about the longer-term effects of strontium and teriparatide on the skeleton.

Are non-pharmacological interventions beneficial?

- Vertebroplasty and kyphoplasty are techniques when bone cement can be injected into cervical, thoracic, and lumbar vertebrae where fractures have occurred.
- Emerging evidence suggests that these techniques are very effective for the relief of pain that has not responded to conventional management.
- This pain relief appears permanent in appropriately selected patients.

Further reading

NICE (2008). TAG 161 Alendronate, etidronate, risedronate, raloxifene, strontium ranelate and teriparatide for the secondary prevention of osteoporotic fragility fractures in postmenopausal women.

National Osteoporosis Guideline Group (NOGG). Guideline for the diagnosis and management of osteoporosis in postmenopausal women and men from the age of 50 years in the UK. ⏚ www.shef.ac.uk/NOGG/NOGG

Assessment tools

How are these used to assess quality of life?

Quality of life questionnaires are being increasingly used in the overall management of osteoporosis and usually incorporate physical and emotional aspects. In many cases the use of assessment tools would include generic and disease specific tools such as those outlined.

There are six major questionnaires that have been developed for patients with osteoporosis. All focus on a combination of physical and emotional functions (Table 3.2).

Table 3.2 Osteoporosis assessment questionnaires

Name	Administration	Number of questions	Domains
OFDQ	Interview	69	General health, back pain, ADL, socialization, depression, confidence
OPAQ	Self-administer	67	Physical function, emotional status, symptoms, social interaction
OPTQOL	Interview	33	Physical activity, adaptations, fears
OQLQ	Interview	30	Physical function, ADL
Quallefo-41	Self-administer	41	Pain, physical function, social function, general health perception, mental function
QUALIOST	Self-administer	23	Physical function, emotional status

OFDQ, Osteoporosis Functional Disability Questionnaire; OPAQ, Osteoporosis Assessment Questionnaire; OPTQOL, Osteoporosis Targeted Quality of Life Questionnaire; OQLQ, Osteoporosis Quality of Life Questionnaire; Qualleffo-41, Quality of Life Questionnaire of the International Osteoporosis Foundation; QUALIOST, Questionnaire Quality of Life in Osteoporosis.

Hip fracture

- Although the quality of life is impaired following hip fracture, the collection of data on the degree of this impairment is problematical.
- Elderly patients may have impaired cognition prior to the fracture, hospital admission, and subsequent surgery. The episode itself may lead to disorientation.
- Visual impairment may limit the use and validity of self-administered questionnaires.
- Patients with hip fracture had lower baseline scores and a significant ↓ in the short form (SF)-36 domains of physical function, vitality, and social function compared to the general population (control).

Vertebral fracture

- Studies frequently fail to consider the impact on quality of life to those demonstrating recent radiographic vertebral fractures.

- The Qualeffo-41 is osteoporosis specific instrument used to assess quality-of-life issues associated with vertebral fracture.
- Patients without back pain or vertebral fracture were compared to those with vertebral fracture. Individuals with vertebral fracture reported overall impairment, and specific impairment in social, mental, physical, and general health.
- The Multiple Outcomes of Raloxifene Evaluation (MORE) used Quallefo-41 as one of its instruments to assess quality of life in 751 postmenopausal ♀ with osteoporosis across seven European countries.
- There was a trend for a greater negative impact on quality of life with an ↑ number of vertebral fractures, particularly associated with ↑ age.
- The differences between those with prevalent fractures and those without vertebral fractures were highly significant in pain, physical function, and general health.
- Lumbar fractures impacted more than thoracic fractures on the domains of pain, physical function, and general health.

The role of the nurse in osteoporosis

All nurses should be able to identify key resources to inform the patient about the lifestyle, disease-specific issues and treatment options. Depending upon the local resources nurses should look for links with:
- GP, community pharmacist, physiotherapist.
- Community falls services, if appropriate.
- Social care if appropriate.
- Patient support groups and telephone advice lines.
- 2° care services.
- Voluntary organization who may offer local exercise or education classes.

See Box 3.5.

Box 3.5 The nurse's role across different specialties.

Practice nurse	• Risk assessment. • Health promotion. • Treatment issues. • Education about the disease.
District nurse	• Nursing care of frail elderly. • Link with residential/nursing care. • Falls prevention. • Treatment issues. • Education of teams and patients.
Health visitor	• Health promotion across lifespan. • Encourage bone healthy lifestyle.
Orthopaedic nurse in trauma wards and fracture clinic	• Acute fracture management of in- and outpatients. • Rehabilitation • Falls prevention. • 2° prevention of fracture including early identification of those 'at risk' of osteoporosis. • Liaise with community services.
Rheumatology nurse in out-patients and in ward	• Risk assessment. • Health promotion. • Treatment issues. • Use of IV bisphosphonates/corticosteroids. • Identification of those 'at risk'.
Care of the elderly nurse in hospital and nursing home	• Nursing care of frail elderly. • Rehabilitation. • Falls prevention. • Treatment issues.
Nurses in other specialities, e.g. endocrinology, oncology	• Risk assessment. • Awareness of specialist therapy on bone health (e.g. glucocorticoids and aromatase inhibitors).
Osteoporosis Specialist Nurse	• Risk assessment. • Clinical assessment. • Interpretation of DXA results. • Possible DXA scanning role. • Initiation and monitoring of treatment. • Wide-based educational role for healthcare. professionals, patients, and general public.

Frequently asked questions

Is loss of height something I should take note of when I see patients I think might be at risk of osteoporosis?

Loss of height >4cm might indicate that vertebral fracture has occurred. If several vertebrae are crushed there may also be curvature of the spine.

If someone has been diagnosed as having osteoporosis should I bother with educating them about diet?

All patients diagnosed with osteoporosis should be encouraged to maintain a well-balanced diet, incorporating 1000mg calcium daily, essential vitamins B, C, K, and also minerals such as magnesium. Regular helpings of dairy produce and fruit and vegetables will provide these essential nutrients.

Is there a good source of information on dietary advice that I can use to help people understand their calcium and vitamin D intake?

The Food Standards Agency[1] is an excellent source of information; just type in 'osteoporosis' and a range of options are available to print off for the patient. You may also find your own organization has a dietician who may be able to provide additional information. The NOS will also be a good source of information.

How can I encourage concordance with bisphosphonates— so many people struggle with taking them?

Providing sufficient information on the benefits is really important particularly if they have few symptoms. Patient-orientated information, both verbal and written, given on initial diagnosis and subsequently reiterated on review visits will be helpful. Some people struggle with remembering a treatment that is once a week. There are plenty of practical tips such as encouraging them to take the medication on the day that has more of a routine. Magnetic fridge timers are available that can be programmed to alarm once a week.

I see a lot of patients who have, over a year, quite a high dose of steroids, for example, regular Depo-Medrone® injections—shouldn't they be on bone protection?

Current guidelines on the management of steroid-induced osteoporosis are based on oral drugs only. However, in clinical practice it is reasonable to consider the cumulative effects of steroids given by alternative routes and to perform DXA measurements if there are other risk factors or fracture history.

Reference

1. Food Standards Agency (UK): www.food.gov.uk

Inflammatory joint diseases

Overview

Inflammatory joint diseases are conditions that have underlying inflammatory component that may be driven by a faulty auto-immune response by the body, often resulting in the body's tissues being attacked by the body's own immune responses. Examples of such conditions include:

- AS.
- PsA.
- RA.
- JIA.
- Connective tissue diseases.
- Crystal-related arthropathies.

These inflammatory conditions are understood to:
- Target specific joints and/or surrounding tissues.
- Have a genetic predisposition—although this does not provide the complete picture to causality.

Prompt diagnosis is essential to differentiate between acute, mild self-limiting conditions from those that can rapidly result in life-threatening, multi-system disorders. Evidence related to inflammatory (polyarticular) joint diseases (IJD) such as RA demonstrate that prompt aggressive and proactive treatment improves long-term outcomes. This is referred to as the 'window of opportunity'.

On initial presentation it can sometimes be difficult even to the trained eye to detect swelling and tenderness on palpation of the joints (Box 4.1).

📖 Also see Assessing the patient, p.62.

Box 4.1 Index of suspicion for inflammatory joint disease requiring referral

- Joint pain.
- Report of joint stiffness >30min in the morning.
- Presence of inflammation (joint swelling) in >3 joints—beware of swollen ankles (oedema).
- Relationship between joint pain and symptoms related to movement—stronger relationship more likely to be OA.
- Presence of fatigue—if associated with poor sleep and widespread pain consider fibromyalgia.
- Raised inflammatory markers (CRP, ESR) and rheumatoid factor (RF) positive (absence of RF positive should not preclude diagnosis or referral).

❶ Individuals presenting with a monoarthritis, particularly if accompanied by red, hot swollen, and tender joint—consider septic arthritis (emergency treatment required).

Key points to consider

- Short-term symptom relief may be achieved by steroids or NSAIDs.
- Initially, signs and symptoms may be sudden or insidious.

- Early presentation of IJD may not fit any classical diagnostic group but early assessment and treatment is paramount.
- Regardless of diagnosis/prognosis indicators, all patients presenting with joint pain should receive appropriate treatment and advice on managing their symptoms.

Also see Classifying joint disease, p.4; Psoriatic arthritis, p.84; Ankylosing spondylitis, p.90.

Rheumatoid arthritis

What is RA?

RA is a symmetrical polyarticular disease that affects ~0.8–1% of the population. The chronic systemic inflammation attacks the synovial tissues of moveable joints causing pannus formation, cartilage and bone degradation to joints, and systemic effects to other tissues. (Figs. 4.1–4.3). Initial presentation of the disease may vary. RA has the potential to reduce life expectancy and result in progressive joint destruction and ultimately changes in function.

• The actual mechanism of triggering RA is unknown.
• A genetic predisposition to developing RA (human leucocyte antigen (HLA) DR class II molecules) has been identified yet, only 17% of both identical twins develop RA.
• RA is a progressive and destructive disease with poor long-term outcomes.

 Also see Rheumatoid arthritis: clinical features, p.60.

Who does it affect?

• RA can present at almost any age although the peak age of onset is between 35–50 years.
• RA affects 3♀:1♂.

How is it diagnosed?

In early disease, joints involved and symptoms may fail to adequately fulfil rigid criteria for established disease. The European League against Rheumatism (EULAR) advocate prompt referral for early arthritis based upon a high index of suspicion for IJD. The squeeze test is a simple pragmatic tool used to elicit synovitis in the commonly affected joints MCP joints of hands or MTP joints of feet (Fig. 4.2). More detailed diagnostic criteria to support clinical examination findings have been devised (see pp.60, 61).

However:
• It can be difficult to diagnose, particularly in the early phases of the disease. May have a rapid or insidious onset.
• Commonly starts with joint pain (usually in the MCPs of the hands or MTPs of the feet). A high index of suspicion of an inflammatory joint disease should warrant prompt and early referral for diagnosis.
• A high positive titre for RF serology is a poor diagnostic tool, particularly in the absence of clinical signs. RA can be diagnosed in the absence of RF.
   • The use of anti-CCP serology test has shown to have a higher specificity and sensitivity than RF serology and is increasingly being used to aid diagnosis and predict optimum treatment pathways because it is seen in patients with more erosive disease. It is present in serum of patients with RA years before signs and symptoms develop.

Further reading

Combe B, Landewe R, Lukas C et al. (2007). EULAR recommendations for the management of early arthritis. *Annals of the Rheumatic Diseases*, **66**, 34–45.

Luqmani R, Hennell S, Estrach C, et al. (2006). British Society for Rheumatology and British Health Professionals in Rheumatology guideline for the management of rheumatoid arthritis (the first two years). *Rheumatology*, **45**(9), 1167–9.

Oliver S (2007). Best practice in the treatment of patients with rheumatoid arthritis. *Nursing Standard*, **21**(42), 47–56.

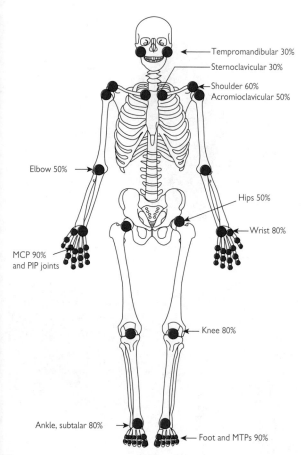

Fig. 4.1 Joints and tissues affected in RA and the percentage of those most commonly affected.

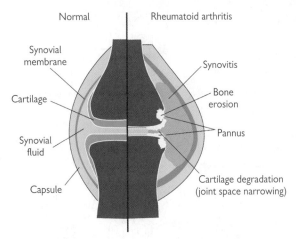

Fig. 4.2. The pathology of RA. Reproduced with permission of Annual Review of Immunology 1996.

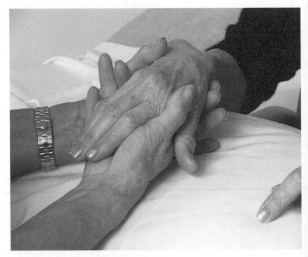

Fig. 4.3 The squeeze test. MCP or MTP joints. Positive squeeze test = if tender/ painful on squeezing across MTPs or MCPs.

Rheumatoid arthritis: clinical features

The predominant features that can be seen in RA are:
- Joint pain.
- Joint swelling.
- EMS.
- Fatigue and lethargy.
- Individuals may also experience low grade fever and weight loss.
- Anaemia of chronic disease.

Also see Box 4.2.

In addition there are changes to joints and surrounding tissues:
- Pannus formation of synovial tissues.
- Erosion of bone and joint space narrowing.
- Damage to tendon sheaths and cartilage.
- Deterioration in joint function and general functional ability.

Extra-articular manifestations of RA
Systemic organ involvement and extra-articular features including:
- Rheumatoid lung and interstitial lung disease.
- Vasculitis, anaemia of chronic disease.
- Occular involvement—episcleritis, scleritis.
- Weight loss.
- Subcutaneous nodules. Exocrine, salivary, and lachrymal glands involvement.
- Cardiovascular disease—pericarditis, myocarditis.
- Hematological—Felty's syndrome, lymphomas.
- Lymphadenopathy.
- Sjögren syndrome.
- ↓ life expectancy and ↑ risk of malignancies.

Prognostic indicators of poorer disease outcomes
- Delayed access to treatment:
  - Longer disease duration at presentation—'window of opportunity'.
  - X-ray evidence of joint damage or erosions at presentation.
  - Poor functional status at presentation.
  - Inflammation of the MCP joints lasting >12 weeks.
  - Evidence of active and sustained synovitis using US or MRI.
- Raised acute phase response (CRP, ESR).
- Shared epitope for HLA type.
- Seropositivity of the RA.
  - Absence of RF does not preclude diagnosis but is a prognostic indicator of aggressive disease with a poorer outcome. Anti-CCP serology has been shown to have a higher specificity and sensitivity than RF.
- Social and psychological factors that may reflect poor outcomes (📖 see Education, social, and psychological issues, pp.318, 320).

Box 4.2 Features of established RA

Signs
- Presence of EMS >30min.
- Symmetrical polyarticular joint pain and swelling. Joints involved could be any of the synovial joints but classically might be :
  - Small joints and or/ knuckles of the hand.
  - Wrists, elbows, shoulders.
  - Knees, ankles, and small joints of the feet.
- Subcutaneous nodules.
- Genetic pre-disposition, e.g. family history of RA.
- Clinical evidence of synovitis or erosions—using x-ray, US, or MRI.
- Raised inflammatory indices, e.g. CRP or ESR.
- Anemia of chronic disease.

Symptoms
- Joint changes—reduction in joint function, mobility, and ROM.
- Fatigue and joint pain.
- Sleep disturbances.
- Changes in mood and self-esteem.
- Short-term symptom relief achieved from NSAIDs or steroids.

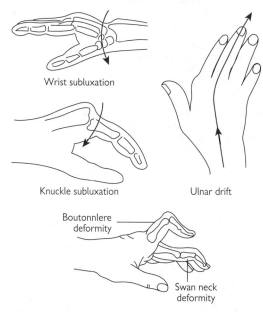

Wrist subluxation

Knuckle subluxation

Ulnar drift

Boutonnlere deformity

Swan neck deformity

Fig. 4.4 Examples of changes in function. a) Wrist subluxation; b) knuckle subluxation; c) ulnar drift; reproduced with kind permission from the ARC. d) Boutonnière and swan neck, reproduced with permission from Davies R, Everitt H (2006). *Musculoskeletal Problems*. Oxford University Press, Oxford.

Rheumatoid arthritis: assessment and management

RA is a long-term condition (LTC) characterized by pain, lethargy, and changes in functional ability. RA is a multi-system disease requiring long-term treatment with disease-modifying drugs. The diagnostic issues are only the beginning of the management plan; there is still much to be done, from a nursing perspective. The natural course of the disease varies and short-term changes need to be considered in the context of the overall assessments.

The clinical assessment will:
- Inform management and guide diagnosis.
- Identify specific prognostic indicators that will define treatment strategies.
- Focus on a patient-centred approach.

Management of early RA requires an assessment to support:

- Time for the individual to discuss their anxieties and needs in the context of a holistic assessment, e.g. adjusting to diagnosis, expectations and beliefs, social support, psychological aspects, other comorbidities, work-related issues, relationships.
- Information, support, and advice about RA, pharmacological and non-pharmacological options, risks, and benefits of treatment and monitoring.
- A Disease Assessment Score (DAS28)—swollen and tender joints (Fig. 4.5).
- An assessment of pain (using a Visual Analogue Scale, VAS) and symptom control.
- Review all investigations:
  - Blood tests including hematology, biochemistry, inflammatory markers (CRP, ESE) and urinalysis.
  - Radiological investigations including chest, hand, and feet x-rays, US, or MRI results.
- Assess current functional ability and need for prompt referral to other members of the MDT—occupational therapy, physiotherapy, podiatry.
- Fertility, sexuality, and relevant relationship issues.
- Immunological status, e.g. vaccinations, recent contact with infectious diseases, previous TB etc.
- 📖 Also see Pregnancy and fertility issues, Chapter 14, p.391; 📖 Pharmacological management, Chapter 16, p.419.

The window of opportunity

Radiographic joint damage, loss of function, and reduction of bone mineral density are evident very early on in IJDs (up to 40% of early RA patients have erosive disease at presentation). Treating within the 'window' aims to:
- Focuses on prompt treatment.
- Improve long-term outcomes by ensuring early aggressive disease control.
- Reduce the risks related to mortality and morbidity.

Clinical distinctions need to be made between the wide spectrums of musculoskeletal disorders in order to:
- Make a firm diagnosis of the disease and optimum treatment.
- Identify the conditions that rapidly deteriorate and may result in life-threatening multi-system disorders.
- Identify acute, mild, self-limiting conditions.

EULAR core data

PAIN

No pain _____ Pain as bad as it could be

Swollen Joints

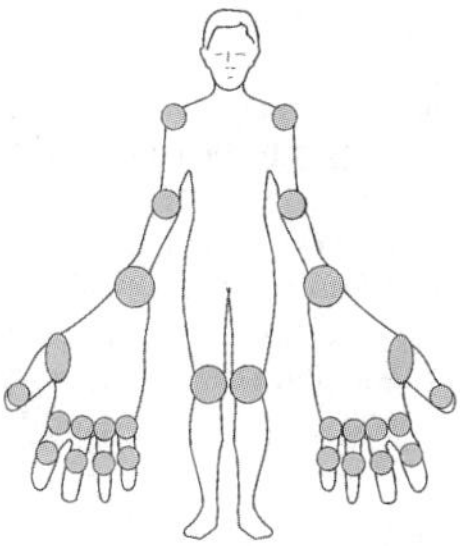

Number ☐☐

ESR ☐☐☐ mm/hr

Tender joints

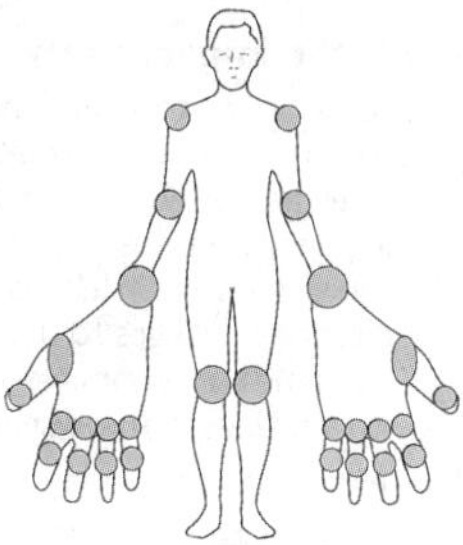

Number ☐☐

C-reactive protein ☐☐☐ g/l

PATIENT'S GLOBAL ASSESSMENT OF DISEASE ACTIVITY

Not active _____ Extremely active
at all

ASSESSOR'S GLOBAL ASSESSMENT OF DISEASE ACTIVITY

(1-5): ☐   1 = asymptomatic; 2 = mild; 3 = moderate; 4 = severe; 5 = very severe.

Fig. 4.5 DAS28. Note: the assessor's global assessment of disease activity and pain VAS are not used to calculate the core DAS28 data. Reproduced with kind permission from Scott DL, van Riel PL, van der Heijde D, *et al.* (1993). *Assessing disease activity in rheumatoid arthritis: the EULAR handbook of standard methods*. Pharmacia: Sweden.

Rheumatoid arthritis: management

The RA management plans should consider:

- Disease-modifying anti-rheumatic drugs (DMARDs). DMARDs include methotrexate (MTX), sulfasalazine, and leflunomide (☐ see Disease-modifying anti-rheumatic drugs, p.424).
- Advice on how to manage treatments, side effects, and flares of RA.
- Guidance on taking combination therapy—use of two or more DMARDs taken consecutively.
- Outline of blood monitoring, where the blood monitoring will take place and what to expect and when to contact the specialist team.
- Advice on of the telephone advice line service.

What is the impact to the patient?

RA is poorly understood and individuals may express concern about the aggressive nature of their symptoms that fail to match their perceptions of what they perceived to be 'arthritis'. They may fear that they must have something 'more serious' such as cancer. RA can have a significant impact on the individual's lifestyle, including the need for long-term healthcare and medications, changes to quality of life, functional ability, and long-term health outcomes. The variable nature of the condition also adds to the stress of adjusting to the disease and the consequences of the disease (Fig. 4.6).

☐ Also see Education, social, and psychological issues, pp.318, 320.

Social and psychological impact of RA

- Perceptions related to 'chronic disease status' and role in society.
- Changes to self-esteem and perceived level of control of life events and ability to manage the problems (self-efficacy).
- Loss of mobility, changes in functional ability and body image.
- The unpredictable nature of exacerbations (sometimes called 'flares') of the disease.

Nurse-led follow-up and review of RA

- A review of holistic needs.
- Documented evidence (outlined above) should be compared and regular disease assessment (including DAS28) and patient-reported outcomes such as functional ability, symptom control (pain VAS).
- Review of treatment regimen, side-effect profile and blood monitoring, x-rays.
- Prompt access for advice and treatment/support for exacerbations of the disease—changes of DMARD regimen according to clinical pathway criteria.
- Referrals to multi-professional team if required.

☐ Also see Ward-based care and referral to multi-disciplinary team, Chapter 12.

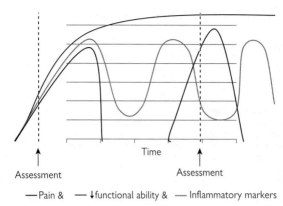

Assessment   Assessment

—Pain &   — ↓functional ability &   — Inflammatory markers

Fig. 4.6 Natural course of disease.

Rheumatoid arthritis: treatment

The key principles of treatment are:
- Control of symptoms.
- Preservation of functional ability.
- Effective control of the disease.
- Empower the individual to manage their condition and understand their treatment.

Control of symptoms

Pain, fatigue, stiffness are common features of RA. Achieving effective disease control is imperative but the drugs used to control the disease can take up to 3 months to control the disease and therefore additional medications may also be required to relieve pain. Pain relief options include pharmacological and non-pharmacological options:
- Simple or compound analgesia
- NSAIDs or COX-2 inhibitors—topical/oral/rectal.
- Corticosteroids—long-term maintenance therapy remains controversial but short-term relief is advocated, e.g. IA injection of joint with active synovitis:
  - Intramuscular (IM) injections.
  - Intra-articular (IA).
  - Intravenous (IV).
  - Oral.

Non-pharmacological symptom relief

- Pacing/energy conservation/rest and relaxation/education and support.
- Joint protection.
- Application of cold packs/hot packs.
- Complementary therapies.

Disease control

DMARDs include traditional DMARDs and the more recent addition of biologically engineered therapies.
- DMARDs may be given in combination or triple therapy, e.g. MTX, sulfasalazine, hydroxychloroquine (☐ see Pharmacological management, p.424).
- Biologic therapies often prescribed with a DMARD, usually MTX:
  - Anti-tumour necrosis factor alpha (anti-TNFα) adalimumab, etanercept, infliximab.
  - B-cell depletion therapies (rituximab).
  - Co-stimulatory modulators (abatacept). Note: NICE did not find abacept cost-effective ∴ was not recommended for RA treatment. However, NICE has proposed early review of this decision. Refer to ⏁ www.nice.org.uk for latest guidance.

Empowerment

- Education and information on condition and treatment options.
- Informed decision making using a patient-centred approach.
- Enhancing patient self-efficacy and perceptions of control—including family, partner, and work-related issues.

- Access to advice and support (telephone advice line) for exacerbation of the disease.

📖 Also see Pharmacological management, Chapters 15,16; 📖 Telephone advice, p.342; 📖 Self-management, p.324.

Rheumatoid arthritis: nursing care issues in management and when to refer

During the lifetime of an individual with RA they will come in contact with a wide range of healthcare professionals (HCP) due to the condition itself or complications of the disease, or treatment side effects, and, in some circumstances, other co-morbidities.

Nurses caring for individuals with RA must:

• Provide adequate pain control.
• Maintain concordance with appropriate drug therapies that provide disease control.
• Monitor potential adverse events related to the treatment or the disease.
• Enable functional ability and independence wherever possible.
• To maintain dignity in all ADL—including use of aids and devices to enable dressing, eating and hygiene:
  • Take into account ward or other routines that may affect those with RA participating effectively –for example EMS affecting the ability to mobilize promptly in a ward environment.
• To provide support and guidance on additional comorbidities and needs in relation to that condition.

The Specialist Nurse: roles and management

Nurse Specialists in Rheumatology have developed significant expertise in the management of those with RA. These include:

• Providing information, education, and support about the diagnosis, treatment options, and managing symptoms.
• Undertaking a holistic assessment of social and psychological needs in relation to the diagnosis and ongoing management of the condition.
• Outlining risks and benefits of drug therapies and documenting informed consent.

Some nurses may undertake additional advanced roles that include:

• Drug monitoring clinics:
  • Reviewing blood, urine, and general health status to ensure safe continuation of treatment.
  • Assessing the effectiveness of disease control.
  • Adding a DMARD or titrating doses of DMARD therapies (as a nurse prescriber or protocol-driven care pathways).
• Nurse-led clinics:
  • Rapid access for flares/exacerbations of the condition.
  • Administering IA joint injections or IM steroids.
  • Manage a caseload.
  • Structured review process on follow-up appointments.
  • Undertake structured DAS for national registers, and regular assessments and reviews in the context of treatment criteria for new therapies.

- Running telephone advice line services:
  - Access to fast-track referrals via the advice line.
- Structured telephone follow-up consultations using telephone review.
- Nurse triage services reviewing early referral and treatment pathways.
- Act as a first point of contact to refer patients when required to the multidisciplinary team (see Box 4.3).

Box 4.3 When to refer to a Nurse Specialist or Specialist Team—occupational therapist (OT) physiotherapist (PT)

Referral should be considered for:
- Poor disease control—either frequent or sustained flares of RA with raised inflammatory markers and active synovitis.
- Poor symptom control including pain, stiffness, and fatigue.
- Inability to tolerate DMARD therapies either from toxicity or general intolerance.
- General trend in blood values that flag cause for concern (📖 see Drug monitoring, p.473).
- Seek guidance on any potential adverse events related to DMARD or biologic therapies—including infections, adverse trends in blood results, new cardiac or respiratory symptoms.
- Guidance on immunization or challenges to immune status of patient particularly contact with infectious disease and conditions such as herpez zoster, chicken pox.
- Rapid changes in functional ability.
- Changes in general health status.
- Index of suspicion for infections, respiratory, or cardiac complications.
- Skin integrity, rashes, and ulcers—seek advice.
- Poor psychological coping.

Referrals to OT and PT for:
- For those admitted to hospital advice from OT or PT on postoperative recovery, mobilization and functional ability, exercises, and management will be beneficial to the patient.
- Access to aids and devices (including chair and bed raisers).
- Guidance on how to best handle patients postoperatively.
- Opportunity to undertake a review of functional issues and exercises including review of splints—where appropriate.

Frequently asked questions: rheumatoid arthritis

I find the RA patients who come into the ward I work in difficult because they want to stay in bed until late in the morning—I feel bad as it looks like we just have ignored them but they are very slow in moving around. Are there any tips to helping them in the morning?

The joint stiffness and pain makes movement difficult particularly after inactivity or first thing in the morning. Medication routines may also be altered by ward routines, especially if they are unable to self-medicate. Ensure the patient has been provided with effective analgesia (and possibly NSAID). If prescribed an NSAID they will need time for the therapeutic benefit before mobilizing (depending upon drug ~30–45min). A hot bath or shower will also help in the morning—relieving the pain and stiffness and make mobility a little easier.

I see a lot of people with RA in my community but don't really have enough time to give them. What quick tips can you give me to focus on key issue?

The important quick points include:

- Observe their functional ability on entering and leaving the room; use of joint movements, guarding, or protecting joints due to active synovitis/pain.
- How long does their EMS last (in minutes)? In general (in the context of all information) a reduction in EMS indicates less disease activity.
- Use a VAS scale for Pain and Global Health—using a ruler to document the scores numerically to capture and track changes over time. The greater the score the worse the pain and disease activity as perceived by the patient.
- Ask how many painful and swollen joints they have.
- An ↑ level of fatigue may indicate poor disease control.
- Review their blood results and inflammatory markers—an ↑ in inflammatory markers usually indicates higher disease activity. A trend towards lower hemoglobin may also indicate poor disease control. ⚠ could also indicate a gastrointestinal bleed
- Check they are concordant with their medications for DMARDs but also regular analgesia if they are experiencing a flare.

When you have the information you might want to discuss the case with the nurse specialist or review the patient notes and discuss with the specialist team or your local GP first. Telephone advice line services frequently provide guidance for community nurses or in many cases there may be a local community-based GP with a special interest (GPwSi) or Clinical Assessment Team.

Juvenile idiopathic arthritis: classification

JIA, is an umbrella term to describe the differing types of arthritis in childhood. The term 'juvenile', referring to pre-16 years, idiopathic as cause unknown.

In 1997, JIA was classified into 6 distinct types by the International League of Associations for Rheumatology (ILAR). This classification primarily for research purposes will be used here to demonstrate the diversity of JIA presentation and its subsequent management. JIA has formerly been known as Still's disease, juvenile chronic arthritis (JCA) and juvenile rheumatoid arthritis (JRA). In the USA all childhood arthritis is still defined as JRA whilst in the ILAR classification JRA is one of the distinct subsets (need to consider if consulting American literature).

Clinical findings

1. Oligo-articular onset (oligo = few): 40–50% of all JIA

- 4 or fewer joints affected in first 6 months of disease—typically affecting knees, ankles, and fingers, often asymmetrically.
- ♀:♂ ratio 4:1; peak incidence 1–3 years.
- Joint swelling often with out pain may have morning stiffness.
- Associated with asymptomatic uveitis (inflammatory eye disease) the risk is higher if antinuclear antibodies are detected (ANA+).

The number of joints can remain constant during the period of follow-up. However, in some children more joints become involved in the first 6 months and if there are >4 joints involved this is called extended oligoarticular JIA.

2. Poly-articular onset (poly = many)

Is further subdivided into rheumatoid negative and rheumatoid positive (RF detected on 2 occasions, 3 months apart).

Poly-articular RF negative

- 5 or more joints involved in first 6 months of disease—typically affecting small joints with symmetrical distribution.
- Can have minimal synovitis and flexor tendon involvement.
- May have constitutional features of lethargy and anaemia.

Poly-articular RF positive

- Similar to adult disease.
- Predominantly affects teenage ♀.
- Severe aggressive erosive disease affecting many joints.
- Group most likely to require joint replacement.

3. Systemic onset (also called Still's disease): 10–20% of all JIA

- Affects ♂ and ♀ equally.
- 2-week history of spiking fevers >39°C. Typically late afternoon/early evening. Occurring rapidly and settling rapidly described. Quotidian describes the daily fluctuation of ups and downs of fever of a 24-hour period.
- Fever associated with a macular rash.

- Generalized lymphadenopathy, hepatomegaly and/or splenomegaly, serositis, and myalgia.
- May mimic malignancy and carries a risk of morbidity and mortality, although outcomes have improved significantly with better treatments. Amyloidosis used to be a cuase of renal failure although now rarely seen.
- Joints affected—typically wrists, knees, hips, and ankles.

4. PsA

- Dactylitis—'sausage' fingers or toes.
- DIP involvement.
- Family history of psoriasis.
- Associated with asymptomatic uveitis.
- Continues into adult life.

5. Enthesitis-related disease (previously defined as spondyloarthropathy)

- Predominantly affects ♂.
- Inflammation at the insertion of the tendons, ligaments, or fascia to the bone.
- Affecting feet and ankles with heel and foot pain.
- Responds poorly to anti-inflammatory drugs.
- Associated with family history of psoriasis and HLA B27-related disease, AS, inflammatory bowel disease.
- ☙ There is also some controversy over whether symptomatic acute or chronic uveitis forms part of this classification.
- Back and sacro-illiac involvement rare in childhood, significant proportion of those affected will develop this in adulthood

Unclassified

Any form of JIA which doesn't fit into the above

Arthritis in childhood has the additional complication that the skeleton is still developing and therefore joint deformity and poor growth can occur either as a result of disease activity, undertreatment, or excessive steroid usage. JIA, other than rheumatoid positive poly-articular arthritis, is clinically distinct from arthritis in adults and will continue to be referred to as JIA in adulthood.

Juvenile idiopathic arthritis: assessment and treatment

JIA is a diagnosis of exclusion based on a good clinical history and physical musculoskeletal examination. Blood tests are not diagnostic but may aid the diagnosis. It is important to exclude some differential diagnoses such as:
- Musculoskeletal non-inflammatory pain.
- Hyper-mobility.
- TB or other infections.
- Malignancy.

Assessment needs to cover physical, social, and psychological issues
- Precipitating factors, symptoms, speed of onset, duration.
- Joint swelling—duration generally persistent lasting for weeks to months.
- Stiffness of joints—morning or after being in one position for a period of time.
- Pain—areas, type, severity, relieving factors.
- Growth—chart height and weight on appropriate growth chart.
- Nutrition—refer to dietician if necessary.
- Effects on activities of living. Use of functional assessment questionnaires such as the Childhood Health Assessment Questionnaire (CHAQ) allows objective comparisons of improvement/deterioration of condition over a period of time.
- School, play, and hobbies.

Physical examination
- Joint examination to identify active inflammation—joint line tenderness, swelling, heat.
- Range of movement.
- Joint deformity, subluxation, bone changes.
- Reduction of muscle bulk.

Guidelines set out the ophthalmology assessments which are required for the detection of uveitis.

Treatment
There is no curative treatment for JIA, therefore the aim of treatment is to achieve and maintain remission.

Children and young people with more than oligo-articular arthritis should be referred to and supported by tertiary paediatric rheumatology centres, with shared care arrangements.
- Should be holistic, family centred, and well coordinated.
- Multidisciplinary approach, ideally including nurse, physiotherapist, OT, psychologist, and social worker.

Aim of treatment

To ensure that each individual achieves their full potential by:
- Control of inflammation.
- Relief of pain—pharmacological and non-pharmacological.
- Preserving range of joint movement.
- Prevention of deformities and disability.
- Minimizing side effects and complications of disease and treatment.
- Promoting normal growth and development.
- Rehabilitation.
- Education of child and family.

Treatment modalities
- NSAIDs—need to be given regularly for 3–4 weeks to relieve symptoms and reach maximum benefit.
- Steroids to expedite disease control by oral, IV, or intra-articular route.
- DMARDS to effect remission. MTX usually drug of choice.
- Biological therapies used in refractory JIA. Etanercept is a licensed, NICE-approved drug for 4–17-year-old age group.
- Joint surgery.

Nursing management
- Age appropriate disease education/management for child, family, carers, and others involved in care.
- Knowledge of treatment modalities and monitoring requirements.
- Ongoing support and management in between clinic visits.
- Liaison as appropriate with 1° care team, education, social services, and voluntary agencies.
- Psychosocial support for child and family/carers.
- Facilitation of effective transition to adult services.

Therapeutic interventions
- Physiotherapy and hydro-therapy—maintenance of normal function, posturing, pacing, and exercise.
- Occupational therapy—functional assessment, aids, adaptations, and splinting of joints as appropriate.
- Orthotics—for correction of foot positioning.
- Psychology.

Further reading

British Society of Paediatric and Adolescent Rheumatology (BSPAR) guidelines for eye screening, available at: ⁂ www.bspar.org.uk.

Glasper EA, McEwing G, Richardson J (2006). *Oxford Handbook of Children's and Young People's Nursing*. Oxford University Press, Oxford.

National Institute of Clinical Excellence (2002). *Guidance on the use of etanercept for juvenile idiopathic arthritis*. Technology appraisal no. 35A. London: NICE.

Juvenile idiopathic arthritis: social and psychological impact

A diagnosis of JIA impacts upon daily activities and functioning of both the affected child and the whole family. Families should to be encouraged to maintain normal activities and routines but will have to adapt to:

- The child's reduced mobility, drug administration, assistance with ADL, and additional exercise programmes.
- The need for parents to take time off work for frequent medical or therapy appointments which may compromise employment.
- Changes in behaviour—the child may deny they are in pain to avoid further treatment, be very moody after or during steroid therapy, or be non-adherent with medication.
- The needs of siblings who may fear that they too will become ill with JIA or resent the attention given to their sibling.

The age of the child will also influence the impact of JIA. Help with ADL is acceptable for a young child but inappropriate for a teenager.

Schooling

Most children can and do attend mainstream nurseries or schools, where they should be encouraged to participate in all aspects of school life. The school nurse and key teaching staff should be made aware of the child's diagnosis, its management, and possible causes for concern. Teachers will need to be flexible to the needs of the child as their condition can fluctuate from day to day, particularly during a flare of their illness.

- EMS may affect physical functioning, e.g. sitting on the floor in assembly, taking part in PE, or getting to school on time.
- If children experience pain, have difficulty in writing, or they need to move about to avoid becoming stiff they can be allocated 25% extra time in exams. In severe cases a scribe or laptop computer may be required.
- Mainstream schools are required by law to appoint Special Educational Needs Coordinators (SENCOS). SENCOs ensure the child's educational needs are met by liaising with teaching staff, the multidisciplinary hospital team, and parents or carers.
- Juvenile arthritis, dependant on severity, can qualify as a Special Educational Need (SEN). Schools apply for a formal assessment called a 'Statement' to provide additional funding for non-teaching staff to assist with physical activities, e.g. getting changed after PE or carrying heavy equipment.
- Individual Education Plans (IEPS) are used to outline the pupil's specific needs, e.g. drug administration in school or being allowed to leave lessons 5min early to avoid the rush in the corridor.
- OTs can undertake formal assessments of seating and hand writing and then provide specialist equipment.

Adolescence

This is a challenging time and JIA impacts on teenage issues:

- Reduced independence—physical limitations, dependence on others, and potentially overprotective parents.

- Awareness of being different—delayed puberty and/or poor growth.
- Limited fashion opportunities—swollen/atypical joints.
- Body piercing/ tattoos—↑ risk when taking immunosuppressant drugs.
- Implications for risk-taking behaviours in relation to treatment, e.g. alcohol and MTX; pregnancy and MTX.
- Visible drug side effects, e.g. weight gain and cushingoid features.
- Lower expectations from parents and teachers—reduced career opportunities.

Frequently asked questions: juvenile idiopathic arthritis

How many children have JIA?

~1 in every 1000 children in the UK.

Will it 'burn itself out?'

Variable clinical course and outcomes of the different sub-types make prediction difficult. Spontaneous remission may occur; however, up to 1 in 3 have active inflammatory disease into adulthood and up to 60% will continue to have some limitation in their ADL.

Does it have a genetic element?

JIA is not 'genetic' although some forms e.g. PsA and enthesitis-related arthritis do have a familial link. Families with a strong history of auto immune diseases may also be at greater risk.

Is there any special diet that would improve the symptoms?

Healthy eating during childhood and adolescence is important particularly for those at risk from osteopoenia or osteoporosis due to disease activity and or drug therapy. Adequate amounts of calcium and vitamin D are recommended.

Further reading

British Society of Paediatric and Adolescent Rheumatology: 🖰 www.bspar.org.uk

Glasper EA, McEwing G, Richardson J (2006). *Oxford Handbook of Children's and Young People's Nursing*. Oxford University Press, Oxford.

Szer, I, Kimura, Y, Malleson, P, et al. (2006). *Arthritis in Children and Adolescents: Juvenile Idiopathic Arthritis*. Oxford University Press, Oxford.

Sero-negative spondyloarthropathies

What is it?

The spondyloarthropathies consist of a group of conditions that are chronic and inflammatory diseases; these have a number of overlapping signs and symptoms that form part of the diagnostic criteria for different types of spondyloarthropathies. The heterogeneity of the conditions adds to the complexities of identifying rigid diagnostic criteria for each of the spondyloarthropathies.

Changes are seen in the insertion of tendons and ligaments to bone with some extra-articular features such as uveitis, cardiac valve disease, and skin changes (such as psoriasis).

Spondyloarthropathies include:

- AS.
- PsA.
- Reactive arthritis—used to be referred to as Reiter disease.
- Enteropathic arthritis: arthritis of inflammatory bowel diseases.
- Undifferentiated spondyloarthropathies.
- Enthesitis related JIA.

Common characteristics of all spondyloarthropathies

- Negative for RF.
- Peripheral inflammatory arthritis—usually asymmetrical.
- Radiological evidence of sacroilitis.
- Enthesopathic pain.
- Strong association with HLA B27—association not fully understood.

Who does it affect?

The prevalence varies among ethnic groups but is considered to be about 1% of the population in Europe. Spondyloarthropathies affect ♂ and ♀, however in AS it is usually at a ratio of (♂: ♀) 3:1 and presents in late teen to early–mid 20s. It can occur occasionally in childhood (adolescent ♂ presenting with a swollen knee).

How is it diagnosed?

Diagnostic criteria are outlined in detail in Hakim et al.[1] However, diagnostic criteria for spondyloarthropathies remain a focus of research interest. There is an association with seronegative spondyloarthropathies and the HLA B27 molecule.

Reference

Hakim A, Clunie G, Haq I (eds) (2006). *Oxford Handbook of Rheumatology*, 2nd edn. Oxford University Press, Oxford.

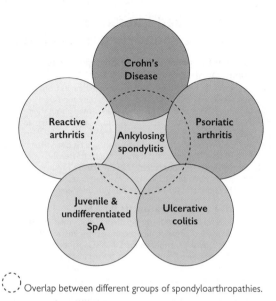

Overlap between different groups of spondyloarthropathies.

Fig. 4.7 Sero spondyloarthropathires—disease overlap. The dotted line indicates the common link of all these conditions with HLA-B27; the strongest association being with 1° AS. If there are no signs of associated spondyloarthropathy for Crohn's or psoriasis then the HLA B-27 association may not be present.

Frequently asked questions: sero-negative spondyloarthropathies

AS affects a lot of young ♂ of working age—does the condition mean they should give up work?

Many people give up work because of negative messages from their healthcare professionals. For the majority of patients they should be encouraged to stay at work as long as their employer is informed about their diagnosis and can be supportive whilst assessment and treatments are made. Teams play a really important role in helping patients stay at work—discuss work issues and put the condition, and how they should be once treatment is instigated, in context. The one difficult group can be those who work in heavy manual jobs although the continued physical activity reduces the stiffness that people with more sedentary roles may experience. Encourage them to see the OT and discuss their condition with their employers.

How effective are the treatments for AS?

The disease itself can vary with some patients having mild disease that will benefit from lifestyle changes, regular exercise regimens, and the occasional use of NSAIDs. However, evidence for DMARDs is not that encouraging for those with aggressive AS and there is no evidence for benefits to the spine. Sulfasalazine (SAS) has demonstrated some benefit for peripheral joints. It is important to assess patients regularly so that they get the most effective treatment options as early as possible. The biologic DMARDs demonstrate significant treatment effects but have rigorous criteria for eligibility of treatment (see NICE[1] for treatment criteria with anti-TNFα therapies).

Who assesses and treats those patients who have skin involvement in PsA?

Patients may go to a dermatologist in the first instance (particularly if their first problems were related to the skin). However, in some places patients are seen in a clinic with dermatology and rheumatology expertise. There are some excellent models of nurses working across both specialties to ensure the patient has both issues (skin and joints effectively assessed and treated). Scoring of skin and nail involvement does require training.

Reference

1. NICE: ⊕ www.nice.org.uk

Psoriatic arthritis: overview

What is PsA?

PsA is a chronic inflammatory joint disease that is strongly associated both with the skin disorder psoriasis and arthritis. The condition follows a variable and heterogeneous clinical course with some patients who experience very mild disease that responds well to treatment and others with erosive and destructive disease that is resistant to treatment resulting in poor long-term outcomes. A form of PsA called PsA mutilans causes severe destruction (Fig. 4.8). In a similar way to RA, PsA follows an erratic course with flare ups and times of quiescence.

Relationship of skin and joints

- Simultaneous skin and joint involvement occur in about 15% of those with PsA.
- 60% have psoriasis before arthritis.
- Severe arthritis can have little or no skin involvement and visa versa.
- The PsA has similarities to RA although there are some important differences which include:
  - PsA is classified as a spondyloarthropathy.
  - Affects ♂ and ♀ equally.
  - Diagnostic criteria differ (🕮 see How is PsA diagnosed?, in this section).
- See Fig. 4.8.

Who does it affect?

- Prevalence of between 0.1–2% of the population.
- 5–7% of psoriasis patients have PsA.
- 40% of those with extensive psoriasis have PsA.
- In specialist services, 40–60% of PsA have erosive and deforming arthritis.

How is PsA diagnosed?

PsA can be a difficult disease to diagnose due to the differing disease presentations with many clinical subgroups of PsA. New diagnostic disease classifications have been published.[1]

Key aspects of disease presentation (Fig. 4.9) and diagnosis include:

- Sero-negative for RF.
- Fewer joints involved and generally asymmetrical distribution.
- Axial manifestations of the disease are associated with HLA B27.
- Clinical features include a heterogeneous pattern of joint involvement.
- Imaging studies confirm the presence of enthesis in PsA but not RA
- Entheses and soft-tissues changes result in dactylitis (sausage-like digit) (Fig. 4.9c,d)
- Affects DIP joints.
- Nail involvement (Fig. 4.9a).

Axial disease

- Shared features with AS:
  - But less severe overall disease severity.
  - Reduce association with positive serology for HLA B27 than AS.
  - Fewer syndesmophytes, cervical involvement, and sacroilitis.
  - Better spinal mobility and sparing of apophyseal joints.

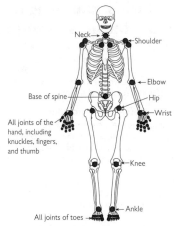

Fig. 4.8 Joints commonly affected by PsA.

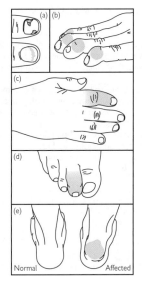

Fig. 4.9 Signs and symptoms of PsA. Adapted with permission from the ARC.

Reference

Kavanaugh, AF, Ritchlin, C, GRAPPA Treatment Guideline Committee (2006). Systematic review of treatments for psoriatic arthritis: an evidenced based approach and basis for treatment guidelines. *Journal of Rheumatology*, **33**, 1417–21.

Psoriatic arthritis: managing the condition, treatment, and when to refer

PsA is a very heterogeneous condition with involvement of joints and disease severity varies. People with mild disease may require treatment to treat symptoms whereas others may have an erosive and progressively destructive disease. For those with aggressive and destructive disease, there are many similarities in the treatment and management with that of RA.

The management of PsA must include:

- Educating and supporting the patient with PsA:
  - Disease, long-term outcomes, and treatment options.
  - Self-management principles and support available.
  - Holistic assessment and management of social and psychological needs.
- Relieving symptoms—joints:
  - Analgesia and, when required, NSAIDs for exacerbations/flares.
  - Active synovitis confined to one or two joints—consider IA steroid injections.
- Relieving symptoms—skin:
  - Topical therapy.
  - Psoralen plus ultraviolet A light (PUVA) or ultraviolet B light (PUVB).
- Treating the disease:
  - For those with erosive and destructive disease—aggressive disease control to prevent long-term disability.
  - Disease-modifying drugs include MTX, ciclosporin A, sulfasalazine, leflunomide.
  - Where the disease fails to be controlled if treatment criteria fulfilled—anti-TNFα therapies adalimumab, etanercept, infliximab.
- Maintaining functional ability for those with erosive disease:
  - Use of aids and devices.
  - Assessment and advice on ADL and joint protection.
  - Exercise and protection of joints and use of walking aids.
  - Podiatry where appropriate for footwear, arch supports, etc.

Disease assessment

- Indices to measure joint, skin, and nail involvement
  (📖 see Indices to measure joint, skin and nail involvement, p.88).
- Inflammatory markers—CRP, ESR.
- Pain and global health VASs.
- Functional ability.

When to refer

- Where the patient experiences numerous flares/exacerbations of the disease.
- Where there are toxicities or poor concordance issues with disease-modifying therapies.
- When symptoms are poorly controlled and require re-assessment.
- For specialist support on functional changes may benefit from OT, PT, or podiatrist.

• For some patients, specific psychological needs may require referral to a psychologist (uniquely issues related to PsA and skin involvement).

What is the impact to the patient?

📖 See Nursing issues p.300 and patient-centred care, p.314.

Psoriasis

Psoriasis is a non-contagious skin condition. There is a link with psoriasis and arthritis in the sero-negative spondyloarthropathies. PsA is a condition with inflammatory joint disease and evidence of psoriasis (📖 see Psoriatic arthritis, p.84).

Epidemiology and incidence

- Psoriasis is a common inflammatory skin disease which affects ~2% of the population in the UK.
- ♂ and ♀ are equally affected.
- Peak age of onset between 20–35 years of age.
- 75% of all cases occur for the first time before the age of 40.
- ~10% develop psoriatic arthritis.

The prevalence varies between races with the highest recorded numbers in the white populations of Scandinavia and Northern Europe and the lowest prevalence in Native American Indians and the Japanese population.

Causes

There is growing evidence that psoriasis is:

- Primarily a T-cell driven disease where the usual process of skin replacement is accelerated.
- In 30% of cases there is a family history of psoriasis.
- Genetics play a role in ~40% of patients.
- Environmental triggers include infection (streptococcal infection accounts for 60% of guttate psoriasis), drugs (e.g. lithium, systemic steroids, and anti-malarial), physical and psychological stress.

History and examination

Important factors to consider in the history are:

- Persistent scaling in the ears and/or longstanding dandruff.
- Anal or vulval itching.
- Joint problems and concomitant or previously diagnosed autoimmune disease.

Clinical features

The regions commonly involved are scalp, elbows, knees, sacrum, and the dorsal aspect of the hands, especially over the knuckles and the nails All psoriasis lesions show varying degrees of three cardinal characteristics:

- Scaling.
- Thickening (induration).
- Inflammation (redness) and are highly symmetrical in most cases.

Types of psoriasis

Psoriasis is a very diverse skin disease which appears in a variety of forms; each form has its own distinct characteristics. It is usual for people to have one type at a time; however, it can occasionally change from one type to another.

There are five main types of psoriasis:

- *Plaque psoriasis:* the most prevalent form of the disease. About 80% of patients have this form of psoriasis. Features typically found on elbows, knees, scalp, and lower back are characterized by raised, inflamed, red lesions covered by a silvery, white scale.

- *Guttate psoriasis* ('guttate' from the Latin word meaning drop): typically starts in childhood or adolescence. Lesions usually appear on the trunk and limbs. Thinner than plaque psoriasis and resembles small, red, individual spots on the skin. Guttate psoriasis frequently appears following an upper respiratory tract or a streptococcal infection.
- *Flexural or inverse psoriasis:* found in skin folds (e.g. armpits, groin, under the breasts, around the genitalia or buttocks). Flexural psoriasis appears as smooth and shiny and is particularly subject to irritation from rubbing and sweating from the skin folds.
- *Pustular psoriasis:* primarily seen in adults and is characterized by white pustules surrounded by red skin. Commonly seen on the palms of the hands and soles of the feet (called palmar plantar pustular psoriasis). Pustules are sterile and not contagious. Cycles of widespread pustular psoriasis covering most of the body can occur with reddening, followed by pustules, and then scaling.
- *Erythrodermic psoriasisis:* the most common form of inflammatory psoriasis affecting most of the body surface. Can occur in association with widespread pustular psoriasis. Characterized by periodic, widespread, fiery redness of the skin with associated itching and pain. Protein and fluid loss can occur, leading to disrupted temperature regulation and severe illness such as infection, pneumonia, and heart failure. In severe cases hospitalization may be required.

Differential diagnosis

Various dermatological conditions resemble psoriasis, including: candidiasis, tinea infection, eczema, contact dermatitis, superficial basal cell carcinoma, cutaneous T-cell lymphoma, and pityriasis rosae. Routine history, physical examination, and laboratory findings required to confirm diagnosis.

Management and treatment

Goals of treatment are to:
- Improve the patient's quality of life and disease control.
- Aim for long-term remission and reduce drug toxicity.
- Evaluate cost/benefit of treatments.

~70% of patients can be managed on topical treatments alone. Time spent educating the patient in the practicalities of topical therapy is crucial to success.
- Topical treatments include emollients to alleviate itching, reduce scale, and enhance penetration of concomitant therapy; keratolytic agents e.g. salicylic acid to reduce scale; topical steroids for severe inflammation and for short periods; vitamin D analogues, coal tar, and dithranol.
- Phototherapy—light therapy using UVB and photo chemotherapy. PUVA where methoxsalen is ingested followed by a measured dose of PUVA.
- Systemic treatments are used for severe psoriasis, when topical therapies UVB or PUVA, have failed or in those where there is a negative impact on quality of life. Drugs include MTX, ciclosporin, retinoids, tacrolimus, azathioprine (AZA), and mycophenolate mofetil (MMF).
- Biologic therapies are used for those who have severe disease and fail to respond to conventional therapy.[1] Drugs include etanercept, adalimumab, infliximab, and efaluzimab.

Reference

1. NICE: ⁀ www.nice.org.uk

Ankylosing spondylitis

AS is a chronic inflammatory condition that causes a progressive, disabling arthritis that affects the axial spine (including the sacro-iliac joints) causing chronic lower back pain and progressive stiffening of the spine. 20–40% of patients can have peripheral joint involvement at some time of the disease duration.

Prevalence is thought to be 13:1000, it is most common in adolescents or young adults, with a ♂:♀ ratio of 3:1.

Clinical features

The inflammation in AS cause the bone to erode. When the inflammation subsides, the bone begins to repair itself but also replaces the previously inflamed elastic tissue of the tendons and ligaments with bone. The bones can slowly fuse and cause restriction of movement. In the spine, the outer annular fibres are replaced by bone and the vertebrae become fused forming a long, bony column known as 'bamboo spine'. AS is characterized by exacerbation and remission of disease activity, it is widely under-recognized, under-diagnosed, and under-treated. See Figs. 4.10, 4.11.

Typical symptoms of AS

- Gradual onset of back pain over a period of weeks or months.
- Fatigue.
- EMS and pain that wears off during the day with exercise.
- Back pain that is worse after rest but better with exercise.
- Pain in the sacroiliac or gluteal region.
- Enthesopathy (bone erosion): Achilles tendonitis, plantar fascitiis, costochondral, and costovertabral abnormalities.
- Weight loss.
- Fever.
- Uveitis (iritis).

Diagnostic criteria

- The Modified New York Criteria provide detailed diagnostic criteria for AS.[1]
- AS is not easily diagnosed; although there is no specific blood test, the gene HLA-B27 is associated with the disease and is positive in many patients. However, it is not a reliable guide to prognosis. Most patients are RF negative. Other blood tests that may indicate AS include CRP—a marker of inflammation, and ESR—which can be elevated during active inflammation.
- AS is not solely a disease of the musculoskeletal system, it can manifest in other organs including the eyes, lungs, and cardiovascular system.

Late clinical features

- Fusion of spine leading to restriction of movement—'bamboo spine'.
- Restriction in the range or movement of the hips and shoulders.
- 50% peripheral joint disease.
- 25% eye involvement e.g. iritis.
- Flexion contractures of hips and knees.
- Reduction in chest expansion—can also appear early in disease.

- Heart valve involvement/aortic incompetence.
- Cauda equina syndrome.
- Amyloidosis.

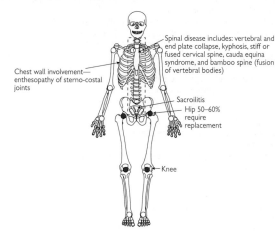

Fig. 4.10 Joints commonly affected in AS. Note: peripheral involvement (knees and hips)—can occur particularly in lower limbs in 20–30% (more severe disease).

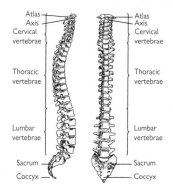

Fig. 4.11 The vertebral column in AS. Reproduced with permission from Khan MA (2002). *Ankylosing Spondylitis: The Facts.* Oxford University Press, Oxford.

Reference

Hakim A, Clunie G, Haq I (eds) (2006). *Oxford Handbook of Rheumatology*, 2nd edn. Oxford University Press, Oxford.

Ankylosing spondylitis: assessment

The most commonly used assessment tools are self-administered questionnaires—these are validated and used throughout the UK in determining treatment therapy.

- Bath Ankylosing Spondylitis Disease Activity Index (BASDAI).[1] Made up of 6 questions relating to the patient's self-reported disease activity.
- Bath Ankylosing Spondylitis Metrology Index (BASMI).[2] This is a way of measuring spinal and hip movement.
- Bath Ankylosing Spondylitis Functional Index (BASFI).[3] Made up of 10 questions relating to the patient's self-reported functional ability.
- Bath Ankylosing Spondylitis Global (BAS-G) score.[4] Made up of 2 questions relating to the patient's self-reported global health.

Management

- Symptomatic relief of pain and stiffness.
- Disease control.
- Baseline assessments and review of changes in disease.

The nurse's role:

- Patient education:
  - Information on the disease.
  - Support patient empowerment/patient-centred care.
  - Self-management principles.
- Exercise.
- Physiotherapy.
- Hydrotherapy.
- Lifestyle modification—smoking cessation, work related issues.
- Support Groups—National Ankylosing Spondylitis Society.[5]

Medications

- NSAIDs are a core treatment for pain relief but they do not alter the underlying mechanism of AS.
- DMARDs if insufficient benefits from NSAIDs, but there is limited evidence of their efficacy, except in patients with peripheral disease.
- Anti-TNFα drugs show significant benefits in maintaining functional ability and symptom control.[6]

📖 Also see Biologics, p.448; 📖 Assessment tools: clinical indicators and disease-specific tools, Chapter 20.

References

1. Garret *et al.* (1994). A new approach to defining disease status in Ankylosing Spondylitis; The Bath Ankylosing Spondylitis Disease Activity Index (BASDAI). *Journal of Rheumatology*, **21**, 2286–91.

2. Jenkinson *et al.* (1994). Defining spinal mobility in Ankylosing Spondylitis (AS): The Bath AS Metrology Index. *Journal of Rheumatology*, **21**, 1694–8.

3. Calin *et al.* (1994). A new approach to defining functional ability in Ankylosing Spondylitis: the development of the Bath Ankylosing Spondylitis Functional Index (BASFI). *Journal of Rheumatology*, **21**, 2281–5.

4. Jones *et al.* (1996). The Bath Ankylosing Spondylitis Patient Global Score (BAS-G). *British Journal of Rheumatology*, **35**, 66–71.

5. National Ankylosing Spondylitis Society: ⌖ www.nass.co.uk.

6. British Society for Rheumatology (2004). *BSR Guideline for prescribing TNFa blockers in adults with ankylosing spondylitis.* BSR, London.

Reactive arthritis, Reiter syndrome, and enteropathic arthritis: overview

Reactive arthritis (ReA) and Reiter syndrome (also called sexually acquired reactive arthritis, SARA)

Clinical features and joints involved

ReA (sometimes referred to as Reiter syndrome) is a systemic sero-negative spondyloarthropathy not solely confined to joints (see Fig. 4.12). ReA is a term used to describe any infection that triggers joint pain (e.g. rheumatic fever following a streptococcal infection). ReA usually develops following an infection within the previous month of presenting symptoms, which may be mild and unnoticed at the time.

The infecting organisms are most commonly related to infections seen in the oral, gastrointestinal (GI), or genitourinary areas.

Features include:

- Strong association with genetic HLA-B27 antigen positive individuals.
- Predominately young (20–40-year-olds) ♂ ≈ ♀.
- Asymmetrical oligoarthritis (usually weight-bearing lower limbs).
- Skin and mucous membrane lesions (mucosal psoriasis, urethritis, balanitis circinata, cervicitis, keratodermia blenorrhagica—rash on soles and palms of hands).
- Eye inflammation (uveitis, conjunctivitis).
- Lower back pain (unilateral sacroiliitis) or abdominal discomfort.
- Dactylitis, enthesopathy, tendonitis, tenosynovitis, and muscle pain.
- EMS.

ReA can present in many ways and mimics many other forms of arthritis. A good clinical history is essential to exclude other diagnoses and identify any potential infective event. See Box 4.4 and Table 4.1.

Enteropathic arthritis (EA)

The condition is not fully understood but has a number of similarities with spondyloarthropathies and ReA. ♂ ≈ ♀. Any age can be affected. Joints commonly affected are knees and ankles.

Signs and symptoms

- Similar to ReA (sacroiliitis, mono or asymmetrical arthritis).
- Enthesitis may be present (sites: elbow, foot, knee).
- Gradual onset.
- Skin lesions (e.g. erythema nodosum).

In EA there are three cardinal features:

- Joint pain and related symptoms follow an onset of bowel disease.
  - Arthritis present in 20% of ulcerative colitis and Crohn's disease.
- In the short term there is a relationship between 'flares' of the arthritis and exacerbations of bowel disease.

- Treatment of bowel condition results in improvement or complete remission of synovitis (STS).

Box 4.4 ReA investigations

- Aspiration of swollen joints for culture to exclude septic arthritis, gout, and HIV-associated arthritis. Microscope analysis to exclude evidence of crystals (gout) if indicated.
  - ❶ Septic arthritis is a medical emergency and requires prompt medical treatment.
- Cultures for urine, blood, and stools as appropriate: check urethral discharge for chlamydia and gonococcal infection.
- Inflammatory markers will be raised (ESR, CRP).

Table 4.1 ReA presentations

Common	Rare
REA incidence ~30–40 per 100,000 adults/year	Radiological signs in early disease
20–40-year-olds	Small children and the elderly
65–96% positive to HLA B27 antigen	Severe destructive disease
Pain on palpation of tendon insertion sites and difficulty in walking	Muscle wasting and severe disability
Ocular involvement including unilateral or bilateral conjunctivitis (sterile), acute uveitis	Glomerulonephritis and IgA nephropathy
Enthesitis especially heel pain (Achilles), metatarsalgia (plantar fasciitis) or 'sausage digits' (dactylitis)	Cardiac involvement

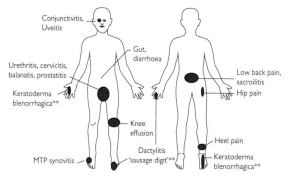

Fig. 4.12 Signs and symptoms of ReA. ** Less common but may be associated with long-term prognosis.

Reactive arthritis, Reiter syndrome, and enteropathic arthritis: management and treatment

Managing the condition and treatment

The onset of the condition and subsequent symptoms require empathy and good nursing support in the first instance at initial presentation when the diagnosis is yet to be confirmed, and subsequently in supporting the patient from social and psychological needs and expectations.

- Education and guidance on treatment, condition, and symptom control is essential and should be reinforced by written information.
- Consider social and psychological impact (💷 see Nursing issues, p.300, 346 and patient centred care, p.314).
- If sexually transmitted disease, counselling and contact tracing must be undertaken.
- Health promotion and disease prevention advice to avoid future infections.
- IA joint injection for swollen joints—consider referral to OT or PT.
- Antibiotics if an infective organism is identified (see local antibiotic policies for guidance on drug of choice).
- If there are no contraindications may require NSAIDs or COX-2 inhibitors.
- Uveitis, topical steroids—refer to ophthalmologist if unresolved >3 days.

Prognosis

- If ongoing synovitis and joint destruction >6 months—DMARD may be indicated (SAS or MTX).
- Complete remission for the majority by 6 months. Almost all have complete remission at 2 years (70%). Poorer prognosis for those who have persistent symptoms and joint damage.

Treatment for EA

- Education and guidance on EA and the underlying bowel condition.
- Consider social and psychological impact (💷 Nursing issues, p.300, 346 and patient-centred care, p.314).
- IA steroids for swollen joints.
- Caution with NSAIDs which may precipitate a flare of the bowel disease.
- Treatment of underlying bowel condition will improve joint problems:
  - For those failing to respond DMARDs may be used (SAS, MTX).
  - Anti-TNFα used to treat Crohn's disease will also resolve arthropathies.
- Surgical removal of the inflamed colon can improve or resolve arthropathy.

Table 4.2 Micro-organisms implicated in SARA

Involvement	Micro-organisms	Susceptibility	Comment
Gastrointestinal	Campylobacter jejuni Clostridium difficile Escherichia coli Gardia Lambia Salmonella Yersinia	HLA B27 antigen positive	May complain of abdominal pain many months after initial attack
Genitourinary	Nisseria Gonorrhea Chlamydia Trachomatis Ureaplasma urealyticum	HLA B27 antigen positive	Mild kysuria or mucopurulent discharge may be present
Oral and other			Lesions—painless, shiny patches occuring on palate, tongue, uvula and tonsilar region

Polymyalgia rheumatica

Introduction

Polymyalgia rheumatica (PMR) is a common condition in the elderly population. It is a clinical syndrome of pain, tenderness, and stiffness in the shoulder and pelvic girdle and is frequently accompanied by fever, weight loss, and fatigue. Onset may be sudden with clear diagnostic features (Box 4.5). An insidious onset with more systemic features may also present. PMR has an estimated prevalence of about 1% and is rare in those <50 years old. The ♀:♂ ratio is 2:1.

Social and psychological impact

Patients can feel anxious and fearful as onset of disability and symptoms are sudden. General health education and instruction on protecting joints and muscles can help overcome anxiety. Relaxation and education indicating steady, gradual, graded exercise can also assist recovery.

Nursing care issues in management

PMR, once diagnosed, will require regular review/follow-up for 2 years (until condition is stable). Management can be undertaken by nurses in either 1° or 2° care. There are specific issues that will need to be considered and documented:

- Nurse specialist should undertake a patient-centred holistic assessment and provide education (verbal and written) about the condition, medications, and managing symptoms.
- Patient's functional ability and ADL are affected (particularly in early phases and during exacerbations).
  - Reported difficulties include rising from a chair, getting out of bed, and difficulties with washing and dressing.
- Physiotherapy or occupational therapy referral may be required to support management of ADL (exercise and use of aids and devices).
- Practical advice on relief of pain and stiffness include the use of warm showers and gentle exercise.
- Nurses in all care settings should advise patients about 'flares' of PMR, which may be related to reducing prednisolone. If there is a relapse of symptoms—particularly aching and stiffness in the shoulder and hip girdles—monitor ESR, review prednisolone dose, and seek specialist help where necessary.

Review

Review the patient after starting initial treatment (Box 4.6) and also shortly after changing prednisolone dosages. Re-check inflammatory markers every 2–6 weeks after changes in treatment to assess response.

Response to treatment

Relapse is most common in the first 18 months of treatment but may recur when steroids are stopped. Steroids should be very slowly tapered down to reduce the risk of relapse. Pain is a predominant feature and will provide a good indicator of reductions in disease activity.

Box 4.5 Diagnosis of PMR

Classical presentation:
- Aching and stiffness in the shoulder and hip girdles.
  - Systemic features: anorexia, weight loss and low-grade fever.
- Elevated ESR ↑40mm/hour
- EMS >1 hour
- A mild normochromic anemia is common.

Diagnostic considerations
- Differential diagnoses e.g. RA, malignancy.
- Does the patient have giant cell arteritis (GCA)?

Investigations
- ESR.
- CRP.
- FBC.
- LFT.

Differential investigations
- RF, ANA.
- Immunoglobulins, protein electrophoresis and Bence Jones urine to exclude myeloma.
- Creatine kinase to exclude myositis.
- Thyroid function test to exclude hypothyroidism.
- Chest x-ray to screen for malignancy.

Box 4.6 Treatment of PMR

- Low-dose prednisolone 15–20mg (often considered diagnostic of PMR).
- When response achieved, reduce dose by 2.5mg every 6 weeks to a dose of 7.5mg (depending on patient symptoms). Maintain for 6 months.
- Dose ↓by 1mg every 6–8 weeks until complete withdrawal of prednisolone (~2 years for most patients).
- For those that fail to achieve dose reductions this may take longer and require a steroid sparing agent (e.g. MTX).
- Analgesia may aid pain relief whilst reducing prednisolone.
- Monitor ESR or CRP—↑ may not necessitate recurrence
- Bone-protective therapy (bisphosphonate and calcium and vitamin D) should be started on commencing prednisolone.

Response to treatment
- 70% global response usually achieved within 1 week.
- Return to normal values in acute phase responses.
- If response not demonstrated—stop treatment and review diagnosis.

▶ Although not indicated as core treatment, an analgesia or NSAID may be prescribed in the short term for pain relief whilst weaning off prednisolone (refer to BNF for cautions and contraindications).

Frequently asked questions: polymyalgia rheumatica

What if the ESR remains elevated after starting prednisolone?
Diagnosis should be reviewed.

What if the patient with PMR is unable to stop prednisolone after 2 years?
Some patients may require a small dose past 2 years or you can try introducing analgesia.

What if you suspect an underlying malignancy?
Refer to a consultant/physician for urgent opinion

What if a patient is unable to tolerate bisphosphonate therapy?
Try strontium ranelate, or raloxifene

Further reading

Hennell SL, Busteed S, George E (2007). Evidence-based management for polymyalgia rheumatica for rheumatology practitioners, nurses and physiotherapists. *Musculoskeletal Care*, **5**(2), 65–71.

Royal College of Physicians (2002). *Guidelines on the prevention and treatment of gluco-corticosteroid induced osteoporosis*. RCP, London.

Giant cell arteritis

There is an association between PMR and giant cell arteritis (GCA). GCA is inflammation of the larger blood vessels commonly affecting the extra cranial branches of the carotid artery. ~1/5 of those diagnosed with PMR may develop GCA. When monitoring PMR ensure screening for GCA:

▶Screening for GCA when monitoring PMR should include:

- Symptoms of unilateral headache or any visual symptoms.
- Scalp tenderness and jaw claudication.
- Review acute phase responses (ESR 30mm/h).

▶ Seek urgent specialist opinion if GCA suspected. If GCA suspected temporal biopsy may be required.

Management of PMR and GCA

GCA will require prednisolone as outlined in the PMR regimen (☐ see Box 4.6, p.99) including gradually reducing the dose when symptoms are effectively managed.

▶ If new visual disturbances are reported seek ophthalmology opinion.

Crystal arthropathies

Crystal arthropathies describe a group of inflammatory joint disorders that develop as a result of micro crystal formation in the joints or in periarticular tissues. Other organs vulnerable to crystal deposition include excretory organs (e.g. liver, kidneys). For incidence and features see Table 4.3

Crystal arthropathies are an important differential diagnosis for conditions such as RA, ReA, and septic arthritis where acute extremely painful joint pains are a presenting symptom. This chapter will provide the essential issues related to crystal arthropathies with a specific focus on gout. For further more detailed information on crystal arthropathies refer to Hakim et al.[1]

Types of crystal arthropathies

Three major crystal arthropathies develop as a result of crystal deposits and these include:

- Monosodium urate monohydrate (MSM) ≈ gout.
- Calcium pyrophosphate deposition (CPD) ≈ pseudogout.
- Calcium hydroxyapatite ≈ acute calcific periarthritis.

Crystal arthropathies can cause:

- Arthritis.
- Tenosynovitis.
- Bursitis.
- Cellulitis.
- Tophaceous deposits (usually late disease—gout only).
- Renal disease.

Presenting features and joints affected

- Symptomatic condition results in an 'acute' attack of arthritis.
- Joints become hot, swollen, and extremely tender to touch.
- The affected joint(s) may appear red and have a shiny appearance.
- Feel generally unwell, may have a fever.

⚠ Also signs of septic arthritis (a medical emergency).

Distribution of joints

The distribution of joints and tissues affected varies according to the type of crystal arthropathy:

- Gout: usually affects peripheral joints (big toe 50–70%; foot 50%; knee 30%; wrists 10%; elbows 10%; fingers 25%).
- Pseudogout: knees, wrists, hips, symphysis pubis, shoulders.
- Hydroxyapatite: central joints usually shoulders, rarely hips, spine, and knees.

Reference

1. Hakim A, Clunie G, Haq I (eds) (2006). *Oxford Handbook of Rheumatology,* 2nd edn. Oxford University Press, Oxford.

Further reading

Kelsey M. et al. (2007) on behalf of the British Society for Rhematology and British Health Professionals in Rheumatology Standards, Guidelines and Audit Working Group. *British Society for Rheumatology and British Health Professionals in Rheumatology Guidelines for the Management of Gout,* **46**, 1372–4.

Table 4.3 Incidence and features of crystal arthropathies

Condition	Gout	Pseudogout
Age of onset:	Mean age of onset >40 years 4 >50 years 5; rare before menopause.	Rare in those <60 years of age
♂:♀ ratio:	Ratio: 4♂:1♀	Ratio: 1♂:1♀
Mechanism:	High levels of serum uric acid (SUA) develop as a result of over production or failure to adequately secrete SUA.	Calcium pyrophosphate crystals (CPPC) released and shed into joint capsule causing inflammatory response (acute episode of pseudogout) CPPC can also deposit in tendons resulting in calcific tendonitis.
Common precipitating factors:	↑ SUA predisposing factor to developing may be combined with : • Family history/genetic factors • Social class ↑ richer dietary protein/alcohol ◆ • Obesity/systemic illness/ trauma/surgery • Alcohol (beer and wine) • High protein ◆	There may be: • No obvious precipitating cause • Injury to joint • Generalized illness (especially if associated with ↑ temperature)
Comorbidities:	Hypertension/hyperglycaemia/ hyperlipidaemia	Strong associations: with • Hyperparathyroidism • Haemachromatosis • Hypomagnesia • Wilson's disease
Exacerbating conditions:	Inherited metabolic conditions— Lesch Nyan deficiency Uric acid overproduction conditions: e.g. myelosuppressive disease Uric acid underexcretion: e.g. renal disease/failure.	
Differential diagnosis:	Septic arthritis RA PsA ReA Exacerbation of OA	Several subcategories of CPPD. Septic arthritis and other inflammatory joint diseases (as for gout)

Gout and pseudogout

Gout and pseudogout are the two most common forms of crystal disease.

Gout

Gout is a condition where urate crystals occur in joints, connective tissues, and urinary tract. Gout is associated with comorbid conditions including cardiovascular disease. The incidence and prevalence are set to rise with the growing elderly, obesity, and lifestyle changes. In the UK ~250,000 people every year consult their GP with a diagnosis of gout (◻ see Table 4.3, p.103). Overall prevalence in UK in 1999 is 1.4%.

The predominant cause of gout is hyperuricemia (SUA concentration >7mg/dL). Uric acid is the end-product of protein metabolism and is usually excreted by:
- Kidneys (2/3^{rds}).
- GI tract (1/3rd).

Precipitating factors for gout

The risk of developing gout ↑ as SUA rises. Hyperuricemia + precipitating factor (e.g. a patient starting diuretics or cytotoxic therapy) = gout. (◻ see Table 4.3, p.103). Gout can be described as either:
- 1°: no known cause or inherited metabolic disorder (e.g. Lesch Nyan syndrome).
- 2°: to conditions that result in ↑ SUA.
  - High SUA can be attributed to either over production or under excretion of UA and in some cases a mixture of both.

The presentations of gout include:

- Acute attacks: sudden presentation of disabling pain (usually during night), red, shiny skin, tender joint (usually big toe 50–70%, or lower limbs). Systemically unwell. Untreated can last days or weeks.
- Recurrent gout: can result in joint damage and residual disability.
- Chronic tophaceous gout: following recurrent attacks tophi are formed from accumulation of uric acid crystal and inflammatory cells forming under the skin and in periarticular tissues (the ear, bursae, and tendon sheaths); rarely tophi can form in the eye and heart.
  - Also seen in elderly patients (usually ♀) on diuretics.

Pseudogout

Pseudogout develops following the shedding of CPPC from articular cartilage and is strongly associated with chondrocalcinosis (calcium crystals in hyaline cartilage e.g. menisci). There are many similarities to gout as well as differences (◻ see Table 4.3, p.103). The presentation of pseudogout is similar to that outlined in an acute attack of gout; however, the long-term course of the condition is usually more benign than gout. Symptoms can develop over a period of 24 hours and the clinical picture can sometimes mimic OA. Precipitating factors include:
- Injury to joint.
- Generalized illness (especially with associated fever).
- Surgery.

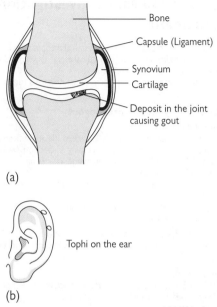

Bone

Capsule (Ligament)

Synovium

Cartilage

Deposit in the joint causing gout

(a)

Tophi on the ear

(b)

Fig. 4.13 Joints affected in gout and pseudo gout. Urate may collect under the skin forning small white pimples ('tophi') but these are not usually painful. Reproduced with kind permission from the ARC.

Crystal arthropathies: investigations and treatments

As with all MSC the diagnosis of a crystal arthropathy relies upon a thorough clinical history and good musculoskeletal examination (📖 see Chapter 8, Assessing the patient, p.272).

⚠ Septic arthritis is an important differential diagnosis (urgent medical treatment required)

Investigations for gout and pseudogout

Joint aspiration and microscopy

Microscopy of the synovial fluid analysis should aid identification of the crystals implicated in the joint pain, including inspection by the naked eye (blood stained, purulent, with high white cell count and crystals). Microscopy should examine for:

- Urate crystals (gout)—negatively birefringent (murky, pus like appearance).
- Calcium pyrophosphate—positive birefringent (may be blood stained).
- Hydroxyapatite—stain with alizarin red.

Failure to identify crystals does not exclude the diagnosis.

⚠ Culture of synovial fluid is important to exclude/confirm septic arthritis.

Blood tests

- FBC—leucocytosis.
- Uric acid (may be normal during an acute attack but does not preclude gout). May be useful for monitoring treatment.
- Acute phase response—usually raised ESR.
- U&E and creatinine—may require additional investigation for renal function if indicated.
- Bloods to consider contributing factors, e.g. alcohol (raised γ GT or LFTs) glucose (diabetes) lipids (hyperlipidaemia).

Radiological investigations—not always required

- X-rays can exclude trauma, fracture or infections.
- In pseudogout may identify additional factors such as OA.
- Soft tissue swelling or periarticular osteoporosis may be evident in gout.

Treatment

- Removal of crystals by aspiration (especially in large joints) and IA steroid injection.
- Immediate relief of symptoms (analgesia, NSAIDs, colchicine, corticosteroids, rest, ice, elevation).
- Exclude/manage exacerbating factors related to 1° or 2° causes of gout.
- Gout—if second or further attack within 1 year instigate prophylactic therapy (1–2 weeks after resolution of symptoms).
- Education and support on condition, self-management strategies and life style changes required—↓ alcohol and purine intake, obesity.
- Nursing care including education, symptom relief.

Box 4.7 Treatment for CPPD

- CPPD management similar to gout at initial presentation.
- Rest, information about the condition, management, and pain control.
- Paracetamol + codeine or NSAID for pain (although a very painful condition—review benefit).
- Colchine—only recommended for recurrent attacks (rare).
- Exercises to reduce muscle wasting/weakness should be advocated when attack has resolved.
- Diet—no specific dietary factors.

⚠ *Important: septic arthritis is a differential diagnosis for acute onset of very painful joints.*

Crystal arthropathies: nursing care issues in management

The commonest crystal arthropathy is gout followed by pseudogout. Gout is an extremely painful condition and requires prompt management to relieve the pain and distress and aid recovery. Individuals who are affected by these conditions initially require very similar nursing support and management, particularly in relation to:

- Pain-relieving strategies.
- Functional limitations.
- Monitoring of the condition and results of investigations.
- Education and support in relation to medications and general health status.

Severity of attacks and resolution will vary from mild (1–2 days) to severe (1–several weeks). The attacks may appear less aggressively in elderly compared to the younger patient.

Aims of management

Treatment and rapid relief of symptoms (Table 4.4)

- Relief from the immediate attack of gout, with a focus on pain relief strategies.
- Analgesia.
- Rest, ice packs, and pressure-relieving devices (e.g. bed cradle).
- Functional limitations.
- Reassurance/education and advice.

Self-management principles

- Education on condition and treatment options.
- Advice on resolution of attacks and managing future attacks.
- Managing medications.
- Lifestyle advice and issues related to concordance.
    - ↓ alcohol (beer especially) below recommend national intake and consider alcohol-free days (gout only).
    - Restrictions on (protein), high purine foods (red meats, shellfish, offal) (gout).
    - Weight loss if appropriate. Avoid crash diets (gout).
    - Encourage fluid intake of ~2L per day.
    - Sensible moderate exercise—avoid intense physical exercise.
    - Recommend discussing herbal/complementary therapies with healthcare professionals before starting any new therapies.

Prevention of future attacks (gout) (Table 4.5)

Management must focus on treating the 1° or 2° causes related to the over production or under excretion of SUA resulting in ↑SUA.

- Urostatic—inhibit production xanthine oxidase inhibitor (e.g. allopurinol).
- Urosuric—promoting renal excretion of urate (sulfinpyrazone):
    - Urosuric drugs are less commonly used.
- Identification contributing factors—related to co-morbidities etc..
- Guidance on managing a future attack—prompt NSAIDs.

Table 4.4 Prophylactic treatment for gout (also refer to *BNF* and full SPC)

Treatment:	• Uricostatic drugs:	• Uricosuric drugs (less
• Do not commence treatment during acute attack • Commence treatment: 1–2 wks after resolution of acute episode	• Xanthine-oxidase Inhibitors • Allopurinol	commonly prescribed) • Sulfinpyrazone • Benzbromarone (unlicensed in UK Prescribing Named Patient Basis). Can ↑ LFTs
Mode + onset of action:	• Requires metabolism by liver (pro-drug) • Half life ~24 hours (depending on renal function)	• Reduces renal re-absorption of SUA
Treatment regimen: ▶Allopurinol should be co-prescribed with low-dose NSAID or colchine (0.5mg bd) as risk of precipitating acute attacks (co-prescribe for ~12 months)	• Aim for SUA <300 mcg/L • Start with allopurinol 50–100mg with 50–100mg/day increments every few weeks adjusted for SUA target and renal function (max. dose 900mg/day)	• Aim for SUA <300mcg/L • Prescribe for under-excretors of SUA. • 200–800mg/day normal renal function • 50–200mg/day mild/moderate renal insufficiency Note: Ineffective generally in patients with mild renal insufficiency.
Side effects:	• Hypersensitivity reactions (rare) • Hepatic toxicity /GI symptoms, CNS • Be aware of drug interactions:	• Avoid in renal insufficiency;/disease or blood disorders/pophyria/ risk of urinary stones • Do not co-prescribe with aspirin/salicylates • GI symptoms (common) Blood disorders (rare)
Monitoring (patient concordance is generally poor (50%), indicating a greater need for education):	• Monitor SUA levels every 3 months in the first year: then annual SUA, creatinine clearance and patient knowledge/ lifestyle	• Ensure adequate fluid intake (2–3L daily) • Monitor SUA levels every 3 months in the first year: then annual SUA, creatinine clearance and patient knowledge/lifestyle

Table 4.5 Treatment during an acute attack (refer to Summary Product of Characteristics and BNF) (◻ also see Symptom control, Chapter 9)

	Pain control	Nursing care	Analgesia	Corticosteroids	NSAIDs/ COX-2	Colchicine (gout only)
Consider contraindications and cautions: GI/CV/ renal/hepatic/elderly	Identify precipitating factors (e.g. diuretics) and refer to clinician. Rest, ice, elevation. Relief of pressure on affected joint(s)/evaluate functional limitations. Consider MDT referral if appropriate	Avoid aspirin-based analgesia (low dose for CV risk can continue). Opiates can be used as adjunct to core treatment. NSAIDs/Cox-2s/ colchicine	IA injections per joint. Consider if confined to 1 joint: or contra-indicated other therapies/refractory to treatment. Aspirate: culture and microscopy. IM injections. See above	Review risk factors: NSAIDs/Cox-2s; contra-indicated: consider steroids or colchicine.	Narrow therapeutic window (efficacy vs. toxicity/side effects). Used whilst initiating prophylactic treatment with allopurinol – for at least 6 weeks (if tolerated)
Onset of action	Review pain scores/ Assessments and review nursing support/treatment required	Consider risk factors, tolerance and pain relief needs Select: compound analgesia or opiate with dosing regimens to add to therapeutic benefit of NSAIDs	Rapid onset of benefit	Select NSAID/Cox-2. Full licensed dose, short half life, rapid onset NSAID: indometacin 50mg tds. Consider: diclofenac, ibuprofen, naproxen, etorocoxib	Alternative for those contraindicated NSAIDs/Cox-2s. Side-effect profile inhibits use.

Treatment regimens				
Regular analgesia Monitor benefit Monitor bloods Observations: fluid intake, pyrexia, skin integrity Education and advice on medications, lifestyle (when appropriate time). Use resources for dietary advice ww.arc.org.uk	Assess risk factors and consider: Compound analgesia: Co-codamol at different dose ranges 1-2, 4-6-hourly Co-dydramol 10/500 1-2 tabs 4-6-hourly. Or select: opiod Tramadol hydrochloride 50-100mg 4-hourly.	IA injection to affected joint: Triamcinolone acetonide (40-80mg) IA or IM methylprednisolone acetate (80-120mg)	Limit treatment to 6 weeks max. Traditional NSAID + PPI Cox-2: if GI but no CV risk ± PPI Select NSAID /Cox-2 in relation to patient individual risk factors.	Start: 500mcg bd (max 6mg per course of treatment) Do not repeat within 3/7days
Benefits				
Essential to aid recovery/ functional ability and encourage positive coping styles.	Adjunct to NSAIDs	IA: aspirate can also be diagnostic. Relieves swelling promptly	Highly effective for pain relief.	Valuable for heart failure patients or those on warfarin
Risks				
Psychological distress Pain, fatigue, and loss of appetite	Constipation Nausea Encourage fluid intake	⚠ Consider: septic arthritis IA: Small risk of infection on injecting. Steroid related side effects:	Side effect profile of NSAIDs/COX-2s Should be lowest optimal dose for shortest duration	Side-effect profile: narrow therapeutic window IV colchicines: **not recommended**

Frequently asked questions: crystal arthropathies

Is gout hereditary?

A genetic predisposition means some people will have a higher chance of developing gout, e.g. people who have a familial hyperuricemia due to an inability to secrete uric acid (~30% of ♂). However, otherwise gout itself is not hereditary.

What is the long-term risk related to having gout?

The long-term damage to joints (such as a chronic arthritis) tends to happen only if there are repeated attacks of gout over a sustained period — however, with current treatments and management this rarely happens.

Complications related to gout tend to occur more in the complex patient with other long-term conditions. These patients do appear to have an ↑ risk related to high blood pressure and possible renal stones if untreated. In addition, another risk to be considered is that for patients who have started treatment for gout they will need to remain on treatment in the long term.

How many people have more than one attack of gout?

The first attack usually occurs between 40–60 years of age and for some people may never experience another attack. It seems that about 62% of patients have another attack within the first year. These attacks can become more frequent in those who receive no long-term treatment for gout. Allopurinol is normally started for those who have >1 attack or have high risk factors but is prescribed after the attack has resolved. Patients should be warned that starting allopurinol may precipitate another attack and that the treatment will need to be long term.

Connective tissue diseases

Systemic lupus erythematosus

Introduction

Lupus (systemic lupus erythematosus, SLE) is an auto-immune disease of unknown aetiology. This is a complex auto-immune disease, that is multi factorial in nature and currently has no know cure. It is the commonest of the connective tissue diseases (CTDs) and follows a pattern of unpredictable activity with quieter phases of the condition.

Genetic, hormonal, and infective causes have all been cited as playing an important part in the development of lupus in any one individual. Lupus is 10–20 times more commonly seen in ♀ than in ♂, and frequently presents in young ♀ of child-bearing age. Although lupus is reported worldwide, certain ethnic groups have a higher incidence (Afro-Caribbean, Chinese) which reflects in epidemiological figures.

Widespread inflammation leads to symptoms ranging from simple joint aches and pains, with fatigue and skin rashes, to life-threatening multi-system organ failure. Organs that can be targeted are the kidneys, the heart, the lungs, and the CNS. Less commonly the inflammatory component of lupus also has the potential to damage other organs including:
- Pancreas.
- GI system.
- Circulatory system.

Classification criteria

Criteria for the classification of SLE were published in 1982,[1] and revised in 1997 (see Box 5.1).[2] These classification criteria, devised by the ACR are of value for clinical trials but play a small part in the clinical diagnostic process. In routine daily practice, a full clinical examination, presenting symptoms, and blood results all enable the clinician to confirm diagnosis.

Prognosis

Lupus still carries with a significant risk of mortality and long-term morbidity despite advances in treatment. Renal lupus remains one of the major causes of death in lupus, however more recently cardiovascular events are increasingly being recognized as playing an important role in improving long-term outcomes.

📖 Also see Diagnosing lupus: the importance of blood and urine tests, p.116, and Pregnancy in Sjögren's syndrome, p.135.

Box 5.1 Revised criteria of the ACR for the classification of SLE.[1]

4 out of these 11 criteria must be present for a diagnosis of SLE.

1. Malar rash.

2. Discoid rash.

3. Photosensitivity.

4. Oral ulcers.

5. Arthritis.

6. Serositis: pleuritis or pericarditis.

7. Renal disorder: proteinuria >0.5g/24 hours at 3+ persistently or cellular casts.

8. Neurological disorder: seizures or psychosis (excluding other causes such as drugs).

9. Haematological disorder:
• Haemolytic anaemia *or*
• Leucopenia or <4.0 x 10^9/L on 2 or more occasions *or*
• Lymphopenia or <1.5 x 10^9/L on 2 or more occasions *or*
• Thrombocytopenia <100 in 10^9/L.

10. Immunological disorders: raised dsDNA antibody binding or anti-Sm antibody or positive antiphospholipid antibodies (abnormal serum level IgG/IgM anticardiolipin antibodies and a positive lupus anticoagulant) or a false positive serological test for syphilis known to be positive of at least 6 months and confirmed by *Treponema pallidum* immobilization or fluorescent treponemal antibody absorption test.

11. Antinuclear antibody in raised titre.

Reference

1. Tan EM, Cohen AS, Fries JF, *et al.* (1982). The 1982 revised criteria for the classification of systemic lupus erythematosus. *Arthritis and Rheumatism*, **25**(11), 1271–7.

2. Hochberg MC (1997). Updating the American College of Rheumatology revised criteria for the classification of systemic lupus erythematosus. *Arthritis and Rheumatism*, **40**(9), 1725.

Diagnosing lupus: the importance of blood and urine tests

Lupus is diagnosed through clinical history and systemic examination. Confirmation of the diagnosis is through positive autoantibody tests. Blood abnormalities are common in lupus, ranging from anaemia, leuco-penia, thrombocytopenia, and other clotting disorders. Iron deficiency and immune mediate anaemia are also common.

Red blood cells (RBCs)

Up to 40% of lupus patients will become anaemic at some point during the course of their disease. There are numerous causes related to the anaemia including iron deficiency, GI bleeding, or medications (steroids and NSAIDs). Anaemia of chronic disease can lead to antibody formation, which target the RBCs leading to a normochromic-normocytic anaemia.

Thrombocytopenia (low platelets) occurs in 25–35% and can respond to low-dose steroids. Coombs positive haemolytic anaemia occurs in 10% of lupus patients. In cases of haemolytic anaemia/thrombocytopenia, high dose steroids with immunsuppression (azathioprine, MMF) are required. Liaison with haematology is essential in those with platelets regularly <100 $\times$ 10^9/L.

White blood cells (WBCs)

Low WBCs are common and can lead to a greater risk of infection. Leucopenia is found in 15–20% and is common in active lupus.

Auto-antibodies

Specific auto-antibody testing is a valuable diagnostic tool in lupus. The commonly presenting auto-antibodies are as follows:

- Anti-nuclear antibody (ANA): over 90% of those with lupus have a positive ANA, above a titre of 1/40. This is not specific for lupus and needs to be considered with other more specific tests. ANA can also be raised in chronic infections.
- Anti-Sm: Sm is a riboneucleoprotein found in the cell nucleus. Highly specific for lupus, present in about 30% of those with lupus.
- Anti-dsDNA: an immunoglobulin that is highly specific for lupus that can fluctuate with disease activity and therefore serial testing is a useful monitoring tool. Associated with a higher risk of lupus nephritis.
- ENA (extractable nuclear antigen) anti-Ro and anti-La: these immunoglobulins are commonly found together and are specific against RNA proteins. Anti-Ro is found in 30% of lupus and 70% of those with 1° Sjogren's. Anti-La found in 15% with lupus and 60% of 1° Sjogren's. Anti-Ro is associated with photosensitivity and both are associated with neonatal lupus

Anti-phospholipid syndrome (APS) 2° to lupus

Anti-phospholipid antibodies should always be checked in lupus, with or without any history of thrombo-embolic disease. These are antibodies that react against phospholipids and are present in up to 50% of those with lupus.

2 separate tests at least 6 weeks apart must be positive to make a diagnosis of 2° anti-phospholipid syndrome, which can also present as a 1° diagnosis. Three separate laboratory tests complete the screening:
- Lupus anticoagulant (APTT, dRVVT and KCT).
- Anticardiolipin antibodies.
- Anti-β2 glycoprotein 1.

Other tests
- *Complement proteins* (C3 and C4): help to mediate inflammation, and are a useful aid to diagnosis in lupus.
- *Inflammatory markers*: general measure of inflammation such as PV and ESR are useful in lupus, although CRP can be normal. A raised CRP in lupus may indicate infection.
- *U&Es, creatinine and LFTs:* routine blood testing must always include U&Es and LFTs. Protein/creatinine ratio is important in suspected renal involvement.
- *Urine testing*: essential at every clinic visit. The routine dipstick alerts the nurse to early signs of kidney disease. Protein and haematuria in those with lupus must always be investigated with blood for protein/creatinine clearance and 24-hour urine collection to quantify protein loss and detect any reduced levels of creatinine clearance.

▶▶ Immediate action must be taken in anyone with lupus that shows signs of early renal disease. This should include referral to a renal physician for potential kidney biopsy to determine the extent and type of inflammation and/or damage.

▶ *Any rise in blood pressure may be an associated sign of renal complications.*

⚠ A flare of lupus is often seen as a rising titre of dsDNA antibodies and PV/ESR, falling complements and lymphocytes, accompanied by systemic symptoms (📖 see Nursing care of lupus patients, p.128).

Lupus: anti-phospholipid syndrome, fertility/pregnancy, and hormone replacement therapy issues

Lupus: anti-phospholipid syndrome (APS)

APS can be either 1° or 2° to lupus. This classically presents as blood clotting (thrombosis) and, in ♀, a tendency to miscarriage. This can be both arterial and venous clotting leading to a wide range of symptoms. It is also described as 'sticky blood' which can be worse during pregnancy when blood viscosity is naturally thicker. This can lead to a higher risk of pre-eclampsia and premature birth.

Classically APS can cause:
- Thrombosis—venous (DVT), arteries (cerebrovascular accident, hypertension) and brain (memory loss, seizures, migraine).
- Recurrent miscarriages.
- Livedo reticularis—blotchy skin rash.
- Thrombocytopenia.

Treatments for APS depend on the history of clotting but can include low-dose aspirin, warfarin, and during pregnancy, low molecular weight heparin. Close supervision is required to enable a healthy fetus to survive. In those ♀ with lupus and APS, who carry the Ro/La antibodies, pre-pregnancy counselling and close nurse specialist support is vital.

Lupus: contraception, pregnancy, and HRT

Lupus is known to be exacerbated by hormones and can lead to flares when the menstrual cycle is due and often postpartum. Oestrogen is known to flare lupus, so contraception and HRT should always be progesterone-only where possible.

Steroid management during pregnancy can be life saving. At the same time it must be recognized that pregnant ♀ with lupus—especially those on steroids—are more likely to develop hypertension, diabetes, hyperglycaemia, and renal complications. Pregnancy itself may also cause the disease to flare. However, many ♀ with lupus have normal pregnancies and these should be encouraged in ♀ when their disease is quiescent.

Pregnancy carries some risks, especially in those ♀ with the anti-Ro/La antibodies and 2° APS. Babies from mothers who carry the anti-Ro/La antibodies can be born with a transient neonatal lupus (see Pregnancy in Sjögren's syndrome, p.135)

The risk of miscarriage is high for those with positive anticardiolipin antibodies and positive lupus anticoagulant. Figures suggest up to a 30% risk of miscarriage with the first pregnancy, and with a history of at least 2 spontaneous miscarriages, up to 70% during the following pregnancy. 50% of miscarriages occur in the 2nd and 3rd trimesters. Aspirin and low molecular weight heparin should replace warfarin and be continued throughout pregnancy and postpartum period.

Where possible, all medications should be to a minimum and drugs such as MTX and mycophenolate must be stopped in advance of conception as they are tetragenic. Medication reviews and pre-pregnancy counselling are a vital part of the nurse's role in giving information about these risks and ensuring where possible, that pregnancies are planned events. A consultant-led hospital birth should be booked and ♀ and their partners allowed time to discuss any issues at length

📖 See Nursing issues, p.300, 346; and Patient-centred care, p.314.

Lupus: musculoskeletal system and the skin

Up to 90% of lupus patients describe musculoskeletal symptoms of flitting symmetrical joint and muscle aches and pains. There is usually little erosive damage to joints but tenosynovitis is common. Subluxation of some joints can occur, which is typically seen as a reversible deformity, though it can be severe and disabling as in the case of Jaccoud's arthropathy.

Investigations of musculoskeletal symptoms

- Plain x-ray to exclude any overlapping erosive disease.
- MRI can reveal characteristic signs of soft tissue changes and bony alterations although this investigation is not indicated routinely.

Management of musculoskeletal symptoms

- Symptoms can be improved by simple NSAIDs or hydroxychloroquine, an anti-malarial.
- DMARDs such as MTX may be required in rare cases of lupus overlap disease with some components of erosive disease.
- Surgical referral to orthopaedics may be necessary in severe cases of tenosynovitis.
- Patients who have lupus with musculoskeletal involvement can see their condition impact on work, home, and social life, ultimately affecting their quality of life.
- Arthralgia can cause a range of functional limitations affecting work and home life.
- Managing children and juggling work and home commitments can lead to high levels of fatigue and subsequent depression.
- Nursing management of musculoskeletal symptoms includes assessment of active disease and patient education relating to understanding the disease process and the importance of balancing exercise and rest.
- Self-management techniques as part of formal education programmes are beneficial, but require high levels of support and resources.[1]
- Referrals to occupational therapy for ADL assessment and physiotherapy for graded exercise programmes are essential to encourage the individual to optimize sometimes limited personal resources.

Lupus and the skin

Cutaneous involvement of lupus is very common, with the classic 'butterfly rash'. The butterfly rash is:

- Seen in about 1/3 of those diagnosed with lupus.
- Is a disc-shaped lesions seen across the face (sparing the nasal folds) and light exposed areas of the skin.
- In discoid lupus (skin only), these rashes can be scarring.
- Sun exposure can trigger systemic disease flares of lupus. Oral manifestations include:
  - Recurrent crops of mouth ulcers (a feature of active disease).
  - Dryness related to a 2° Sjögren's syndrome, affecting the eyes, mouth, skin, and vagina.

Management of lupus skin problems

Again, hydroxychloroquine can be helpful, with mepacrine and thalidomide as options for severe rashes. Collaborative workings with a dermatologist are essential for those with severe rashes.

Nursing advice is important in order to help patients successfully manage skin flares of lupus. Nursing advice includes:

- Use of high factor sun cream (above SPF50) on a regular basis all year round.
- Sun Sense and Uvistat both provide comprehensive ranges or other high quality products that also include moisturizer and tint for the face.
- Simple advice such as avoiding the midday sun, using sun hats for protection, wearing sun protective clothing, and choosing an appropriate holiday resort will help to prevent skin flares.
- Referral to the British Red Cross cosmetic camouflage service enables successful covering of scars.

Also see Nursing care of lupus patients, p.128.

Reference

1. Brown S, Somerset ME, McCabe CS and McHugh NJ (2004). The impact of group education on participants' management of their disease in lupus and scleroderma. *Musculoskeletal Care*, **2**(4), 207–217.

Lupus: fatigue and psychological manifestations

Nurses play a vital role in enabling individuals to share their feelings and provide support during difficult phases of the condition and symptoms experienced. Fatigue is one of the most frequently reported symptoms of lupus, and is the most challenging to treat. Fatigue can lead to:

- Frustration and anger. These symptoms can be compounded by the despair experienced in the protracted processes involved in achieving a diagnosis.
- A sense of helplessness fuelled by the fatigue and inability to undertake normal ADL.
- Problems with personal relationships and in working life.
- Associated fibromyalgia can worsen fatigue.
- Depression is common, is complicated by fatigue, and requires careful management and support.

General management issues

- Psychological effects can worsen symptoms, and it is important for the nurse to be alert to any signs of potential psychological repercussions.
- In some cases the treatments such as hydroxychloroquine may help improve feelings of fatigue
- For those requiring additional psychological support initiation of anti-depressive treatment and referral to psychology teams should be considered in severe cases.
- Contact with others patients with lupus may enable individuals to share common feelings. Local support groups and access to national support should be available and are often provided by national organizations such as Lupus UK.[1]

📖 Also see Nursing care of lupus patients, p.128. 📖 Education, social, and psychological aspects of a new diagnosis, pp.318, 320.

Reference

1. Lupus UK website: ⚲ www.lupusuk.com

Lupus: cardio-pulmonary, renal, and central nervous system

Lupus and the cardio-pulmonary system

All cardiac and pulmonary symptoms should be taken seriously and referral to a cardiologist and a pulmonary physician to undergo thorough investigations. These can include pulmonary function tests (PFTs) (including gas transfer), echocardiogram, HRCT of the chest, and right-heart catheterization where pulmonary hypertension is suspected. Cardio-vascular disease is becoming the leading cause of death in lupus. Cardiac/cardiovascular abnormalities include:

- Pericarditis with a rub.
- Myocarditis (in up to 15%) with combinations of tachycardias and dysrhythmias, systolic murmurs, and endocarditis.
- Accelerated atherosclerosis; due to the chronic inflammatory nature of the disease and the use of steroids to control inflammation.
- ↑ risk of myocardial infarction (MI). Screening for those at high risk is an important part of the clinic consultation.

Pulmonary abnormalities

Pulmonary involvement of lupus is often described as sub clinical, with late presentation sometimes limiting treatment.

Pulmonary hypertension in lupus is rare, and is usually pulmonary arterial hypertension which is managed with targeted therapies such as endothelin receptor antagonists (bosentan, sitaxentan). Immunosuppresin may need to be reviewed in the light of evidence of a flare of lupus. PH can also be 2° to lung fibrosis or pulmonary emboli as a result of antiphospholipid antibodies.

- Pulmonary arterial hypertension.
- Pulmonary fibrosis.
- Pleurisy—the most common respiratory problem and pleuritic chest pain is a common feature.

Managing cardio-pulmonary systems

- Cholesterol should be measured (aim to be <5), blood pressure, weight, BMI, and dietary intake should all be addressed.
- Cessation of smoking is imperative to reduce the ↑ risk of cardio-vascular events.

The role of the nurse is to enable the patient to make informed choices about their risks and treatment options in the context of the individual's lifestyle. Nurses should also be informed about detecting changes in cardiac and pulmonary function and alerting specialist teams.

Lupus and the kidneys

Renal involvement is one of the most life-threatening complications of lupus. Regular investigations at *every clinic visit* must include blood test for renal function, urinalysis for protein, and blood pressure. Renal biopsy can be helpful in guiding treatment. Treatments include:

- High dose steroids.

- Immunosuppression with cyclophosphamide and/or mycophenolate mofetil/azathioprine.
- Diuretics and anti-hypertensives as needed.
- Or anti-B cell ablation with the anti CD-20 monoclonal antibody, rituximab.

Lupus and the CNS

This is the most worrying complication for the individual with lupus. Symptoms can be vague and somewhat difficult to distinguish from other diseases. There is no one single diagnostic test. Symptoms can range from:
- Headaches and seizures.
- Mood swings.
- Depression/psychosis.
- Cranial or peripheral neuropathy.

If these symptoms occur they can result in extreme fear and distress for the patient. Nurses play an important role by providing:
- Relevant information, anticipating concerns, and helping the individual and their family to develop coping skills, allowing time and attention to all involved. Support from and referral to local psychiatric services may be required.
- ▶ Nursing support in identifying early referral to specialist teams.
- This support is often achieved by providing a first point of access with a telephone advice lines. Vigilance in identifying fluid retention, weight gain, lethargy, hypertension (with proteinuria), raised creatinine or other signs indicating renal failure or fluid and electrolyte imbalance can limit damage
- 📖 Also see Nursing care of lupus patients, p.128.

Assessment tools to evaluate lupus activity

Evaluating lupus activity is divided into:
• Disease activity.
• Disease severity.

These measures are system based and calculate a score based upon evidence reviewed through clinic assessment over the last 6 months. There are currently >60 indices available for disease activity, but the BILAG (British Isles Lupus Advisory Group Classic) and the SLEDAI-2000 (Systemic Lupus Erythematosus Disease Activity Index) are the most commonly used. A further BILAG-2004 is currently being validated.

There is only one damage specific index—the SLICC (Systemic Lupus International Collaborating Clinics). Health status is usually measured using the SF-36.

📖 See Assessment tools, Chapter 21.

Prognosis

Lupus still carries a significant risk of mortality and long-term morbidity despite advances in treatment. Renal lupus remains one of the major causes of death in lupus; however, more recently cardiovascular events are increasingly presenting. Knowledge of the impact of premature atherosclerosis must be at the forefront of the nurse's mind when managing lupus patients, where prevention is the key. Early management and intervention of any atherosclerosis will improve long-term prognosis in those who survive the early years of the illness.

📖 Nursing care of lupus patients, p.128.

Nursing care of lupus patients

Nursing care management of lupus is aimed at enabling individuals to make informed choices through access to up-to-date information and support. From the patient perspective they have invariably been referred to numerous specialists over time, with significant delay in receiving a diagnosis. This delay can vary from a number of months to many years of 'non-specific' symptoms, and can often depend on a chance referral to an enlightened specialist for correct diagnosis

Treatments are aimed at managing acute periods of potentially life-threatening illness, minimizing the risk of flares when disease is quiescent, and controlling day-to-day symptoms.

Some specialist rheumatology units have access to lupus nurse specialists who can offer:

- Specialist support through consultations and telephone advice lines.
- Education—vital to those newly diagnosed who need to recognize potentially serious symptoms and know how to gain early access to specialist treatment.[1] The key areas for nursing input in lupus are in providing education, support, information, and counselling in helping individuals to work towards accepting lupus as a chronic illness that is with them, in some shape or form, for the rest of their lives. The difficulty for nurses is balancing the right level of information without causing distress or worry to the lupus patient.
- Proactive support to the patient to prevent common problems related to the condition such as fatigue and depression. Diagnosis can depend on a chance referral to an enlightened specialist. Delay in diagnosis impacts on the individual's ability to cope with their diagnosis, its treatment, and potential complications. Furthermore, lupus can also be misdiagnosed, and is known as a mimic of other diseases such as multiple sclerosis or syphilis.
- Knowledge of the impact of premature atherosclerosis must be at the forefront of the nurse's mind when managing lupus patients, where prevention is the key. Early management and intervention of any atherosclerosis will improve long-term prognosis in those who survive the early years of the illness.
- Nursing interventions include explanation of the significance of the blood and urine tests and giving education to ensure patients attend the surgery for regular tests when they are known to have systemic manifestations of lupus. Alerting specialist teams when developing symptoms such as ↑ fatigue and bruising/bleeding may enable early intervention
- Medication reviews and pre-pregnancy counselling is a vital part of the nurse's role in giving information about these risks and ensuring where possible, that pregnancies are planned events

Nursing care of the lupus patient: key points

- Education about the disease process, early warning signs, recognizing and managing a flare, knowing when to contact the specialist team.
- Assisting in adjusting to physical and psychological changes, encouraging lifestyle and self-management skills.

- Empathy and support: enabling contact with specialist teams and self-help groups such as Lupus UK.[2]
- Availability by telephone for on-going support between consultations.
- Body image problems: addressing worrying concerns such as rashes or scarring.
- Pregnancy advice and pre-pregnancy counselling.
- Setting realistic achievable goals in maintaining best level of health and optimise resources.
- Balancing the need for information, relevant to the individual and their lupus, without causing distress or worry.

References

1. ARMA (2007). *Standards of care in connective tissue diseases.*

2. Lupus UK website: ⌖ www.lupusuk.com

Sjögren's syndrome: overview

Introduction

Sjögren's syndrome (SS) is a systemic autoimmune disease of unknown aetiology. It is a chronic condition that can have a significant impact on an individual's quality of life and working capacity and is characterized by lymphocyte infiltration of the exocrine glands leading to dry mouth (xerostomia) and dry eyes (keratoconjunctivitis sicca). Inflammatory cells target both the salivary and lachrymal glands, resulting in atrophy of the glands and subsequent dryness of not only the eyes and the mouth, but in severe cases the vulva/vagina, pharynx, oesophagus and skin. SS affects:

- 9 times more women than men. Incidence figures vary, but it has been reported as affecting between 3–4% of the UK population.
- Tends to occur between the ages of 40 and 50 (but can affect children and the elderly).
- One of the complex connective tissue diseases, SS has some genetic, environmental, and infective causes although there is currently no clear evidence to support any one cause. It has been associated with certain viruses, in particular the Epstein–Barr and retrovirus. There is no cure for SS, and treatments aim to reduce symptoms and preserve organ function.

Diagnosis

Box 5.2 outlines the revised international criteria for diagnosis of SS.[1] Diagnosis is also supported by excluding other diagnoses or medication related symptoms (e.g. sarcoidosis can mimic the clinical picture of SS). SS can be either a 1° or 2° diagnosis:

- **1° SS is** associated more with more systemic (extra glandular) disease and carries with it a 40-fold relative risk of lymphoma (although the absolute risk is very small). 1° SS patients often report significant fatigue, fever, Raynaud's phenomenon, myalgias, and arthralgias
- **2° SS** is reported in 10–20% of those with lupus and RA.

Tests of reduced tear/salivary secretion can be useful, but not wholly diagnostic of SS, as keratoconjunctivitis sicca occurs in many different conditions. Extraglandular features are seen in about 1/3 of SS patients. Most frequently seen extra glandular features include:

- 60% with arthritis/arthralgias.
- 40% with Raynaud's phenomenon.
- 14% with lymphadenopathy.
- 14% with lung involvement.

The importance of blood tests

As SS is a syndrome (that can appear in many different forms) it can be difficult to diagnose and there are no specific simple diagnostic tests. Blood tests to aid diagnosis include:

- ANA—89% positive in SS.
- Anti-Ro/La antibodies on testing of extractable nuclear antigen (ENA).
  - Anti-Ro (SSA) seen in 70%.
  - Anti-La (SSB) seen in 60%.

- Up to 60–90% of Europeans who are Ro/La positive also carry the HLA DR3 association.
- Raised PV/CRP/ESR, acute phase response to inflammation.
- Always exclude other diagnoses. Clinicians should always test for hepatitis C, AIDS, pre-existing lymphoma, sarcoiditis, and graft-versus-host disease.

Box 5.2 Classification criteria:[1] diagnosis of SS confirmed if 4 out of the following 6 criteria are met:

1. Ocular symptoms: a positive response to at least 1 of the following questions:
- Have you had daily, persistent, troublesome dry eyes for >3 months?
- Do you have a recurrent sensation of sand or gravel in the eyes?
- Do you use tear substitutes >3 times a day?

2. Oral symptoms: a positive response to at least 1 of the following questions:
- Have you had a daily feeling of dry mouth for >3 months?
- Have you had recurrently or persistently swollen salivary glands as an adult?
- Do you frequently drink liquids to aid in swallowing dry food?

3. Ocular signs: positive Schirmer's test without anaesthesia ≤5mm in 5min or Rose Bengal score ≥4 according to van Bijsterveld's scoring system.

4. Histopathology: in minor salivary glands, focal lymphocytic sialoadenitis with a focus score ≥1.

5. Salivary gland involvement: objective evidence defined by a positive result in at least one of the following:
- Unstimulated whole salivary flow <1.5mL/min.
- Parotid gland sialography showing presence of diffuse sialectasias.
- Salivary scintigraphy showing delayed uptake, reduced concentration and/or delayed excretion of tracer.

6. Auto antibodies: presence in the serum of the following auto antibodies: antibodies to Ro (SSA) or La (SSB) antigens, or both.

Reference

1. Vitali *et al.* (2002). Classification criteria for Sjögren's syndrome: a revised version of the European criteria proposed by the American-European Consensus Group. *Annals of the Rheumatic Diseases*, **61**, 554–8.

Sjögren's syndrome and the glands

Symptoms of glandular involvement can be very non-specific, making diagnosis difficult and sometimes protracted. Dry eyes are commonly the first presentation and intensity of symptoms can worsen over time. Other conditions and medications can also be responsible for presenting symptoms and they should always be excluded as part of the screening process for SS.

Oral signs and symptoms

Lymphocytic infiltrate of the exocrine glands can result in significant symptoms. Enlargement of the parotids can be episodic or frequent and occurs in 50% of those with 1° SS, leading to chronic enlargement. The 1° symptom that causes most problems is dryness (xerostomia), leading to symptoms such as:
- Difficulty in swallowing food.
- Difficulty in holding a conversation, an inability to speak continuously.
- Experiencing disturbed sleep.
- Dental caries, periodontitis, and gingivitis.
- Oral thrush.
- Change in taste sensation.
- Pain and burning.

Treatment for oral symptoms using simple remedies, such as:
- Sips of water frequently.
- Avoiding sugared drinks or highly sugared foods.
- Chewing sugarless chewing gum to stimulate salivary production.
- Saliva sprays—Saliva Orthana® or Luborant® (contain fluoride) or Glandosane® (fluoride free).
- Biotene range including gels, gums, and toothpastes.
- Spoonful of natural sugar free Greek yoghurt before bed.

Ocular signs and symptoms

This is the major glandular manifestation that can lead to significant eye infections and possible corneal and conjunctival damage. Symptoms described include:
- Gritty, burning sensation in the eye.
- Redness and itchiness in the eye.
- Photosensitivity.

Schirmer's test evaluates tear secretion and is measured through a filter strip of paper 30mm long, that is placed on the lower eyelid. The result is positive if ≤5mm is wet in 5min. A further measure of tear secretion is the Rose Bengal test where a dye is applied to the ocular surface which is taken up by devitalized epithelial cells. Positive staining is consistent with SS.

Treatments for ocular symptoms include:
- Simple lubricants such as hypromellose drops (preservative free), with longer acting agents such as viscotears or celluvisc if necessary.
- Ointments such as lacrilube are helpful at night.
- If there is mucus stranding, then mucolytics are prescribed such as acetylcysteine eye drops.

- Punctal occlusion should be considered in those with severe symptoms, with temporary performed first.
- Ciclosporin and tacrolimus eye drops have been used with variable effect.

Treatment for chronic enlargement of parotids can require:
- Antibiotics for chronic recurrent flares of parotid enlargement.
- Pilocarpine can be useful in some cases of parotid enlargement but the use of the drug is often limited by the side effects (use slow titration to develop tolerance level).
- Steroids in severe cases.

Sjögren's syndrome and extraglandular manifestations: systemic disease

Systemic disease is seen in 1/3 of those with 1° SS. Most commonly presenting symptoms include fatigue, arthralgias, myalgias, and low-grade fevers. Raynaud's phenomenon is also present in up to about 35% and this symptom can predate sicca symptoms by many years. Digital fingertip ulceration is not a feature. Treatments depend on severity of systemic damage, with immunosuppression often required using high dose steroids, DMARDs and newer agents such as rituximab and other B-cell targeted therapies currently producing promising results.

Musculoskeletal symptoms

70% of 1° SS patients report arthralgias, with 25% of those developing arthritis. In those with Raynaud's, they are more likely to develop a non-erosive arthritis. Arthralgias and fatigue respond well to hydroxychloroquine, and in those who have erosive disease, other DMARDs such as MTX would be appropriate. The use of steroids would be reserved for those with significant flare of musculoskeletal symptoms, including chronic recurrent glandular enlargement.

Skin

The skin can be very dry leading to symptoms of stinging, itching, and patchy alopecia. Hypersensitivity vasculitis can also develop. The dryness can also affect the vulva and vagina, and can lead to major complications in sexual relationships. Treatments of dry skin include use of non-lanolin based products for washing (such as Aqueous Cream), tissue nourishment with moisturizers—either ointments or creams—and avoiding highly scented products. Vaginal dryness can impact on a sexual relationship and most women with SS will be using simple lubricants regularly. Hormonal moisturisers or oestrogen creams and HRT are sometimes needed when symptoms are severe.

Pulmonary and renal involvement

Interstitial lung disease with dryness of the trachea can lead to a dry cough and airways obstruction due to dryness in the pleura. 25% will develop pulmonary abnormalities. Steroids are effective in reducing inflammation and can be used effectively with DMARDs such as AZA.

Renal disease is found in about 10% of those with 1° SS. Glomerulonephritis is uncommon, but would need to be treated with steroids and DMARDs such as AZA, MMF, or cyclophosphamide if present.

Neurological complications and neuropathies

Neurological complications present in many different ways, from diffuse sensorimotor neuropathy to a multiple sclerosis-like illness. Diffuse sensory motor neuropathy: occurs in up to 20%; sensory symptoms predominate. Mononeuritis multiplex is seen in 1–3% of these with SS and often presents as a lateral popliteal nerve palsy. This is associated with vasculitis and responds well to high dose steroids and DMARDS such as cyclophosphamide.

Lymphoma

There is a 40-fold higher relative risk of developing lymphoma in SS. Persistent parotid gland enlargement, lymphadenopathy, splenomegaly, and glomerulonephritis are all associated with higher risk of developing lymphoma. SS patients must be screened when first diagnosed, at frequent intervals when there is any suspicion. Nurses must be available to counsel patients about this diagnosis and offer support and information on an individual basis as needed.

Pregnancy

♀ with SS who carry the Ro and/or La antibodies will need to be counselled for pregnancy-related complications. Antibodies pass through the placental barrier during pregnancy:

- Can lead to a transient neonatal lupus rash in the newborn (approx. 5%).
- A lower risk of congenital heart block is less than 2% of first pregnancies.
- Risk increases in subsequent pregnancies to about 12%.

Women should also be screened or antiphospholipid antibodies. Birth plans need to be hospital based, with an obstetric led birth and frequent scans. Pregnancies need to be planned during an inactive phase of the underlying SS.

📖 Also see Disease-modifying anti-rheumatic drugs, p.424; 📖 Rituximab, p.454.

Sjögren's syndrome: fatigue and psychological manifestations

Fatigue affects the majority of those diagnosed with SS and can be extreme, causing incapacitation influencing daily activities, and work, social, and personal relationships. Hydroxychloroquine can help in some, with mastery of self-management techniques influencing an individual's ability to cope with this frustrating chronic illness. Symptoms are difficult to treat in SS and can result in physical changes that can affect a personal relationship. These difficult symptoms are often little recognized and result in depression, isolation, and anger.

Support for symptoms of fatigue

- Counselling and psychology services should be accessed early to prevent any further distress, encouraging the individual with SS to develop positive strategies to manage their symptoms.
- Referral to occupational therapy and physiotherapy is essential and a MDT approach benefits the patient immensely.
  - Pacing and planning advice, balanced with assessment of individual needs and the introduction of a graded exercise programme can enable an individual to find purpose and direction.
- Access to nurse specialist support is essential both in the consultation settings and between appointments through the telephone advice line.

Evaluation tools

No gold standards for assessment have been accepted in SS to date, although a recent research has developed a disease activity measure for use in clinical trials in 1° SS, The Sjogren's Systemic Clinical Activity Index (SCAI).[1] This study confirmed the view that the commonest systemic symptoms in 1° SS are fatigue, Raynaud's phenomenon, and musculoskeletal symptoms.

The SCAI scores assess activity in the past 4 weeks and is a system based score, which requires further testing for sensitivity. Other objective tools exist to assess the severity of clinical sicca features.[2]

References

1. Bowman SJ, Sutcliffe N, Isenberg DA, *et al.* (2007). Sjögren's Systemic Clinical Activity Index (SCAI)—a systemic disease activity measure for use in clinical trials in primary Sjögren's syndrome. *Rheumatology*, **46**, 1845–51.

2. Asmussen KH, Bowman SL (2001). Outcome measures in Sjögren's syndrome. *Rheumatology*, **40**, 1085–8.

Nursing care in Sjögren's syndrome

Nursing care management is aimed at enabling the patient with SS to have access to evidence based information in order to manage their symptoms effectively. In common with other CTDs care is aimed at reducing organ failure and maintaining periods of remission from disease flare.

Patients need to know how to access specialist resources and when to call for help. SS is commonly seen in rheumatology units, often as a 2° diagnosis, and for many the symptoms are overlooked in favour of the underlying 1° conditions. It is these frustrating sicca symptoms that can lead to poor sleep patterns, exhaustion, severe fatigue, and, ultimately, significant depression when not addressed and treated appropriately. ♀ are the predominate group affected and as such these symptoms can impact on home, work, and relationships. Relationships suffer due to physical sicca changes and fatigue, and this affects their ability to have a comfortable physical relationship. There is no one treatment that is beneficial all round to treat these difficult symptoms.

Nurses provide a key role to SS patients through education and support, information, and counselling. Some specialist rheumatology units have access to a nurse specialist who can offer:

- Education: most important in times of a new diagnosis, when the disease is flaring, when complex treatment regimens are being initiated, and in helping an individual to come to terms with the psychological effects of living with a chronic illness. Education about SS is balanced on individual need, but individuals need to understand that SS is a multi-system autoimmune disease, where symptoms are manageable with early intervention to prevent systemic failure.

- Information: importance of blood results and autoantibody status is crucial in the young ♀ with SS, where pregnancy must be discussed and should be a planned event where possible.

- Support: nurses are able to refer patients to self-help groups such as the British Sjögren's Syndrome Association (BSSA), which are vital to enable patients to have to opportunity to meet others with similar symptoms and problems.[1]

- Counselling: this should be available for those requiring support and in times of distress. In particular, for ♀ with personal sexual problems to enable them to manage a reasonable physical relationship with their partner (🕮 see Sexuality, p.398).

- Symptom management: sicca symptoms are challenging to live with and nurses can support patients, offering simple measures that can have effective results. Patients should be encouraged to develop a close relationship with their dentist and hygienist in maintaining good oral health.

- Advocate: nurses become the advocate of the SS patient, giving them appropriate information to help them to manage their disease more effectively and encouraging them to make lifestyle choices that will have a positive impact on their health and well-being. Self-management should be encouraged to enable individuals to gain control and lead fulfilling lives.

Nursing care of the Sjögren's patient: key points

- Simple management of sicca symptoms.
- Pacing and planning, with exercise to help with fatigue symptoms.
- Pregnancy advice and pre-pregnancy counselling.
- Support via telephone advice line in between clinic appointments.
- Providing clear information about risks of lymphoma and systemic disease in 1° SS.
- Empathy and support: contact with specialist teams and groups such as BSSA.
- Balancing the need for information, relevant to the individual and their SS, without causing distress and worry.

📖 Also see Diagnosis, p.130; 📖 Outcome measures, Chapter 20.

Reference

1. British Sjögren's Syndrome Association website: 🖰 www.bssa.uk.net

Further reading

Arthritis and Musculoskeletal Alliance (ARMA) (2007). *Standards of Care for Connective Tissue Disease*. ARMA, London.

Bowman SJ, Sutcliffe N, Isenberg DA, *et al.* (2007). Sjögren's Systemic Clinical Activity Index (SCAI)—a systemic disease activity measure for use in clinical trials in primary Sjögren's syndrome. *Rheumatology*, **46**, 1845–51.

Vitali C, Bombardieri S, Jonsson R, *et al.* (2002). Classification criteria for Sjogren's syndrome: a revised version of the European criteria proposed by the American-European Consensus Group. *Annals of the Rheumatic Diseases*, **61**, 554–8.

Scleroderma: overview

Scleroderma is an uncommon auto-immune CTD. The word comes from two Greek words; 'sclero' meaning hard and 'derma' meaning skin. Scleroderma occurs when immune dysfunction leads to damage of the small blood vessels and production of excess collagen. This in turn causes fibrosis of the skin and its underlying structures, and in the systemic form affects the internal organs.

Scleroderma spectrum of disorders

Although the term scleroderma is often used as if it were a single disease, it is a generic or umbrella term for a family of diseases (Box 5.3). The two forms of systemic scleroderma—limited scleroderma and diffuse scleroderma—together make up 90% of all cases of scleroderma.

Epidemiology

Scleroderma:
- Occurs worldwide but more frequently in the US than in Europe or the UK.
- Has a prevalence of ~8 per 100,000 and ♀ are 5 × more likely to be affected than ♂.
- Can develop at any age although typically presents between the ages of 30–60.
- Systemic scleroderma is almost unseen in children <12 years

Cause

The cause of scleroderma is unknown. Scleroderma is characterized by extensive fibrosis and damage to the blood vessels. Although the disease is driven by activation of an auto-immune mechanism the triggers for this process are not clear. It is likely that several factors combine to cause scleroderma which may include:
- Genetic predisposition.
- Hormonal changes e.g. pregnancy, childbirth, menopause.
- External trigger e.g. exposure to infection or chemicals.

Prognosis

Prognosis varies depending on the type and severity of the disease. A patient with localized (i.e. not systemic) scleroderma is unlikely to have their life expectancy shortened. Systemic scleroderma has a poorer prognosis; however, again it varies depending on the extent and type of organ involvement. The overall 5-year survival rate for systemic scleroderma is in excess of 80%.

Box 5.3 The scleroderma spectrum of disorders

- Raynaud's phenomenon:
  - 1° Raynaud's phenomenon.
  - Auto-immune Raynaud's phenomenon.
- Systemic:
  - Limited cutaneous systemic sclerosis.
  - Diffuse cutaneous systemic sclerosis.
  - Scleroderma sine scleroderma.
- Localized:
  - Morphoea plaque—single or multiple.
  - Generalized morphoea.
  - Linear scleroderma.
  - En coup de sabre.

📖 Also see Scleroderma: clinical features and investigations, p.142.

Scleroderma: clinical features and investigations

Clinical features (also see Box 5.4)

- Raynaud's phenomenon: circulatory disorder causing colour changes to the digits and often the first presenting feature of scleroderma.
- Skin: tight thick skin, sclerodactyly (thickening of fingers), inflammation and itching, digital pitting, telangiectasia, hyper/hypopigmentation, calcinosis, microstomia, digital ulcers.
- Musculoskeletal system: fibrosis, arthritis, myositis, joint contractures, synovitis, tendon friction rubs, compression neuropathies e.g. carpel tunnel syndrome.
- GI system: reflux oesophagitis, dysmotility, gastric antral vascular ectasia, which may cause bleeding into the GI tract, bacterial overgrowth, diarrhoea and constipation, incontinence, nutritional failure.
- Sicca symptoms (dry eyes, dry mouth).
- Viscera pulmonary fibrosis pulmonary arterial hypertension, myocarditis, pericardial effusion, renal disease
- Other: fatigue, sexual problems, changes to appearance and body image issues.

⚠ Any patient showing signs of renal crisis—sudden rise in blood pressure, headaches, vomiting, nose bleeds, blurred vision, breathing difficulties or seizures—should be reviewed immediately by a doctor.

Investigations and diagnosis

Scleroderma is often quite difficult to diagnose as symptoms vary in prevalence and severity in each individual. In the majority of cases, Raynaud's phenomenon or skin tightening and swelling are the initial presenting features. A wide range of clinical tests are used in scleroderma for initial diagnosis as well as ongoing review of the disease to assess the extent of organ involvement and the efficacy of some treatments.

▶ Early diagnosis is critical to allow implementation of treatment and to reduce complications and level of potential disability.

Autoantibodies

Specific autoantibody testing is a valuable diagnostic tool in scleroderma and can indicate potential organ involvement. The autoantibodies most commonly found in scleroderma are:

- ANA: a positive ANA can be a non-specific indicator of immune system dysfunction and is found in almost all people with scleroderma. Two patterns of ANA are associated with scleroderma:
  - Anti-topoisomerase (also called anti-Scl-70): this antibody is specific for scleroderma and indicates that a patient may be at risk of developing interstitial lung disease.
  - Anti-centromere antibody (ACA): this antibody is specific for the limited subset of scleroderma and is associated with the development of pulmonary arterial hypertension.

Tests used in diagnosis and investigation of scleroderma
- Blood tests: FBC, ESR/CRP, biochemistry and muscle enzymes, autoantibody screen, thyroid function.
- Urine: urinalysis, microscopy, 24-hour creatinine clearance, GFR.
- Lungs: chest x-ray, PFTs, HRCT.
- Heart: ECG, ECHO (particularly pulmonary arterial pressure and left ventricular ejection fraction), cardiac catheter.
  Others: capillary microscopy, infrared thermography, joint x-rays, barium swallow, laser Doppler, investigations of small and large bowel, muscle biopsy/EMG.

Box 5.4 Classification of systemic sclerosis

Pre-scleroderma
- Raynaud's phenomenon.
- Nail-fold capillary changes and evidence of digital ischemia.
- Specific autoantibodies—Scl-70, ACA, anti-RNA polymerase I and III.

Limited cutaneous scleroderma
- Raynaud's phenomenon for years, occasionally decades.
- Skin involvement limited to hands, face, feet, and forearms.
- Dilated nail-fold capillary loops, usually without capillary drop-out.
- Significant late incidence of pulmonary hypertension with or without skin calcification, GI disease, telangectasia, or interstitial lung disease.
- Renal disease rarely occurs.
- ACA in 70–80%.

Diffuse cutaneous scleroderma
- Raynaud's phenomenon followed, within 1 year, by puffy or hidebound skin changes.
- Truncal and acral skin involvement—tendon friction rubs.
- Nail-fold capillary dilatation and drop-out.
- Early and significant incidence of renal, interstitial lung disease, diffuse GI, and myocardial disease.
- Anti-Scl-70 (30%) anti-RNA polymerase-I, II, or III (12–15%) antibodies.

Scleroderma sine scleroderma
- Presentation with pulmonary fibrosis or renal, cardiac, or GI disease.
- No skin involvement.
- Raynaud's phenomenon may be present.
- ANAs may be present.

Scleroderma: treatment and follow-up care

There is no cure for scleroderma; however, treatments are available which aim to slow down disease progression.

Immunosuppressants

The choice of immunosuppressant used depends on the extent of skin, joint or organ involvement. Immunusuppressants in most common use are:

- MMF.
- Cyclophosphomide.
- MTX.
- AZA.

Most immunosuppressant drugs require regular monitoring of kidney and liver function and FBC. Low dose corticosteroids are used sparingly in lung involvement or acute inflammation as they are thought to precipate renal crisis.

📖 Also see Pharmacological management, Chapter 16.

Symptom-specific medications

- PPIs (e.g. omeprazole, lansoprazole) to treat reflux oesophagitis due to sclerosis of the gastro-oesophageal junction.
- Pro-kinetics (e.g. metoclopramide, domperidone) used when sclerosis of the GI system results in reduced peristalsis and stomach emptying.
- Rotational antibiotics (e.g. ciprofloxacin, metronidazole) to treat bacterial overgrowth in the small bowel.
- Vasodilators (e.g. diltiazem, losartan) to ↑ blood flow to the extremities thereby treating and preventing digital ulcers and improve symptoms of Raynaud's phenomenon.
- Antibiotics (e.g. flucloxacillin) to treat infected digital ulcers.
- Anti-histamines (e.g. chlorphenamine) helpful in reducing itching in the early stages of diffuse scleroderma when skin can be very inflamed.

Follow-up care

Patients with suspected scleroderma should be referred to a specialist centre as soon as possible with initial diagnosis and treatment implementation taking place under the guidance of the specialist team.

Much follow-up care can take place at the patient's local hospital with less frequent visits to the specialist team. Follow-up care, which will continue for life, may include:

- Regular follow-up appointments with the rheumatologist and team.
- Annual ECHO and lung function tests.
- Blood tests whilst on immunosuppressant therapy.
- Psycho-social support.
- Referrals to appropriate specialists if further organ involvement develops.

Nursing issues in management of patients with scleroderma

As scleroderma is a complex and unpredictable condition nurses have a key role in helping patients to manage their condition (Table 5.1).

Nursing care is aimed at offering a holistic and individualized approach to each patient. The key issues in nursing management are:
- Enabling patients to make informed choices by providing ongoing information, advice, and support.
- Providing a continuing programme of education to empower patients to take responsibility for their own health and become active participants in their care.
- Teaching self-management strategies to help the patient recognize and manage common symptoms and avoid complications of the disease and its treatment.
- Enabling patients to understand the diagnosis, prognosis, and chronic nature of the condition.
- Acting a liaison to ensure appropriate MDT involvement e.g. PT, OT, social worker, podiatrist, counsellor, palliative care team.

⚠ *Patients should be taught to recognize the symptoms of, and seek immediate medical attention for:*
- Infected digital ulcers.
- Hypertension/renal crisis.
- Digital gangrene.

Patients with scleroderma may have an assessment of the skin thickening on their body. This gives an indication of the severity of the skin involvement; however, most importantly, serial assessments at each visit allow evaluation of whether skin thickening is deteriorating further or responding to treatment. The extent of skin involvement may, although not always, be an indicator of disease severity.

The assessment tool used is the modified Rodnan Skin Score Tool. The body is broken down into 17 smaller areas and each area is pinched to assess skin tightening and thickening and given a score between 0 (no skin involvment) and 3 (hidebound skin). The total is then calculated.

Table 5.1 Nursing care plan

Patient problem	Nursing management	Expected outcome
Raynaud's phenomenon	Advice about keeping warm. Stop smoking. Natural remedies	Reduction in frequency and severity of attacks.
Digital ulcers	Recognize infection. Dry dressing	Expedite healing of ulcers, reduce likelihood of further recurrence.
Calcinosis	Paraffin wax baths	Exit of calcinotic lumps through skin.
Tight dry skin	Paraffin wax baths, massage, moisturizers	Moisturize skin to improve tightness
Joint problems	Exercises, refer to physio/ OT, heat and ice, waxing	Relieve pain and stiffness, increase flexibility, mobility.
Foot problems	Refer to podiatrist	↓ pain and ↑ mobility
Breathlessness	Coping strategies	Increase ability to manage ADLs independently
Itchy skin	Moisturizers, anti-itch creams, antihistamines	Decrease pruritis to improve quality of life
Telangestasia	Camouflage make up, refer for laser treatment	Camouflage or remove telangectasia reducing psycho-social burden
GI problems	Practical coping strategies, dietary advice, refer to dietician	Reduction in severity of symptoms improving nutritional intake and quality of life
Dry eyes	Practical measures, over-the-counter eye drops	Relieve dry eyes
Oral problems	Advice about good mouth care, over-the-counter remedies for dry mouth and ulcers, mouth exercises. Referral to specialist at dental hospital if required	Reduce need for future dental intervention
Emotional problems	Provide support, refer to counsellor, social worker, ensure awareness of national patient groups and helplines.	Patient to feel supported in managing condition
Fatigue	Coping strategies. OT referral	↑ ability to manage ADLs
Sexual problems	Identify problem—refer to gynaecologist, urologist or counsellor as appropriate	Maintain sexual activity at desired level

Frequently asked questions: scleroderma

What causes scleroderma?

The exact cause of scleroderma is unknown however it is thought to be a combination of abnormal immune activity, genes, hormones, and an environmental trigger (e.g. viral infection, exposure to chemicals).

Can complementary therapies help in scleroderma?

Complementary therapies can be beneficial, particularly in helping to manage Raynaud's phenomenon and digital ulcers. As always they should be used to complement medical treatment and only used with the knowledge of the specialist.

Will scleroderma reduce life expectancy?

In some cases life expectancy may be reduced due to scleroderma however this depends on the type and extent of organ involvement.

Can patients be seen at their local hospital rather than traveling to the specialist so frequently?

Most patients with scleroderma can be seen at their local hospital for follow-up appointments with only yearly visits to a specialist; however, it is advisable to be seen by a specialist for initial diagnosis and treatment advice.

How do you prevent/treat digital ulcers?

Treatment for digital ulcers is by vasodilation thereby improving blood supply to the affected areas. Calcium channel blockers (e.g. diltiazem) and angiotensin-II receptor antagonists (e.g. losartan) are the most commonly used medications. A maintenance dose can be used permanently, or during cold weather, and the dose ↑ if an ulcer does occur.

What is iloprost?

Iloprost is a prostacyclin analogue which is given intravenously over several days in order to induce vasodilation to treat or prevent digital ulcers.

Will my scleroderma ever get better?

There is no cure for scleroderma. Many people find that skin and musculoskeletal symptoms are worst for the first 2 years and then slowly improve. However a person will remain at risk of developing organ involvement throughout the rest of their lives.

Can anything be done about changing facial features?

Changes in appearance are common in scleroderma and may be significant. There is little that can be done however a consultation with a plastic surgeon familiar with scleroderma may be helpful.

Where can patients get ongoing information and advice between doctors' appointments?

There are patient groups for patients with scleroderma which can provide valuable information, advice, and support. Most specialist centres for scleroderma also have nurse-led telephone helplines for the use of patients and other healthcare professionals.

Do patients need to take medication for life?

Immunosuppressant therapy is taken until the disease is under control, usually for a period of several years. Management of ongoing complications such as reflux or Raynaud's or organ involvement is likely to require ongoing treatment.

How can patients alleviate skin itching?

Skin itching can be severe in the early stages of diffuse scleroderma and is caused by the inflammatory response. Keeping skin well moisturized is very important and anti-itch creams (available over-the-counter) can be beneficial. Antihistamine tablets can help and in very severe cases a small dose of corticosteroid may be prescribed.

Will physiotherapy help?

Physiotherapy is valuable in scleroderma and regular exercises will significantly improve range of movement both in the joints of the fingers and hand and in larger joints. In the childhood forms of localized scleroderma, physiotherapy has a very important role to play in treatment and referral should be prompt to prevent problems with growth and development. Hand waxing is also very helpful in helping to maintain and improve skin condition and joint suppleness.

Why do I need to keep having the same tests done?

It is important to have regular organ tests to ensure that any deterioration in function is detected early in order to implement treatment if it may be required.

Is it right that treatments prescribed are usually used for cancer patients?

Immunosuppressant medications used in scleroderma are the same as those sometimes used for cancer. They are given in lower doses in scleroderma and often produce only minimal side-effects.

Does scleroderma affect pregnancy?

Scleroderma has a varied effect on pregnancy. It is not advisable to get pregnant whilst the disease is active or whilst on immunosuppressant medications; however, once the disease is under control pregnancy (under close medical supervision) is likely to be safe both for mother and child although it is possible a flare may occur due to pregnancy. Sometimes pregnancy seems to trigger scleroderma in a ♀ who had previously been healthy.

Primary systemic vasculitis and the nurse's role

The 1° systemic vasculitides (Wegener's granulomatosis (WG), Churg–Strauss syndrome (CSS), microscopic polyangiitis (MPN) and polyarteritis nodosa (PAN)) are a group of rare, potentially life-threatening conditions, characterized by inflammation and necrosis of blood vessel walls.[1]

It is often difficult to diagnose these conditions as early presentation is often non-specific and may mimic other diseases.

- Non-specific features.
- Malaise.
- Fever.
- Weight loss.
- Arthralgia.
- Arthritis.
- Headache.

These features are common to many other diseases but especially infection and malignancy. Specific clinical features such as a vasculitic rash which is often purpuric, needs to be differentiated from other causes of purpura such as thrombocytopenia and cutaneous vasculitis, this can also be a feature of infectious disease such as bacterial endocarditis. Necrotic lesions in the skin due to vasculitis are also seen in thrombotic disorders such as APS and the whole spectrum of systemic upset, purpura, and sometimes skin infarcts can be seen in the rare but important condition atrial myxoma (Figs. 5.1, 5.2)

Vasculitis should be considered with presentation of unexplained multisystem disease, pyrexia of unknown origin, rash, and renal involvement. 1° systemic vasculitis affects small to medium blood vessels. The annual incidence is 20 per million adults per year, with a median age of onset of 65 years in the United Kingdom.[2]

Diagnosis

Often made when all other causes are excluded, i.e. infection and malignancy. It is the combination of presenting symptoms and clinical features, the pattern of organ involvement, and the results of blood tests, urinalysis, and x-rays, coupled with anti-neutrophil cytoplasmic antibody (ANCA) status and tissue biopsy results that lead to a diagnosis of 1° systemic vasculitis (PSV). The three most common types—WG, CSS, MPN/PAN—will be presented.

The nurses' role in the management of PSV

The treatment of PSV is usually overseen by a consultant with a special interest in vasculitis who leads the MDT. A holistic patient-centred approach to care must be considered in the context of the nurses' role. One of the main responsibilities of the nurse in caring for the patient with PSV will be the administration of IV cyclophosphamide. Cyclophosphamide is a cytotoxic agent used to treat cancer and a number of other conditions. It can be administered either orally daily or as an IV pulse regimen.

📖 Also see Pre-treatment assessment of thalidomide and cyclophosphamide, p.166.

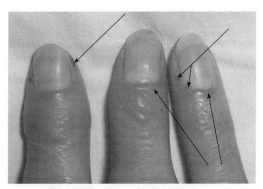

Fig. 5.1 Nail-fold infarcts. Image reproduced with permission of Norfolk and Norwich University Hospital NHS Foundation Trust.

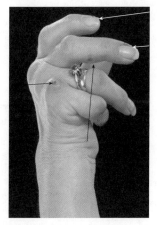

Fig. 5.2 RA vasculitis. Image reproduced with permission of Norfolk and Norwich University Hospital NHS Foundation Trust.

Reference

1. Watts RA, Scott DGI (2003). Overview of the inflammatory vasculitides. In Hochberg MC, Silman A, Smolen JS, et al. (eds), *Rheumatology*, 3rd edn, pp.1581–91. Mosby, London.

2. Watts RA, Lane S, Scott D (2005). What is known about the epidemiology of the vasculitides? *Best Practice Research Clinical Rheumatology*, **19**: 191–207.

Wegener's granulomatosis

WG is a rare, potentially life-threatening disease that classically affects the upper and lower airways and kidneys but can affect other systems (Table 5.2). It is more common in caucasians than other ethnic groups, peak age of onset 60 years, with equal sex distribution. It is a small-to-medium vessel vasculitis characterized by inflammation, and necrosis of these vessels and frequently accompanied by granuloma formation, particularly in the upper airway. The antibody associated with WG is the anti-neutophil cytoplasmic antibody which usually stains with cytoplasmic staining (c-ANCA) with specificity against proteinase 3 (Pr3).

Table 5.2 Clinical features of Wegener's granulomatosis

Clincal features		
Systemic	**ENT**	**Lung**
Fever	Sinusitis	Cough
Night sweats	Nasal crusting	Haemoptysis
Malaise	Oral ulcers	Pleuritis
Arthralgia	Subglotic stenosis	Nodules—chest x-ray
Weight loss	Epistaxis	Fixed infiltrates (>1 month)
	Hearing loss	
	Late clinical presentation	
	Saddle nose deformity	
Kidney	**Skin**	**Eye**
Haematuria	Rash	Epi /scleritis
Proteinurea	Purpura	Proptosis
↑ creatinine		
Nerve		
The commonest is a mild peripheral neuropathy/ but mononeuritis multiplex is the most classical form of vasculitis (commoner in CSS, than in WG or MPA)		

Common presentations
- Bleeding from the nose.
- Deafness.
- Haemoptysis.
- Haematuria.
- Proteinurea.

Investigations

Blood tests, urinalysis, x-rays and tissue biopsies are all used to aid diagnosis, exclude differential diagnosis, assess organ involvement, and disease severity.

Blood tests

- FBC may reveal anaemia (low Hb), raised platelets, and a raised WBC (as the consequence of any chronic inflammatory response).
- A mild eosinophilia is common in allergies and other inflammatory diseases, but a very high eosinophil count is particularly characteristic of CSS (>1.5×10^9/L). But mild eosinophilia is also not uncommon in WG.
- U&Es, creatinine useful in assessment of kidney fuction/impairement. ESR and CRP raised in inflammation and ANCA status.

Urinalysis

Dipstick urinalysis for haematuria and proteinurea is essential for detection of renal involvement. Send MSU for C&S.

▶ Red cell casts indicate renal involvement; this is one of the most serious outcomes in WG.

▶▶ It is important to recognize this as early as possible, so that appropriate treatment can be given.

Biopsies

Tissue biopsies from various organs can be helpful in reaching a diagnosis, the most common sites are:
- The skin.
- Kidney.
- Nose.
- Lung.

Typical appearances are those of necrotizing vasculitis in the skin, focal segmental necrotizing glomerulonephritis in the kidney (indicating small vessel vasculitis), and tissue from the upper airways reveals non-specific changes and granuloma is sometimes seen but this is rare. Needle biopsies of the lung also often reveal non-specific changes but an open biopsy will often show granuloma in WG.

X-rays

Chest x-ray may show lung inflammation, nodules, or cavitating nodules that are associated with WG. Sinus x-rays often show evidence of inflammation/infection with fluid levels but chronic disease causes bone destruction which also may be seen on x-ray.

Key nursing issues

It is vital that routine TPR, blood pressure, and urinalysis are carried out and any abnormalities discussed with medical staff. A rise in creatinine, haematuria, and proteinurea should be discussed with medical staff. Skin rashes should be observed and monitored.

Churg–Strauss syndrome

CSS consists of asthma, eosinophilia, fever, and accompanying vasculitis of various organ systems. It is associated with antibodies to ANCAs, usually pANCA (perineuclear), with specificity against myleoperoxidase (MPO) seen in ~50% cases.

Clinical features

- Asthma.
- Nasal polyps.
- Allergic rhinitis.
- Eosinophilia.
- Sinusitis.
- Rashes.
- Palpable purpura.
- Haematuria/proteinurea.
- Hypertension.
- Malaise.
- Loss of appetite.
- Weight loss.
- Mononeuritis multiplex.
- Neuropathy.

Classic pulmonary feature is of a flitting pulmonary shadowing on chest x-ray (which is similar to eosinophilic pneumonia). Pulmonary haemorrhage is much more commonly seen in MPA.

Asthma is one of the essential features of CSS. Asthma symptoms may begin long before the onset of vasculitis—e.g. many years before any other symptoms arise, and long before the diagnosis of CSS is made. Other early symptoms/signs include nasal polyps and allergic rhinitis.

Peripheral nerve involvement includes pain, numbness, or tingling in extremities (neuropathy/mononeuritis multiplex).

Investigations

- FBC.
- U&Es.
- CRP/ESR.
- ANCA.
- Chest x-ray.
- Eosinophilia is characteristic of CSS (>1.5 × 10^9/L).
- Biposy results show a necrotizing granulomatosis and eosinophilic vasculitis.

Key nursing issues

It is common for the heart to be affected, so any chest pain, shortness of breath (SOB), hypertension, dependent odema, or an abnormal pulse rate or rhythm should be reported to medical staff.

Polyarteritis nodosa

Classic PAN is a non-granulomatosis vasculitis of medium-sized arteries. It is rare in the UK with a mean age of onset of 50 years with equal distribution between the sexes. ANCA negative, rarely involves the kidney.

Clinical features

- Tiredness.
- Fever.
- Malaise.
- Weight loss.
- Loss of appetite
- Hypertension.
- Testicular pain.
- Frank haematuria—indicates severe renal disease.
- Abdominal pain—mainly due to gut infarction with a very poor prognosis.
- Skin rash. The most common are skin ulceration/gangrene (due to infarction) and livedo reticularus (a reticular discolouration pattern generally seen peripherally). Diagnosis of livedo reticularus is confirmed by biopsy. In addition, occasionally angiography will show microaneurysms under the skin which can rupture, causing haemorrhage, as well as infarction due to blockage of similar-sized blood vessels. Angiography more commonly is used to show these changes in the visceral circulation (coeliac axis and renal vessels)

Investigations

- FBC.
- U&Es.
- CRP/ESR.
- ANCA.
- Chest x-ray.
- Eosinophilia is characteristic of CSS (>1.5 × 10^9/L).
- Biposy results show a necrotizing granulomatosis and eosinophilic vasculitis.

Key nursing issues

- It is essential that BP is monitored as hypertension is common.
- Any abdominal pain should be reported to medical staff (to rule out gut infarction).
- Haematuria should be discussed with medical staff.

Microscopic polyangiitis

MPA is a small-vessel vasculitis which occasionally can affect medium and or large vessels, involving the skin, lungs, digestive system, and kidneys. Renal involvement is common. It is associated with antibodies to ANCAs usually p-ANCA with specificity against MPO.

Clinical features

- Tiredness.
- Fever.
- Malaise.
- Flulike symptoms.
- Myalgia.
- Weight loss.
- Haematuria.
- Proteinurea.
- Breathlessness.
- Skin rash.
- Haemoptysis.
- Pulmonary haemorrhage.
- Cough.
- Peripheral neuropathy.
- GI bleeding.
- Abdominal pain.

Inflammation of the kidney (glomerulonephritis) is a common presentation, symptoms/signs include tiredness, haematuria/proteinurea, elevated creatinine. The speed of renal involvement is unpredictable, ranging from slow to rapid progression necessitating a need for close monitoring of creatinine levels.

Investigations (see Table 5.3)

- Chest x-ray may show evidence of haemorrhage with widespread shadowing; this contrasts to WG which shows fixed infiltrates or granulomas with fluid levels, and in CSS where there are transient shadows more suggestive of pneumonia.
- Skin biopsy shows leucocytoclastic vasculitis.
- Bronchoscopy may confirm pulmonary haemorrhage.
- Lung biopsy may also show a small-vessel vasculitis.
- Renal biopsy:
    - In all ANCA-associated vasculitis, the changes are identical with the characteristic change being a pauci immune focal segmental nectrotizing glomerulonephritis.

The characteristic feature differentiating MPA from other auto-immune kidney conditions is the relative absence of immunoglobulin and compliment deposition in the kidney (pauci-immune.)

Key nursing issues

- It is vital that routine urinalysis is performed. Any haematuria/
  proteinurea and/or elevated creatinine must be discussed with medical
  staff.
- Any SOB and haemoptysis should be reported to medical staff.

Table 5.3 Blood and immunology investigations

Test	Result	Indication	Disease
FBC	↓ Hb (anaemia)	Chronic disease/ pulmonary haemorrhage	CSS, WG, MPA
	↑ platelets > 400 × 10^9/L	Inflammatory response (note: seen with active disease)	CSS, WG, MPA
	↑ WBC >11.0 × 10^9/L	Infection (note: also seen as an effect of steroids)	All
	↓ WBC <4.0 × 10^9/L	Drug induced: cyclophosphamide, MTX, AZA	All
	↓ neutrophils <2.0 × 10^9/L	Drug induced: cyclophosphamide, MTX, AZA	Withhold all cytotoxic drugs (cyclophosphamide), recheck bloods, screen for infection
	↑ eosinophils > 0.4 × 10^9/L	Allergy, inflammation	CSS (>1.5 × 10^9/L) Smaller ↑ in WG
	ESR >15mm/hour	Non-specfic indicator of inflammation	All
	CRP >10mg/L	Inflammation/infection	All
U&Es[*]	Creatinine <150micromol	Mild kidney inflammation/ early disease	MPA, WG, CSS
	Creatinine >150 but <500micromol	Generalized/kidney failure	MPA, WG, CSS
	Creatinine >500micromol	Severe kidney failure/ life threatening	MPA, WG, CSS
ANCA	Negative	Does not exclude vasculitis	All
	Positive c-ANCA	PR3 specificity	Strongly associated with WG
	Positive p-ANCA	MPO specificity	Associated with MPA, CSS

[*]Renal involvement: renal function can change rapidly and results need to be interpreted carefully in respect of previous values. Any abnormality of urinalysis, even with apparently normal creatinine can indicate glomerulonephritis—always discuss renal function tests with medical team in these circumstances.

Treatment for primary systemic vasculitis

Treatment should commence as early as possible to avoid irreversible organ damage. Assessment of the target organs involved and the severity of the disease is vital, as this determines the immunosuppressive regimen. The severity of the disease can be categorized into 3 groups and the BSR guidelines for management of PSV should be followed.[1]

▶▶Treatment should not be delayed when waiting for biopsy confirmation in those with organ/life-threatening disease (Table 5.4).

Table 5.4 Treatment for PSV

Classification	Treatment
Localized/early Creatinine <150micromol/L	Prednisolone + MTX Or cyclophosphamide
Generalized/ threatened organ Creatinine < 500micromol/L	Prednisolone + cyclophosphamide
Severe/ organ threatening Creatinine >500micromol/L	Prednisolone + cyclophosphamide + plasma exchange

Cyclophosphamide (always given together with corticosteroids)

- Administered orally or intravenously.
- Oral dose is 2mg/kg daily; maximum dosage 200mg daily.
- Given for 3–6 months.
- IV dosage is 15mg/kg; maximum dosage 1500mg.
- Given as 2–3-week pulses.
- Dosage should be adjusted for age and renal impairment.
- For those on IV pulse regimen 2-mercaptoethane sulfonate (mesna) should be considered as this may protect against bladder toxicity.
- Initial treatment is aimed at inducing remission, this can take 3–6 months.
- Then switch to maintenance therapy.

Maintenance therapy

Cyclophosphamide should be stopped and replaced with either AZA or MTX plus prednisolone. Maintenance therapy should last 2 years, except for ANCA positive Wegener's patients who should continue treatment for up to 5 years.[1]

Reference

1. Lapraik C, Watts R, Bacon P, et al. (2007) BSR and BHPR Guidelines for the management of adults with ANCA associated vasculitis. *Rheumatology*, **46**, 1615–16.

Administration of IV cyclophosphamide

An N59 chemotherapy course is often required for nurses administering cyclophosphamide, although some units stipulate that the minimum should be a training day in the safe handling and administration of cytotoxic agents and adherence to local policy on the administration and disposal of cytotoxic agents. Staff who may be pregnant should not administer cyclophosphamide. See Table 5.5.

📖 Also see Nursing issues patient-centred care, pp.300, 314, 346.

Further reading

Dougherty L, Lister S (eds) (2006). *The Royal Marsden Hospital Manual of Clinical Nursing Procedures*, 6th edn. Blackwell Publishing. Oxford

Nursing and Midwifery Council (2004). *Nursing and Midwifery Council Code of Professional Conduct; standards of conduct, performance and ethics.* NMC, London.

Table 5.5 Pre-cyclophosphamide check list

Patient education/consent	Yes/No	
FBC, U&Es, LFT's, CRP within last 24–48 hours	Yes/No	If no bloods stat
WBC >4..0	Yes/No	WBC <4.0 discus with Dr
Neutrophils >2.0	Yes/No	Neutrophils <2.0 withold cyclophophamide, discus with Dr
Exposure to chicken pox/shingles	Yes /No	Yes check varicella status, inform Dr
Varicella titre (if lst dose and not previously screened)		
Ckeck for signs of infection: wounds, urinary catheter, leg ulcer, cough, cold	Yes/No	If yes, discus with Dr
TPR, blood pressure, urinalysis	Yes/No	
♀ pregnant Date of last menstrual period	Yes/No	If yes, withhold treatment, discus with Dr
Infertlity—discus sperm banking	Yes /No	
Chest and heart examination by Dr	Yes/No	
Dose calculated 15mg/kg, with reduction if indicated for age or renal impairment		
Check drug allergies, especially sulphonamides	Yes/No	
Mesna and anti-emetic prescribed	Yes/No	
Septrin prophylaxis prescribed	Yes/No	
Bone prophylaxis prescribed	Yes/No	
Future invasive procedure planned	Yes/No	

Behçet disease/syndrome

Introduction

Behçet disease is characterized by oral and genital ulcers, eye inflammation, and arthritis. The dominant features of oral/genital ulceration are vasculitic in nature. Blood vessels are sometimes affected with frequent features such as:

- Phlebitis indicating inflammation of the veins.
- Arteritis and the development of aneurysms involving large arteries as well as small arteries.

Other non-vasculitic symptoms include:

- Arthritis.
- Specific types of Behçet disease such as neuro Behçet's, when there is an aseptic meningitis and ocular Behçet's when there is inflammation, rather than vasculitis within the eye.

Behçet disease is not uncommon in the UK (incidence is suggested as similar to SLE) but is much commoner in Eastern Europe and the Middle East. Many of the large series of patients come from Turkey where Behçet's was first described. Other areas where Behçet's is seen frequently include Greece, South East Asia, and Japan. It is rare in children <16 years, peak age of onset is 20–40 years with an equal distribution between ♂ and ♀.

Clinical features and presentation

See Box 5.5 and Table 5.6.

Box 5.5 Common presentation of Behçet disease

- Recurrent painful oral ulcers (almost 100% of patients).
- Genital ulcers (90%):
  - On the scrotum in ♂.
  - On the outer labia and cervix in the ♀.
- Eye manifestations—uveitis (70%).

In severe disease
- Young males 20–25 years old.
- Eye involvement.
- CNS involvement (up to 10% in some series).
- Pulmonary artery aneurysm (associated with a high mortality).

⚠ Eye manifestations can be serious and must be treated; complications are frequent and can cause blindness if untreated; commonest cause of blindness in Middle and Far East.

Table 5.6 Clinical features of Behçet disease

Mucosal surfaces	CNS	Eyes
Multiple episodes of oral ulcers	Headaches	Multiple episodes of uveitis
Multiple episodes of genital ulcers	Memory loss	Blurred vision
	Stroke	Retinal vasculitis
	Impaired balance	Hypopyon (pus in anterior chamber)
Skin	**Other**	**Vasculature**
Erythema nodosum	Fatigue	DVT
Papulopustular lesions	Arthritis	Haemoptysis
Acneiform or paupulopustular rash	GI ulceration	Pulmonary artery aneurysm
	Epididymitis	Thrombophlebitis
	Aseptic meningitis	

Classification criteria for Behçet syndrome[1]

Must have recurrent oral ulceration plus 2 of the following:
- Recurrent genital ulceration.
- Eye manifestations.
- Skin lesions.
- Positive pathergy test.

The classification criteria[1] was developed for research purposes and in clinical practice diagnosis is made by presenting symptoms and clinical features and exclusion of other differential diagnosis such as:
- Herpes simplex virus.
- Sweets syndrome.
- Reiter syndrome.
- AS.
- Crohn's disease.
- Oral aphthous ulcer.

Reference

1. International Study Group for Behcet's disease (1990). Criteria for diagnosis of Behçet disease. *Lancet*, **335**, 1078–80.

Behçet disease: investigations and treatment

As there are no specific diagnostic tests, diagnosis is made using:
- Clinical examination and an assessment of the degree of inflammation.
- Blood tests such as FBC, ESR/CRP, U&Es, and LFTs.
- Pathergy testing has been used in Middle East, but has not been of use in the UK population.
  - A pathergy test involves using a sterile 20–22-gauge needle, to obliquely pierce the skin to a depth of 5mm; a positive is determined if an erythematous papule develops at the test site after 2 days
- Genetic tests for HLA-B51 can be helpful when positive but again is not a helpful diagnostic test usually in a Caucasian population.
- For recurrent oral or genital ulceration where diagnosis is in doubt:
  - Tissue biopsy is important if diagnosis of recurrent oral or genital ulceration is in doubt.
  - Virology—to exclude other causes particularly of genital ulcers.

▶The differential diagnosis includes inflammatory bowel disease which may need investigating separately.

Treatment of Behçet disease

Treatment is aimed at the dominant clinical problem, usually advised by the appropriate specialist i.e. ophthalmologist, dermatologist, rheumatologist, or neurologist.

Eye manifestations

Evidence supports the treatment of severe eye disease with AZA and ciclosporin. Short courses of steroids maybe needed as an adjunct therapy (🕮 see Pharmacological management: ciclosporin and azathioprine, p.428).

Arthritis

Treat with NSAIDs and as any inflammatory arthritis.

Skin

- Treat ulcers with topical steroids.
- Systemically unwell patients will require treatment with steroids/immunosuppression.
- Oral ulcers may require treatment with colchicine.

For a small minority of patients who fail to respond to the above treatment, there is an emerging role for TNFα blockade.

Thalidomide

Is an unlicensed drug in the UK, that can be used to treat serious oral and genital ulcers but should only be used in severe disease or when other treatment modalities have failed.

Dosage: 50–100mg daily, then reduce to 50mg every 2 or 3 days once in remission. Thalidomide must only be prescribed by a consultant who

is experienced in its use. Special assessment and monitoring of patients is required due to the 2 most serious side effects:
• Teratogenic effects.
• Peripheral neuropathy.

A prescription can only be issued for 28 days and repeat prescriptions only issued on each monthly visit after a negative blood pregnancy test (where appropriate).

▶Doctors and pharmacists must be registered in the thalidomide Pharmion Risk Management Programme (PRMP) to prescribe and dispense the drug. Patients must also register with the programme and comply with its requirements to receive the drug.

⚠ Particular care is necessary in women with child-bearing potential
📖 Also see Treatment with thalidomide and cyclophosphamide: the nurse's role, p.166.

Monitoring—requires hospital supervision
• Monthly follow-up:
  • Signs of peripheral neuropathy, pins and needles, stop drug immediately.
• 6-monthly nerve conduction tests or after each 10g.
• Monthly pregnancy test.
• Routine blood teats e.g. for leucopenia.

Must take contraceptive precautions for 3 months on stopping thalidomide

Further reading

de Wazieres B, Gil H, Magy N et al. (1999). Treatment of recurrent ulceration with low doses of thalidomide. Pilot study of 17 patients. *Rev Med Interne*, **20**, 567–70.

McDonald DR, Lee C, Fowler RA, et al. (2007). Behçet's disease. *Canadian Medical Association Journal*, **176**, 1273-4.

Powell RJ, Gardner-Medwin JM (1994). Guidelines for the clinical use and dispensing of thalidomide. *Postgraduate Medical Journal*, **70**, 901–4.

Saenz A, Ausejo M, Shea B, et al. (1998). Pharmacotherapy for Behcet's syndrome. *Cochrane Database of Systematic Reviews*, Issue 2.

Wu J, Huang DB, Pang KR, et al. (2005) Thalidomide: dermatological indications, mechanisms of action and side-effects. *British Journal of Dermatology*, **153**, 254–73.

Treatment with thalidomide and cyclophosphamide: the nurse's role

Thalidomide

Patients being considered for thalidomide must be screened and counselled about the risks and benefits of treatment (Table 5.7). Nurses *must* ensure that:

- The patient fully understands the teratogenic effects of thalidomide.
- Information, counselling, and advice is provided to ensure that the patient is taking reliable contraception.
  - If a patient becomes pregnant they must inform the hospital immediately and stop the drug. An urgent referral to an obstetrician will be essential for specific counselling and advice.
- If patients complain of a painful red eye and reduced visual acuity urgent referral to an ophthalmologist should be made (exclude a potential diagnosis of acute iritis prior to referral).
- It is important to advise patients on good dental hygiene and stress the need for regular dental check ups.

Table 5.7 Thalidomide—pre-treatment assessment check list

Patient education/consent	Yes/No*
Patient registered PRMP	Yes/No *
Pregnancy test within last 24 hours	Yes/No*
♀ pregnant	Yes/No Inform Dr immediately if pregnant ⚠ Must not commence thalidomide
Baseline nerve conduction studies Yes /No	If no: ensure these are arranged
Education re. possible side effects Advise that they must not donate blood	Essential
Teratogenic effects explained	Yes/No*
♂ must use condoms during sexual activity (even if previous vasectomy) ♂ should not donate sperm	
Leucopenia Yes /No	If yes: do not commence treatment
Do not breastfeed	

Cyclophosphamide

Patients receiving cyclophosphamide must be screened and monitored closely to observe for potential side effects (e.g. bone marrow suppression, haemorrhagic cystitis, or ↑ risk of bladder cancer).

Administration of IV cyclophosphamide

An N59 chemotherapy course is usually required for nurses administering cyclophosphamide. In some organizations the minimum amount of training (e.g. safe handling and administration of cytotoxic agents) together with adherence to local policy on the administration and disposal of cytotoxic agents may be acceptable (Table 5.8). Staff who may be pregnant must not administer cyclophosphamide.

Table 5.8 Cyclophosphamide—pre-treatment assessment check list

Patient education/consent	Yes/No
Chest and heart examination by doctor	Yes/No
TPR, blood pressure, urinalysis	Yes/No. Report any abnormalities
Check drug allergies especially sulphonamides	Yes/No
Exposure to chicken pox/ shingles	Yes/No. If Yes check varicella status: discuss with Dr.
Varicella titre	If 1st dose and not previously screened
Check for signs of infection: wounds, urinary catheter, leg ulcer, cough, cold	Yes/No. If present: discuss with Dr.
FBC, U&Es, LFT's, CRP within last 24–48 hours	Yes/No **If no bloods stat**
WBC >4..0	Yes/No **WBC<4.0 discuss with DR**
Neutrophils >2.0	Yes/No. Neutrophils <2.0 withold treatment - discuss with Dr
Females pregnant Date of last menstrual period	Yes/No. If pregnant or uncertainty re pregnancy: withhold treatment and discuss with Dr.
Infertlity—discuss sperm banking	Yes/No
Dose calculated 15 mgs/ kg, ↓dose if indicated for age or renal impairment	
Mesna and anti-emetic prescribed	Yes/No
Septrin prophylaxis prescribed	Yes/No
Bone prophylaxis prescribed	Yes/No
Future invasive procedure planned	Yes/No

Ⅲ Also see Post-cyclophosphamide treatment, p.168; Ⅲ Nursing issues patient-centred care, p.300, 314, 346.

Further reading

Dougherty L, Lister S (eds) (2006). *The Royal Marsden Hospital Manual of Clinical Nursing Procedures*, 6th edn. Blackwell Publishing. Oxford.

Nursing and Midwifery Council (2004). *Nursing and Midwifery Council Code of Professional Conduct; standards of conduct, performance and ethics.* NMC, London.

Post-cyclophosphamide treatment

- Patients must drink at least 3L fluid to reduce bladder toxicity.
- Empty bladder frequently.
- Ensure patient knows when to have follow-up bloods and when to take mesna and co-trimoxazole.
- Avoid live vaccines for 3 months after stopping immunosuppressive treatment .

Follow-up care

These diseases can relapse at any time and require regular follow-up to assess the extent of organ involvement, progression of the disease, and toxicity of treatment especially infection.

Assessment and monitoring

- Regular bloods.
- FBC and differential count.
- U&Es.
- ESR/CRP.
- ANCA status.
- Urinalysis: dipstck for haematuria and proteinurea. Red cell casts indicative of significant kidney inflammation. Cyclophosphamide can cause haemorrhagic cystitis and ↑ risk of bladder cancer (>30-fold). Routine blood monitoring of AZA/MTX.
- The Birmingham Vasculitis Activity Score (BVAS) can be used to assess disease activity and severity of disease and the Vasculitis Damage Index (VDI) can be used to monitor long-term outcome.

▶ It is important to note that ANCA titre is not always associated with disease activity; however, a positive ANCA should alert the clinician to assess the patient more frequently due to a possible imminent relapse.

▶▶Early detection of relapse and prompt treatment is essential, minor relapse (no threat to vital organs) is treated with an ↑ in prednisolone and a major relapse (threated vital organs) is treated with cyclophosphamide.

Further reading

Bacon PA, Luqmani RA, Moots RJ, et al. (1994). Birmingham vasculitis activity score (BVAS) in systemic vasculitis. *QJM*, **87**, 671–8.

Frequently asked questions: vasculitis

What is vasculitis?
Inflammation of blood vessels.

What causes PSV?
We still do not know.

What is the prognosis?
PSV: early mortality is 10%, thereafter prognosis for WG/CSS is good with a 5-year survival rate of 80%. For MPA there is a worse prognosis because of renal involvement; mortality is 50% at 5 years.

What is the risk of bladder cancer from cyclophosphamide?
Up to a 30-fold but highest with long-term cyclophosphamide, probably much less with short-term intermittent (<6 months).

Should patients with PSV be given the influenza and pneumococcal vaccine?
Yes.

Can CSS be diagnosed without a biopsy?
Yes, it is preferable to have biopsy evidence, however this is not always possible but the diagnosis can be made from clinical signs and symptoms, blood tests and anca serology.

How many patients with CSS have asthma?
95%.

Cyclophosphamide can be given orally or as an IV pulse, is there a difference?
No, there is no difference in time to remission but using the IV route allows for a reduction in total dose of cyclophosphamide administered.

Can patients who are ANCA positive become ANCA negative?
Yes, many will become ANCA negative during treatment.

What advice should we give patients?
Aim for a blood pressure of 120/80; do not smoke; eat a healthy balanced diet; and control body weight.

Is Behçet's a sexually transmitted disease?
No, there are no links to sexually transmitted disease and Behçet disease.

Can patients receive vaccinations?
Yes, unless they are immunosuppressed when they should avoid live vaccines.

Chronic non-inflammatory pain

Chronic musculoskeletal pain

Over 80% of the population will consult a GP for musculoskeletal pain. Widespread pain, fibromyalgia, and regional pain have a similar occurrence and shared risk factors which suggest they are all part of the same spectrum of chronic pain. Chronic musculoskeletal pain has several key attributes:

• Pain persists over time.
• Pain affects physical, psychological, and social function.
• Often there is no identifiable pathological cause for the pain.
• The individual is not able to carry out their normal activities.

Consequently the aim of management is not the abolition of pain but to help individuals optimize their function and learn how to cope with the pain.

Defining pain

The most widely used definition of pain is from the International Association for the Society of Pain which regards pain as 'an unpleasant sensory and emotional experience associated with actual or potential tissue damage or described in terms of such damage'.[1] As there is no objective marker to measure pain McCaffery reminds us that 'pain is what the person feelings it says it is'.[2]

The difference between chronic and acute pain

Acute pain is a short-lived experience whereas chronic pain is ongoing occurrence (see Table 6.1).

Chronic non-inflammatory conditions
• Fibromyalgia.
• Osteoarthritis.
• Whiplash.
• Chronic pain syndromes.

Table 6.1 Differences between acute and chronic pain

Acute pain	Chronic pain
Duration is transient	Duration is persistent
Location usually single site	Location is generalized
Identifiable cause	Often no identifiable cause

References

1. International association for the study of pain (1994). *Classification of chronic pain, description of chronic pain syndromes and definitions of pain. Terms.* Second edition. IASP: Seattle, WA.
2. Mc Caffery M, Beebe A (1989). *Pain Clinical Manual for Nursing Practice.* Mosby: St Louis, CV.

Chronic pain syndromes: understanding pain mechanisms

- In the 17th century pain was seen as purely a physical phenomenon with a direct relationship between the amount of damage or 'nociception' and the pain experienced. What this theory did not explain was the variation in the pain experience for a given stimulus or injury (e.g. why do some patients take longer to recover from whiplash than others?) or the persistence of pain beyond the time of tissue healing.
- In 1965 Melzack and Wall revolutionized our understanding of pain mechanisms with the gate control theory of pain. This theory demonstrated that the transmission of pain messages could be modulated within the spinal cord via descending messages from the brain (our cognitions and emotions) or altered by activating another source of sensory receptor (exercise to release endorphins).[1]

Pain receptors

Pain receptors are situated in the tissues, especially the skin, synovium of joints, and arterial walls. These receptors are activated by various stimuli including:

- Mechanical changes, e.g. excess weight on a particular area.
- Temperature changes.
- Inflammatory changes—the release of prostaglandin, bradykinin, histamine and serotonin.

The peripheral sensory nerves transmit a signal of pain from the peripheries to the CNS to enable identification of the stimulus, e.g. pain in the wrist. The Alpha delta fibres (thin and myelinated) transmit the sharp pain of an acute injury and the slower C-fibres (unmyelinated) produce the dull aching pain of a more persistent problem. When these fibres are stimulated the 'pain gate' opens and messages pass to the brain to be perceived as pain. When large fibres become activated (Alpha beta) they close the 'pain gate'. Alpha beta fibres transmit the sensation of touch: consequently acupuncture and electrical nerve stimulation work on the same principle and excite large fibre activity. Nerve impulses that descend from the brain can also operate 'the gate' (Fig. 6.1).

Reference

1. Wall PD, Melzack R (1999). *Textbook of Pain*, 4th edn, pp.165–81. Churchill Livingstone, Edinburgh.

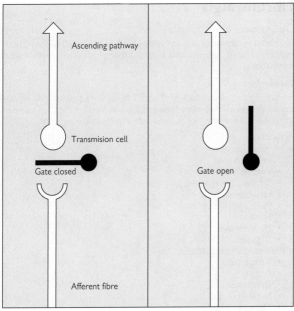

Synapse between nociceptor and transmision cell in the dorsal horn
Gate closed = no transmission at the synapse
Gate open = activity inafferent neuron excites dorsal horn cell

Fig. 6.1 Gate control mechanism. Reproduced with permission from Clinical Skills Ltd.

Fibromyalgia

Definition

A condition characterized by widespread musculoskeletal pain, non-restorative sleep, fatigue, and a host of other physical and psychological associations.

Incidence

Fibromyalgia occurs in 0.5% of ♂ and 3.4% of ♀. The onset in ♀ usually occurs between 25–45 years (Box 6.1). Fibromyalgia is a common cause of joint pain and the condition is often seen in a rheumatology clinic.

Associations

- Physical associations:
  - Irritable bowel.
  - Irritable bladder.
  - Temperature changes.
  - Paraesthesia.
  - Perception of swelling.
  - Headache.
  - Muscle spasm.
  - Dizziness.
- Psychological associations:
  - Panic attacks.
  - Anxiety.
  - Depression.
  - Irritability.
  - Memory lapses.
  - Word mix-ups.
  - Reduced concentration.
  - Atypical facial pain.

Causes

Fibromyalgia usually affects people with no other conditions where is is termed 'primary'. It can be associated with other MSC such as RA or lupus where it is referred to as 'secondary fibromyalgia'. No single pathophysiological causative mechanism has been identified and it would appear that fibromyalgia is a multifactorial syndrome.

Possible causes of fibromyalgia include:

- Abnormal pain processing.
- Sleep disturbance.
- Genetic predisposition to pain sensitivity.
- Neurohormonal dysfunction.
- Neuroendocrine disturbances.
- Neuro transmitter regulation.
- Physical trauma—road traffic accident, whiplash.
- Emotional trauma.

Diagnosis of fibromyalgia

In 1990 the ACR developed criteria for fibromyalgia for diagnostic purposes (□ see Diagnosis of fibromyalgia, p.178). In clinical practice the diagnosis is made on the basis of the clinical history and examination.

Examination

The main finding is the presence of symmetrical tender/painful sites around the body (See Fig. 6.2). In patients without fibromyalgia these sites are uncomfortable to firm pressure but in patients with fibromyalgia the same pressure causes the patient to cry out and withdraw the area being examined. When patients try to stretch out a limb they find that the pain prevents them achieving full extension but when the clinician exams the same area they can achieve full extension but the patient finds it uncomfortable.

Investigations

Limited investigations are required to exclude other causes for the symptoms, including PMR, spondyloarthropathy, and hypothyroidism—all of which can also give rise to similar symptoms.

Investigations include:
- FBC.
- Inflammatory markers e.g. ESR and CRP.
- Biochemical profile—serum calcium, alkaline phosphatase, creatine kinase, blood sugar.
- Thyroid function tests.

It is important to make a diagnosis of fibromyalgia after the clinical history and examination and explain to the patient that the blood tests are simply to ensure there is no underlying condition. Radiological investigations are not required.

Box 6.1 A typical patient

This will often be a ♀ aged 40 who experienced neck pain 5 years ago which never resolved and now has pain all over the body. She will experience fatigue on waking, feels 'worn out with the pain', and is tearful during the consultation. She has seen a number of other consultants in the past for various symptoms including her migraines and irritable bowel symptoms. She feels no one believes how much pain she is in and she is very anxious about her condition. She is no longer working and is finding it difficult to carry out her household chores. Physical examination reveals multiple tender hyperalgesic sites

Diagnosis of fibromyalgia

See Box 6.2.

Box 6.2 ACR diagnostic criteria for fibromyalgia

- Widespread musculoskeletal pain in all 4 quadrients of the body and some axial pain—cervical spine, anterior chest, thoracic spine or low back.
- Pain present for at least 3 months.
- Hyperlagesic points on digital pressure of 4kg in 11 out of 18 sites on the body.
- The points are all bilateral and situated in sub-occipital muscle insertions at the base of the skull.
- Low cervical spine C5–C7 interspinous ligaments.
- Trapezius muscles at the midpoint of the upper boarder.
- Supraspinatus origins above the scapulae spines.
- 2nd costochondral junctions on upper surface lateral to junction. 2cm distal to lateral epicondyles.
- Upper outer quadrient of buttock in anterior folds of gluteus medius.
- Greater trochanters posterior to trochanteric prominence.
- Medial fat pads of knee proximal to the joint line.

Clinical features from the history

- Widespread musculoskeletal pain.
- Pain is a constant feature.
- Tired all the time.
- Joint stiffness.
- Non-restorative sleep.
- Difficulty carrying out normal activities.

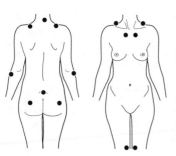

- Tenderness of skin overlaying trapezius
- Low cervical spine
- Midpoint of trapezius
- Supraspinatus
- Pectoralis, maximal lateral to the second costochondral junction
- Lateral epicondyle of the elbow
- Upper gluteal area
- Low lumbar spine
- Medial fat pad of the knee

Fig. 6.2 Some of the tender points in fibromyalgia. Reproduced with permission from Hakim A, Clunie G, Haq I (eds) (2006). *Oxford Handbook of Rheumatology*, 2nd edn. Oxford University Press, Oxford.

Management of chronic pain conditions

There are similarities between patients with fibromyalgia, repetitive strain injury, chronic back pain, and chronic fatigue syndrome. Therefore a common approach to management can be applied. The main goals of management include:

- To optimize physical, psychological, and social function.
- To help patients develop self-management/coping skills.

Chronic pain conditions

Back pain

Back pain is frequently seen in adults between 35–55 years of age. Most episodes settle within 6 weeks but 7% of people will go on to develop chronic pain. Specific guidelines for the management of back pain can be found at the Royal College of General Practitioners' website.[1]

Chronic regional pain syndrome (CRPS)

This syndrome is characterized by variable dysfunction of the musculoskeletal systems. It is a condition that is not fully understood and can be difficult to diagnose. CRPS typically affects the hand or forearm, foot, ankle, or knee.

There are 2 types of CRPS. In type 1, symptoms occur in the absence of injury to the nerves whereas in type 2 there is a nerve injury.

Causes

In a quarter of causes there is no identifiable cause although it sometimes occurs following:

- Trauma.
- Emotional stress.
- Pregnancy.
- Prolonged immobilization.
- Neurological events such as a stroke or meningitis.
- MI.

Signs and symptoms include:

- Pain, often 'burning' in nature, that can occur even after light touch.
- Tenderness.
- Rash.
- Warmth over the affected area.
- Sweating.
- Soft tissue swelling.
- Sleep disturbance.
- If symptoms last for several months then the affected area can change and become cool, with altered colour and abnormal sensation.
- If symptoms continue to progress then wasting (atrophy) of the skin and subcutaneous tissue can occur.

Investigations

The diagnosis is made from the clinical history and examination. Radiological investigation may reveal osteoporosis. The use of technetium scintigraphy can show abnormal blood flow.

Management

- Reassure the patient that they can manage their own symptoms through graded exercise, pacing, minimizing anxiety, developing a structure for the day, and adopting a sleep routine.
- Due to the importance of maintaining and improving function of the affected area as soon as possible, the PT is usually involved and hydrotherapy is a useful option for patients struggling to exercise due to the pain.
- To improve sleep and help with the pain low dose (10–50mg) tricyclics may be used.
- Regional sympathetic or ganglion blocks may also be considered in extreme cases.

All chronic pain conditions have the same management principles which are discussed in this chapter.

The Arthritis and Musculoskeletal Alliance (ARMA), British Society of Rheumatology, and the Pain Society have all produced evidence-based guidelines which can be accessed at the websites.[2–4]

The use of a biopsychosocial approach ensures that all factors contributing to the pain experience will be explored.

Factors contributing to the pain experience

- Physical factors, e.g. ↓ in physical activities results in muscle wasting, muscle fatigue, and ↑ joint stiffness.
- Psychological factors, e.g. low mood and anxiety.
- Cognitive factors, e.g. how a patient feels about their pain; if a patient is fearful that movement could cause damage they are less likely to engage in exercise.
- Social factors, e.g. how the pain is impacting on work, leisure and relationships.

📖 Also see Education, social, and psychological issues, pp.318, 320; 📖 Assessing pain, p.292; 📖 Symptom control: pharmacological and non–pharmacological, Chapter 9.

References

1. ᗡ www.rcgp.org.uk
2. ᗡ www.arma.uk.net
3. ᗡ www.rheumatology.org.uk
4. ᗡ www.britishpainsociety.org

Further reading

Hakim A, Clunie G, Haq I (eds) (2006). Miscellaneous conditions, Chapter 18. *Oxford Handbook of Rheumatology*, 2nd edn. Oxford University Press, Oxford.

Education in chronic pain management

The patient will often need guidance, support, and motivation from a health professional before feeling able to take an active role in the management of their symptoms. Useful patient websites include:

- 🔗 www.healthtalkonline.org
- 🔗 www.britishpainsociety.org/patient_home.htm
- 🔗 www.expertpatients.nhs.uk
- 🔗 www.arc.org.uk

Patient-centred management goals need to be realistic, achievable, and meaningful for the patient to engage in. Patients who utilize active rather than passive coping strategies report less pain-related disability and distress, better general health, and use fewer healthcare services and medications.

Active strategies are those that involve some action by the individual to manage their pain through their own efforts, whereas passive strategies refer to an individual who is more reliant on the efforts of others or depend on medications.

The current evidence advocates the use of behavioural strategies including:

- Graded exercise.
- Pacing.
- Cognitive behavioural therapy (CBT).
- Goal setting.
- Relaxation.
- Stress management.

Some of these strategies are covered in chronic disease management courses such as the EPP.

There is no evidence that one specific behavioural approach is more effective than another but treatment is likely to be more effective if it:

- Includes more than education alone.
- Includes teaching patients skills based on rehearsal or practice.
- Is aimed at changing behaviour and improving function.

CBT

- This is a widely used form of psychotherapy which aims to identify and change maladaptive patterns of thought and behaviour.
- CBT can help patients adjust to their illness and acquire skills that can be used in their daily lives.
- CBT can improve a patient's sense of control regarding their symptoms.
- CBT for persistent pain should be applied early in the development of problems with daily functioning and not as a last resort.
- More intensive courses of CBT are more effective. The choice between less intensive, unidisciplinary, outpatient-based courses versus intense, multidisciplinary, residential- or hospital-based courses should be made on the basis of the impact of the condition. If a patient has been out of work for an extended period, lost the structure of the day, and if their mood and symptoms predominate and dictate their activities, an intense course of multidisciplinary input would be beneficial.

Improving sleep

Patients often experience a disturbed sleep pattern and feel unrefreshed on waking. This ↑ the perception of pain, leading to low mood, reduced cognitive functioning, and a reduced ability to manage the symptoms. Self-help measures should be advocated, including:

- Developing a sleep routine, including going to bed at the same time each night and avoiding day-time sleeping.
- Avoiding stimulants such as caffeine.
- Carrying out relaxation techniques to clear the mind.
- Ensuring that the bedroom is quiet and well ventilated.

Tricyclics can improve sleep quality by improving non-rapid eye movement (REM), sleep which is restorative sleep. Numbers needed to treat are n = 4. The most commonly prescribed tricyclic is amitriptyline. This is prescribed in small incremental doses ranging from 10–50mg and should be taken 2–3 hours before settling. The decision regarding dosage will be based on efficacy and side effects. Tricyclics should help to improve sleep within 2–3 weeks but take 3–4 months before modifying pain perception.

Exercise

Many patients become less physically active due to pain and are fearful that movement will ↑ the symptoms of pain and fatigue. Graded exercise is advocated to recondition the body and to improve muscle stamina, strength, stiffness, and generalized fitness. Graded exercise involves gradually ↑ activity over a period of time. Several sessions of supervized exercise by the PT may be required to provide motivation, education, reassurance, and feedback.

Relaxation

Patient can be taught relaxation techniques to help with:
- Muscle tension.
- Anxiety.
- Sleep.
- Foster a sense of control over symptoms.

Pacing

Pacing involves breaking down everyday activities into achievable components. Patients tend to exert themselves on a 'good day' and under-exert on a 'poor day'. If patients can plan their activities, e.g. cleaning 1 room in the house a day instead of doing all the rooms in one go, they will still achieve their goal and be active every day. Patients should always be encouraged to remain in the workplace and apply the principles of pacing in the work situation.

📖 Also see Non-pharmacological therapies, Chapter 19.

Managing depression in chronic pain syndromes

Symptoms of depression are common in chronic musculoskeletal pain conditions:

* For mild depression, CBT, exercise, relaxation, and pacing techniques can all be considered.
* For moderate-to-severe depression the serotonin-specific reuptake inhibitors (SSRIs) should be the first option. Citalopram 20mg daily is often considered the drug of choice as it is well tolerated, has few side effects, and few drug interactions. Patients should be told that it will take 2 weeks before the drug becomes effective. Antidepressants also have analgesic effects which can be very useful when treating this group of patients although no anti-depressant is currently licensed for the management of chronic musculoskeletal pain in the UK. If a patient does not respond to antidepressant treatment then a psychiatric referral should be considered.

Other pharmacological options for the management of chronic musculoskeletal pain

* Paracetamol may be useful for joint pain in OA but for non-organic pain such as fibromyalgia there is often a poor response.
* If paracetamol is not effective add in codeine phosphate.
* If codeine is not tolerated or ineffective try meptazinal. Some epileptic drugs are used to reduce chronic pain, e.g. pregabalin, which has been shown to reduce pain, fatigue, and improve sleep.
* Nefopam or tramadol may be considered but there is little evidence to support the use of strong narcotics. Tramadol should be used with caution in patients who have a history of dependence or addiction. It can also interact with the SSRIs and the tricyclics to cause convulsions

Complementary/alterative medicine (CAM)

While few studies have examined the benefits of CAM, patients often use numerous types of CAM including massage therapy, chiropractic treatment, and acupuncture.

Roles of the MDT

* Nurse or OT pacing, relaxation, goal setting, education, and self-management.
* Nurse/OT or psychologist for CBT.
* PT for graded exercise.
* Doctor/nurse or therapist prescriber for drug therapy.

📖 Also see Pharmacological management: pain relief, Chapter 15, p.403;
📖 Symptom control: pharmacological and non-pharmacological, Chapter 9, p.289.

Further reading

Rohrbeck J, Jordan K, Croft P (2007). The frequency and characteristics of chronic widespread pain in general practice. *British Journal of General Practice*, **57**, 109–15.

Ryan S, Campbell A (2007). Fibromyalgia syndrome. In Adebajo A (ed), *ABC of Rheumatology*, 4th edn. BMJ Publishing, London.

Frequently asked questions: chronic pain syndromes

How can you be sure that I have got fibromyalgia?

You have described all the classic symptoms, you are tender in all the designated sites, and your blood tests confirm that you haven't got anything else going on.

You want me to take amitriptyline—do you think this is all in my mind?

I have no doubts that the pain you are experiencing is real and amitriptyline is more useful than traditional pain killers in improving sleep and pain. Although the information leaflet included with these tablets mentions that it is used as an antidepressant, you are not being given it in an antidepressant dose but in a dose that will help to improve the quality of your sleep to make you feel more restored on waking. Drugs do have different actions when given in different doses.

Will the pain get better?

We know that patients who carry out regular exercise, have a structure to the day, develop a sleep routine, and keep active are more able to cope with the pain.

When I try to exercise will I make my pain worse?

When you start to use muscles and joints that have not been used for a while you will experience more pain and fatigue; as your body becomes more used to you exercising, the muscle discomfort will ↓ and you will be able to ↑ the amount of exercise that you are doing.

Regional musculoskeletal conditions: overview

A systematic classification of musculoskeletal disorders that comfortably includes everything is difficult to achieve. The scope of MSC is so wide and diverse as it has to cover everything from CTDs to traumatic injuries, inflammatory to degenerative diseases, systemic, and local conditions.

A chapter on regional MSC might therefore be expected to cover a lot of the problems that don't fit into any of the other big disease categories. Don't be fooled however into thinking that the conditions outlined in this chapter are somehow less important. Many of the commonest musculoskeletal problems that occur in the community, and present in a 1° care setting, will be outlined in this chapter. Musculoskeletal problems are presented in ~25% of consultations with health professionals in 1° care. The average GP will see at least one case of back or neck pain every day, and will see at least one case of shoulder or knee pain every other day.

This chapter has set out to focus on the most common problems that you are likely to come across in daily practice but should complement the additional text outlining the less commonly seen conditions that are discussed in this handbook.

The neck and spine are discussed in 📖 Neck and spine, Chapter 6, p.212, 214 and Chapter 8, p.288.

The shoulder: common problems and adhesive capsulitis

Shoulder pain is common and has the potential to significantly impact upon the individual's quality of life and ability to participate in work activities. The pain may be due to disease or injury of structures surrounding the shoulder joint itself, or referred from other sites (Box 6.3).

The most common problems are those caused by disease or injury of the tendons, muscles, ligaments, and capsule of the joint. The majority will be due to either capsulitis or rotator cuff tendon problems. These conditions can often be differentiated by means of a careful history and examination. Possible diagnoses include:

- Adhesive capsulitis.
- Rotator cuff tendonitis and sub acromial impingement.
- Acromio clavicular joint dysfunction.
- Biceps tendonitis.
- Rupture of long head of biceps.

Box 6.3 Shoulder pain: common problems and differential diagnoses

Pain arising from disease or injury of shoulder structures
- The joint capsule, e.g. capsulitis.
- Synovium, e.g. inflammatory arthritis.
- Bursitis.
- Tendon and muscle, e.g. rotator cuff tendonopathy.
- Bone e.g. bony malignant metastases.

Shoulder pain referred from other sites
- Neck problems, e.g. cervical spondylosis.
- Cervical disk disease.
- Structures innervated by C3, C4, C6 segments, e.g. diaphragm (characteristically pain from an inflamed gall bladder may refer to the right shoulder)

Adhesive capsulitis (frozen shoulder)

Epidemiology

Capsulitis presents with pain and global restriction in shoulder movements. The cause is unknown, but the onset of symptoms is often associated with a previous minor injury or may follow a period of immobility of the limb. Presentation usually includes:

- Most commonly seen in 40–60-year-olds.
- Commoner in ♀ and diabetics.
- Bilateral in 15% of cases.
- Following a period of immobility such as:
  • Following a fracture which has lead to immobilization.
  • After hemiplegic stroke.

The natural history of this condition is for symptoms to resolve slowly over 18 months to 2 years. However, even after this time there may be residual joint restriction.

Diagnosis

- Active *and* passive movements are restricted in all directions.
- Lateral rotation at the shoulder shows most restriction as the joint capsule has least laxity anteriorly.
- Passive movement of the shoulder into lateral rotation by the examiner will not only demonstrate restriction but a hard 'end feel' to the joint movement. This helps to differentiate this condition from a rotator cuff injury, but it is important to remember that the two conditions may co-exist.

▶ Differentiate this condition from rotator cuff injury—although the two conditions may co-exist.

Management

The history and examination should be directed at excluding other causes of shoulder pain, in particular bony pain and referred pain.

▶ Don't forget to think about PMR in the elderly person with bilateral shoulder pain and stiffness.

The principles of management include:

- Pain relief:
  - Non-pharmacological measures, heat pads, TENS.
  - Simple analgesia.
  - NSAIDs—short courses where no contraindications exist.
- Mobilization:
  - Avoid using a sling.
  - Advise simple exercises, e.g. Codman's pendular exercises.
  - Refer to physiotherapy if necessary.
  - IA corticosteroid injection.
  - IA corticosteroid injected into the gleno-humeral space may result in both pain relief and improved range of movement. The procedure may need to be repeated, but is not always successful.

▶ It is helpful to demonstrate the exercises to the patient and provide written information. Explain that pain relief is necessary to allow them to perform the exercises, which in turn will aid recovery.

📖 Also see Primary care: common musculoskeletal problems, Chapter 6, p.208; 📖 Primary care: first steps in the assessment of shoulder problems, Chapter 6, p.220.

Shoulder problems: rotator cuff, subacromial, clavicular, and biceps problems

Rotator cuff tendonitis and sub acromial impingement

The 'rotator cuff' is the name given to the muscles and tendons that surround the shoulder joint. The shoulder is the most mobile joint in the body, and therefore relies heavily on the surrounding muscles and tendons for stability. The tendons of the rotator cuff muscles pass through the small space below the acromion, and may cause shoulder pain if they become inflamed, damaged, or torn.

Sub acromial impingement is the term used to describe the pattern of pain and symptoms produced by a number of problems affecting the structures of the rotator cuff. These include:

- Rotator cuff tendon damage or tears.
- Sub acromial bursitis.
- Glenohumeral instability.
- Ostephytes affecting the inferior aspect of the acromioclavicular joint.

All of these will result in pain, characteristically localized to the upper arm; so-called 'military badge pain' which is aggravated by specific rotational or elevational movements of the arm.

Epidemiology

This is the commonest type of shoulder pain in adults. The diagnosis might be suggested by a history of trauma (e.g. a sports injury) or repetitive, forceful, overhead shoulder movements, and may therefore present in particular occupational groups such as painters and decorators and plasterers. The commonest tendon of the rotator cuff to be affected is the supraspinatus tendon, which is responsible for initiation of shoulder abduction. Occasionally calcium deposits may be found within the tendon (so-called calcific tendonitis). This often presents with a more severe acute pain with associated heat and redness.

Diagnosis

Movement will generally be most restricted and painful in one particular plane of movement. Classically pain is maximal through the mid part of shoulder abduction ('mid arc pain') Passive movements are usually not as painful, but each rotator cuff tendon can be tested by loading them individually with resisted movements, which will reproduce the pain.

Management

The initial management is similar to that for adhesive capsulitis and involves:

- Analgesia and rest in the acute phase (avoid overhead movements).
- Passive mobilization exercises may assist recovery.
- A sub acromial IA steroid injection is often useful in severe cases which fail to respond to conservative treatment.
- Occasionally arthroscopic decompression of the sub acromial space may be performed.

- For acute tendon rupture a surgical repair or tendon transfer
  procedure may be necessary.

📖 Also see The shoulder: common problems and adhesive capsulitis,
p.188.

Acromio clavicular joint (ACJ) dysfunction

The ACJ is prone to traumatic subluxation, dislocation, and subsequent
osteoarthritic change, and may sometimes be the source of significant
shoulder pain. The pain is often localized to the site of the ACJ, and results
in pain particularly in the last 20° of shoulder abduction, and in movements which involve adduction the arm across the body, thus compressing
the ACJ. This is the basis of the 'scarf test', which can be helpful in identifying ACJ dysfunction. Significant ACJ problems may also co-exist with sub
acromial bursitis and rotator cuff problems. Symptoms are often chronic
and ongoing, but some relief may be obtained by an IA corticosteroid
injection into the ACJ, or, in severe cases, surgical excision of the lateral
end of the clavicle.

Biceps tendonitis and rupture of long head of biceps

The tendon of the long head of biceps traverses the shoulder joint and
travels through the bicipital groove between the greater and lesser tuberosity of the humerus. It is enclosed in a synovial sheath throughout its
length, and may give rise to pain in the anterior shoulder and the anterior
upper arm, aggravated by repetitive lifting. The pain can be reproduced
by resisted elbow flexion. Treatment is with rest and analgesia, including
NSAIDs if tolerated. Local corticosteroid injection into the tendon sheath
can also be carried out. The tendon may rupture. This is more likely in
older individuals, and is associated with a 'snapping' sensation and the
appearance of a swelling in the upper arm which represents the contracted muscle belly. No specific treatment is required although residual
weakness on elbow flexion is to be expected.

The elbow

The elbow joint enjoys good bony stability, and is often relatively spared in many of the commoner form of arthritis. However, elbow pain may often present from structures around the elbow. The commonest cause of pain around the elbow is medial and lateral epicondylitis, often referred to as 'tennis elbow' and 'golfers elbow'. These two problems will be dealt with together as they represent a common pathological process

Medial and lateral epicondylitis ('tennis elbow' and 'golfer's elbow')

The medial and lateral epicondyles are the bony extensions at the distal end of the humerus. The medial epicondyle acts as an anchor point for the flexor muscles of the forearm, which flex both the wrist and fingers. This point of attachment is often referred to as the common flexor origin. Similarly, the lateral epicondyle is the anchor point for the extensor muscles of the forearm and is referred to as the common extensor origin. The point at which muscles and tendons attach to bone is called the 'enthesis'. The enthesis must withstand tremendous traction forces, particularly during activities which involve frequent, forceful, repetitive gripping, twisting, or wrist flexion and extension. Thus some occupations may be predisposed to this condition (painters and decorators, plasterers, joiners, electricians, or sports-related activities) or it may occur after particular unaccustomed activity. A history of any repetitive forceful forearm activity is therefore significant.

Diagnosis

The pain may be reproduced by resisted wrist extension (lateral epicondylitis) or flexion (medial epicondylitis) with the elbow held straight. There may also be tenderness over the epicondyle.

Management

- Rest, the application of ice, and a short course of NSAIDs may help, but often the symptoms may recur with resumption of activity.
- Physiotherapy and the use of an epicodylar splint may sometimes alleviate symptoms and promote resolution.
- Advice on reviewing grip size of racquet or golf clubs may be helpful as condition may be exacerbated by the wrong grip size.
- Local corticosteroid injection around the enthesis is often beneficial, but the symptoms may still recur, and repeated successive injection at this site carry a high risk of subcutaneous lipoatrophy.
- In instances where none of these measures produce benefit surgery may be considered. Enthesotomy can be carried out as an arthroscopic procedure.

Olecranon bursitis

The olecranon bursa overlies the bony prominence at the point of the elbow. This structure is usually neither visible nor palpable, but in certain circumstances may fill with fluid and present as a large fluctuant lump on the point of the elbow. Causes to consider include:

- It may arise following trauma such as a direct blow to the point of the elbow. In these circumstances a fracture must be excluded.
- Sepsis may also occur in the bursa giving rise to a painful, hot, tender swelling.
- Occasionally an olecranon bursitis may occur in gout.

Aspiration with fluid analysis is frequently necessary and must be undertaken prior to local corticosteroid injection and may reveal:

- Often reveals blood stained fluid.
- Gout—uric acid crystals may be seen on polarized light microscopy of the aspirate.
- ⚠ Although uncommon, septic arthritis needs to be considered as a possible diagnosis. A culture may reveal the organism although septic arthritis is an acute medical emergency requiring prompt referral to 2° care. Usually if there is an index of suspicion of a septic joint referral is made to 2° care and antibiotic therapy may start after aspiration but before the culture results are available.
- A septic bursitis is obviously not as catastrophic as a septic arthritis, but still has to be managed cautiously. Following aspiration these bursae frequently recur, and occasionally surgical bursectomy may be considered.

Ulnar neuritis

The ulnar nerve is in a somewhat vulnerable position as it passes through a grove behind the medial epicondyle, the so-called cubital tunnel (symptoms relating to this nerve are experienced when we refer to 'hitting our funny bone'). The nerve may be vulnerable to more persistent entrapment at this site leading to paraesthesia and numbness affecting the palmar aspect of the 5th digit and the ulnar side of the 4th digit. Tapping over the ulnar nerve with a finger as it passes through the cubital tunnel (Hoffman–Tinel test) may precipitate or exacerbate the symptoms, thus assisting diagnosis.

Treatment includes:

- Rest and attention to posture or activities that may be contributing towards the development of the symptoms.
- Occasionally, corticosteroid injection or surgical decompression may be required.

Wrist and hand

Carpal tunnel syndrome (CTS)

CTS, similar to ulnar neuropathy, represents a nerve entrapment syndrome that occurs as the median nerve passes beneath the flexor retinaculum at the wrist. It is common, and results in an easily recognizable pattern of symptoms which include abnormal unpleasant sensations, often described as 'pins and needles in the distribution of the sensory branch of the median nerve in the hand—palmar aspect of the middle 3 fingers and the base of the thumb.

- Often worse at night and may cause wakening from sleep and described as affected hand as being 'dead' or 'asleep', and often try to gain some relief by shaking it vigorously.
- Pain may be referred proximally up the forearm, and in some cases even to the shoulder.

No cause may be found, but there is an association between the development of symptoms and any condition that may cause swelling or compression in the wrist, e.g.:

- Previous Colles' fracture, OA, or synovitis at the wrist.
- Pregnancy, hypothyroidism, acromegaly, and diabetes.

If the condition is untreated and progresses further the symptoms may become constant and motor symptoms may develop with weakness of the adductor pollicis and flexor pollicis brevis muscles, resulting in weakness of thumb apposition.

Examination

- Tinel's test refers to the provocation of symptoms by tapping over the median nerve as it runs through the wrist.
- Phalen's test again provokes or reproduces symptoms by asking the patient to rest their arm on a table or chair, allowing their hand to hang unsupported with the wrist flexed. In more advanced cases wasting of the thenar and hypothenar eminences may be apparent.
- Further investigation with nerve conduction studies may help to confirm the diagnosis, but this facility is not always readily available, and a reliable diagnosis can often be made on clinical grounds alone.

Management

- Rest and splintage may be helpful.
- Contributing conditions such as hypothyroidism or inflammatory arthritis should be treated appropriately.
- Diuretics are rarely of benefit.
- Local corticosteroid injection into the carpal tunnel may produce improvement in symptoms for ~70% of sufferers.
- Surgical decompression may be required in some cases.

📖 Also see The elbow, p.192.

De Quervains tenosynovitis

This occurs when there is inflammation of the tendon and tendon sheath of the extensor pollicis longus tendon as it runs under the extensor retinaculum at the radial styloid. The anatomical landmarks are usually easily identified. Symptoms include:

- Main presenting symptoms is of pain, often more proximal pain than the pain produced by 1° OA affecting the 1st carpometacarpal joint, which is the main differential diagnosis.
- Pain may occasionally be accompanied with swelling and crepitus.
- Finklestein's test is positive and involves forced adduction at the wrist with the thumb flexed.

Treatment includes rest using a thumb spica splint, or corticosteroid injection of the tendon sheath.

Oarsman's wrist (tenosynovitis of extensor carpii radialis longus and brevis) This produces pain swelling and crepitus over the radial aspect of the wrist proximal to the radio carpal joint, and is almost always associated with unaccustomed overuse, as the name suggests. In the authors' experience it is more often seen in weekend gardeners than oarsmen.

Treatment includes: rest, splintage, and NSAIDs (if not contraindicated).

Ganglia

These are fluid-filled swellings of the tendon sheaths usually seen over the dorsum of the wrist. They are often asymptomatic and the patient may present simply because they are curious to find out what they are. The traditional treatment was to hit the swelling with a heavy object such as a book. This presumably ruptures the swelling and achieves a good functional and cosmetic response. Some patients may report this gratifying result when the swelling is exposed to accidental trauma. The swelling may be aspirated, but if ganglia has been present for a long time the fluid is often gelatinous and difficult to aspirate through a standard 21-gauge green needle. Following aspiration it may often recur. Surgical excision can be considered, but if asymptomatic it is often best to do nothing.

Trigger finger/thumb (flexor tendon nodule)

This condition is more commonly seen in inflammatory conditions such as RA, and in diabetes, but may occur in anyone. The precipitating cause is often trauma to the tendons, but this may often be trivial and not recollected by the patient. A firm tender nodule can be palpated which moves with movement of the affected finger. If the nodule is located close to one of the anular ligaments of the fingers, the nodule may get trapped within the tendon sheath, causing the affected finger to remain in the flexed position when the rest of the fingers of the hand are extended. The finger may be extended forcibly but this is often painful. Treatment: Responds well to injection of corticosteroid into the tendon sheath.

Lower limb: hip problems

Lower limb symptoms may arise as part of a more widespread systemic rheumatic disease, or may be referred from other sites such as the lumbar spine or sacro-iliac joint. The commonest presenting complaint will be of pain in the limb or some part of the limb. Other common symptoms are abnormal sensation (numbness, burning etc.) often of a neurological origin, weakness, and clicking from around a joint.

Hip

Patients may complain of pain in the hip; this pain may arise from the joint itself, from structures around the joint, or be referred from other sites such as the back. Red flags should be excluded. High index of suspicion should be considered if:

- Previous history of malignancy.
- Systemic illness including weight loss, or persisting nocturnal bony pain. The hip joint itself enjoys good bony stability and is deeply situated. Pain arising from the joint is usually felt in the groin and deep within the buttock.

 Also see Neck and spine, Chapter 6, pp.212, 214; Red and yellow flags, pp.294, 335; Osteoarthritis of the hip and knee, Chapter 2, p.14.

Bursitis

There are 3 bursae around the hip which may give rise to periarticular pain. These are the:

- Trochanteric bursa.
- Ischial bursa.
- Ileopsoas bursa.

Trochanteric bursitis

The commonest to be seen and causes pain over the lateral aspect of the hip. It is often painful to lie on the affected side, giving rise to complaints of disturbed sleep. Pain may be exacerbated by adducting the hip and asking the patient to attempt to abduct the hip against resistance. Maximal tenderness usually over the trochanter

Treatment: often responds to local corticosteroid injection.

Ischial bursitis

Causes pain on sitting. The ischial bursa is located deep to the gluteal muscles. Pain may also arise on hip flexion when standing, as in stooping forward.

Treatment: rest and analgesia, preferably with a NSAID if not contraindicated. Local corticosteroid injection can also be considered in resistant or prolonged cases.

Ileopsoas bursitis

Rare and causes groin pain. It is most often seen in association with sports, particularly jumping. It may be associated with groin strain.

Treatment: muscle sprains usually respond to rest and simple analgesia (if necessary consider short course of NSAIDs if not contraindicated).

Lower limb: injuries affecting the knee

Injuries that result in regional conditions affecting the knee include:
Injuries affecting regional knee conditions:
- Ligament strain and rupture: collateral and cruciate ligaments.
  - Meniscal injury.

Causes of knee effusion include:
- Trauma—haemarthrosis if bleeding occurs into the joint.
- Inflammatory:
  - Inflammatory arthritis.
  - Crystal arthritis.
  - OA.
  - Sepsis.

📖 Also see Osteoarthritis of the hip and knee, Chapter 2, p.14.
▶ All knee effusions (irrespective of possible cause) should be have aspirate collected for fluid analysis—culture and Gram stain for bacterial organisms and polarized light microscopy for crystals.

Collateral ligament strain

The medial and lateral collateral ligaments are of great structural and functional importance.
- Injury usually occurs through direct trauma to the knee, particularly where the joint is subjected to excessive lateral force.
  - The joint will be unstable, and there may well be an associated effusion. If symptoms occur after trauma an additional injury may be apparent depending on the force of the trauma.
- May be associated with OA knee, particularly where there is asymmetric arthritis affecting the medial and lateral compartments of the knee joint resulting in an angular deformity, or genu valgus deformity (leads to knock-kneed appearance) and asymmetry of biomechanical forces.
- May also be associated with an anserine bursitis (📖 see Anserine bursitis, p.202).
- A rare complication of trauma to the medial collateral ligament is painful calcification occurring within the ligament, extending distally from the medial condyle of the femur, otherwise known as Pellegrini–Steida syndrome.

Examination
The collateral ligaments are palpable. The medial collateral ligament is a broad band-like structure, whereas the lateral collateral ligament is more cord-like. The pain may be reproduced on applying lateral force to the knee, and the ligament may be tender to palpation.

Treatment
- If ligaments ruptured they may require surgical reconstruction.
- Ligament strain will often resolve with rest, ice, and compression, followed by rehabilitation, under the supervision of a PT.
- Local physiotherapy treatments such as US may help.
- A knee brace for use during sport may also be of benefit.
- Short-term NSAIDs (when not contraindicated) and simple analgesics may help initially.
- Local corticosteroid injection again may be useful in resistant cases.

Cruciate ligament injury

Cruciate ligaments are usually the result of injury and trauma, commonly on the sports field. Cruciate ligament rupture is a significant orthopaedic injury and will usually require surgical repair. A positive anterior or posterior drawer test is pathognomonic of this condition (Fig. 6.3).

Meniscial injury

The menisci are prone to injury during sports activity. The mechanism is usually a twisting injury to the knee, and contact sports such as football and rugby particularly give rise to this injury, where the foot is fixed in position in the studded boot, and the body rotates excessively over the joint. Similar injury can occur in snow sports or water skiing. Acute presentation may be associated with an effusion and haemarthrosis. Following initial injury symptoms may settle, but the hallmarks of previous meniscial injury are recurrent episodes of knee locking and the knee giving way without warning.

Examination

There may be joint line tenderness on palpation, and occasionally a loose cartilaginous body may be palpated along the joint line. The commonest site for meniscial damage is anteromedially. McMurrays test will often demonstrate a positive response (Fig. 6.4). MRI scanning is the investigation of choice.

Treatment: arthroscopic repair of the menisci is the preferred option.

Anterior draw test

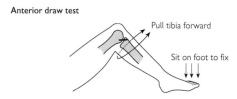

Pull tibia forward

Sit on foot to fix

Fig. 6.3 Anterior drawer test. Reproduced with permission from Hakim A, Clunie G, Haq I (eds) (2006). *Oxford Handbook of Rheumatology*, 2nd edn. Oxford University Press, Oxford.

McMurray's test

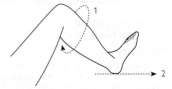

Action:	Hold the knee and the heel.
	Internally rotate the lower leg (1) then extend it (2)
Positive test:	(Palpable) clunk at joint line

Fig. 6.4 McMurray's test. Reproduced with permission from Hakim A, Clunie G, Haq I (eds) (2006). *Oxford Handbook of Rheumatology*, 2nd edn. Oxford University Press, Oxford.

Lower limb: knee problems

▶ All knee effusions (irrespective of possible cause) should have aspirate collected for fluid analysis—culture and Gram stain for bacterial organisms and polarized light microscopy for crystals.

Also see Lower limb: injuries affecting the knee, p.232; Hip and knee, p.234.

Baker's cyst

A Baker's cyst is simply a cyst of the synovial sac in the knee which can be felt in the popliteal fossa (posterior aspect of the calf).

- May be associated with OA in the knee.
- Occur spontaneously—rupture causes pain and swelling in the calf, mimicking DVT. If diagnosis is uncertain an arthrogram may be helpful.

If associated knee effusion, aspiration from knee joint often helps resolve the problem. Direct aspiration of a Baker's cyst is rarely recommended, and should only be undertaken with guided US control, to avoid damage to important structures (e.g. popliteal artery).

Anserine bursitis

The pes anserinus (or the 'goose's foot') is the name given to the area where the 3 tendons of grascilis, semitendinosus, and sartorius muscles join and insert into the medial aspect of the tibia ~3-4cm below the joint line. A bursa underlies this insertion and can be the site of pain; often associated with a genu valgus deformity and OA (see Collateral ligament strain, p.198). It is also common to note a degree of ankle and foot pronation or 'flat footedness'. The pathology may be a bursitis or simply an enthesitis at the insertion of the pes anserinus.

Treatment

- Local corticosteroid injection may help, but the condition often recurs if underlying abnormal biomechanical loads are not addressed.
- Orthoses and arch supports may benefit where there is excessive ankle and foot pronation, and advice to lose weight if the patient is obese.

Pre-patellar/infra-patellar bursitis (housemaid's knee, pasons knee)

This is akin to the olecranon bursitis at the elbow. It presents with a large fluid-filled swelling which is palpable and lies in front of the patella. It is often associated with kneeling (hence the lay term housemaid's or clergyman's knee.). Nowadays it is more often seen in tradesmen who kneel as part of their occupation, particularly carpet fitters.

Treatment

- Aspiration of the bursa. If infection appears to be present steroid injection must be deferred and antibiotic treatment instituted.
- Bursitis may recur and can be reduced by injection of corticosteroid into the bursa.

Chondromalacia patellae

Knee pain is common in teenagers and young adults. There are a number of possible causes which appear to be related to the degree of patellar maltracking. Knee pain which occurs on climbing or descending stairs in young ♀ is suggestive of chondromalacia patellae. This is thought to be more common in ♀ because of the wider pelvis and greater 'Q angle' between the femur and the tibia. The resulting biomechanical forces cause the patella to track towards the medial side of the intercondylar groove of the femur. The cartilage on the posterior surface of the patella becomes degenerate and roughened.

Treatment

Physiotherapy, particularly focusing on strengthening of the Vastus medialus oblique muscle to a greater medial pull on the patella during movement. Taping techniques may also be used to encourage medial tracking of the patella, and may offer some pain relief particularly during sporting activities.

Patellar tendonitis

Commonly seen in sports that involve kicking (e.g. football). The knee on the dominant side is most often affected. There is anterior knee pain localized below the patella, and the lower pole of the patella is tender. Crepitus may be palpable over the tendon.

Treatment

Rest, compression, ice, and anti-inflammatory drugs are the treatment of choice. Occasionally local corticosteroid injection may be considered.

Osgood–Schlatter disease

The pathological term given to this is a 'traction apophysitis or periostitis'. It is seen in teenage ♂ and is related to kicking sports (e.g.rugby and football). The infra patellar tendon attaches to the tibia at the tibial tubercle. Trauma and separation may occur at this point particularly if excessive strains are applied to the area before complete fusion of the epiphysis. Attempted healing occurs through bony reaction and overgrowth at the site of injury resulting in the appearance of a tender, firm, bony mass at the tibial tubercle.

Treatment

Advise rest. Pain often resolves as the patient gets older but the unsightly lump often remains. X-rays are rarely of value except to exclude rare diagnosis such as osteosarcoma of the tibia. Surgical intervention may help in some cases.

Ankle problems

Ankle and foot problems often occur in conjunction with knee, hip, and back pain, and may contribute to such symptoms; therefore when undertaking an assessment consider ankle problems consider the contributing MSC (e.g. inflammatory joint disease or OA). Examples of ankle problems outlined in this section include:

- Achilles tendonitis and retro calcaneal bursitis.
- Tarsal tunnel syndrome.
- Ankle ligament strains.

📖 Also see Walk-in clinics, Chapter 6, p.186, 208, 210; 📖 Inflammatory or Osteoarthritis, Chapter 3, p.54 or Chapter 2, p.10.

Achilles tendonitis

Tendonitis of the Achilles tendon is often related to overuse, particularly in the presence of poorly cushioned footwear. It presents as a localized tender swelling over the tendon. Pain is felt on dorsiflexion of the ankle or where plantar flexion is attempted against resistance as in the propulsion element of the stance phase of normal gait. Degeneration within the tendon occurs as a result of tendonitis and may predispose to tendon rupture.

Treatment

Corticosteroid injection alongside the tendon may improve symptoms, but can increase the risk of tendon rupture (injection should never be directly into the tendon). Advise the patient to rest the limb for 48 hours and avoid strenuous activity for 2 weeks following injection. Following resolution of symptoms an irregular swelling may remain over the tendon which may never resolve.

Occasionally pain and swelling may occur at the insertion of the Achilles tendon into the os calcis resulting in formation of a painful bony lump at the insertion site. Similar to Osgood–Schlatter disease as it is a traction apophysitis of the tendon insertion and may be referred to as Sever's disease. The symptoms may eventually resolve spontaneously but a bony lump may remain on the os calcis which may interfere with the wearing of normal footwear.

Retro calcaneal bursa

The retro calcaneal bursa can be identified on US scanning and lies deep to the tendon on the triangular space bounded by the tendon, the superior surface of the os calcis, and the posterior margin of the tibia. Tenderness in this space may suggest a bursitis which will often respond to local corticosteroid injection.

Tendon rupture presents with sudden severe pain at the back of the heel, may be described as 'being kicked', and may be accompanied by a snapping sound. Complete rupture results in weakness of plantar flexion. The patient cannot rise onto tiptoe on the affected side and limps when walking. A palpable gap is often present in the tendon. With the patient lying prone on a couch, squeezing the calf muscles will cause a degree of plantar flexion at the foot if the tendon is intact, but no movement will be seen in the foot if the tendon is ruptured.

Treatment: surgical repair or immobilizing the foot in partial plantar flexion in a cast.

Partial rupture: in some circumstances the tendon may remain intact but may have a partial tear of the gastrocnemius muscle. This may present in a similar way to tendon rupture but the area of tenderness is more proximal, at the musculo-tendinous junction or in the belly of the muscle. Bruising may be apparent at the site of the rupture and may track distally under gravity to appear as bruising around the ankle joint.

Treatment: acute treatment is with 'RICE' (rest, ice, compression, and elevation). Physiotherapy should be started promptly after these measures to reduce the rare but present risk of myosistis ossificans (calcification occurring within the damaged muscle).

Tarsal tunnel syndrome

This condition is similar to the more frequently diagnosed carpal tunnel syndrome in the wrist. It is an entrapment of the posterior tibial nerve as it passes deep to the flexor retinaculum on the medial aspect of the ankle, behind the medial malleolus. Symptoms are of numbness and burning pain in the sole of the foot, often made worse by standing, and eased by rest and massage. Tinel's test may be positive over the posterior tibial nerve. It may occur as a complication of ankle injury, sprain, or fracture, or in association with inflammatory or OA at the ankle.

Treatment: orthotics and local corticosteroid injection frequently provides benefit.

Foot problems

Ankle and foot problems often occur in conjunction with knee, hip, and back pain, and may contribute to such symptoms. Primary generalized nodal OA will often affect the 1st MTP joint, as will gout. Plantar fasciitis and Achilles tendonitis may occur as part if a sero-negative spondyloarthritis or psoriatic arthropathy. Foot problems include:

• Plantar fasciitis.
• Pes planus (flat feet, fallen arches) pes cavus.
• Metatarsalgia.
• Morton's neuroma.
• Hallux valgus and hallux rigidus.

Plantar fasciitis

This is a common cause of hindfoot pain. The pain is often worse first thing in the morning with the first few steps after getting out of bed. The underlying problem is thought to be excessive traction forces where the plantar fascia inserts into the os calcis. X-rays are often performed but are not recommended as they do not assist in making a diagnosis. A heel spur may be seen on x-ray but this is usually an incidental finding.

Treatment should be conservative and involves addressing biomechanical factors such as excessive weight, and correction of ankle and midfoot pronation with arch supports. Well cushioned footwear should be encouraged, with a low heel and broad forefoot, and secure means of fastening such as laces or Velcro straps (trainers are often ideal). Referral to podiatry may assist in obtaining the best footwear advice. Exercises to stretch the Achilles tendon and the plantar fascia are encouraged. PTs may sometimes employ taping techniques in an attempt to offload the fascia. Local corticosteroid injection into the heel can be considered if conservative measures fail, but it is a painful procedure, and carries a risk of atrophy of the heel fat pad which probably has some shock absorbing function and may predispose to recurrence of symptoms.

Pes planus and pes cavus

Flat feet and high-arch feet are probably variations of normal anatomy and rarely require intervention if they do not cause pain. Flat footedness is particularly common in children. The arch should be restored when the patient is asked to stand on tip toe. Treatment is usually with arch supports and exercises to try to encourage strengthening of the intrinsic muscles of the foot, such as picking up a pencil off the floor with the toes.

Pes cavus (high arch) may arise as a complication of neurological conditions such as polio or spina bifida, but is often idiopathic. It is rarely of significant importance but may lead to clawing of the toes and premature OA of the metatarsal heads or the mid tarsal joint. It can be difficult to obtain appropriate accommodating footwear—podiatry assessment may be helpful in this regard and may be able to slow progression of clawing metatarsal subluxation. Occasionally, orthopaedic intervention may be required to straighten clawing of the toes.

Metatarsalgia

The term metatarsalgia is not a diagnosis but simply descriptive of fore-foot pain. It is commonly due to abnormal pressure on the metatarsal heads when weight bearing. Strain of the intrinsic muscles may contribute to pain, as may inflammation of interdigital bursae. This may be 2° to a number of other conditions including pes cavus, rheumatoid foot deformities, and OA. Management is with the use of orthotics to offload the fore-foot. Occasionally surgical correction of established foot deformities may be useful.

Morton's neuroma

This is caused by entrapment of the interdigital nerve usually between the 3rd and 4th metatarsal heads. This causes attacks of pain and paraesthesia while walking. On examination the symptoms may be reproduced by 'metatarsal squeeze' and there is often an exquisitely tender area between the 3rd and 4th metatarsals. Treatment is with insoles. Local corticosteroid injection around the neuroma is sometimes helpful. Rarely surgical excision may be considered but is not always curative.

There are other conditions related to OA such as hallux valgus and hallux rigidus.

📖 Also see Osteoarthritis, p.7

Primary care: common musculoskeletal problems

Musculoskeletal episodic history taking

Musculoskeletal problems are frequently seen in walk-in 1° healthcare settings. Those presenting musculoskeletal problems can typically be placed into two diagnostic categories:

- Acute minor injuries.
- Acute inflammatory problems including 'overuse' conditions.

A fundamental activity for nurses assessing patients with musculoskeletal problems in 1° healthcare settings is to determine the exact nature of a patient's presenting problem(s) and a detailed history, together with identification of the areas affected. It may not be clear from a patient's opening statement if they have:

- Sustained an injury.
- Have an inflammatory overuse problem or symptoms relate to an exacerbation of a long-term MSC.

Further diagnostic musculoskeletal questions should include:

- The nature of the pain—exacerbating or relieving factors (e.g. does the pain ↑ on movement or not?)
- History of previous musculoskeletal problems of the affected area.
- The patient's use of any over-the-counter or prescription-only oral or topical analgesia and its perceived effect on their presenting problem.
- Any associated neurological symptoms, such as muscle weakness and paraesthesia in the both the affected joint and the area distal to the site of inflammation or injury.

All of the above history enquiries should be considered in conjunction with background history questions such as past medical history, drug history, allergies, social history, and where relevant, family history.

The nurse should then identify:

Has the patient sustained an injury?

Ask the patient to specify exactly where the affected area is and if they can recall any recent history of trauma or do they have any underlying conditions?

- Patients presenting with acute musculoskeletal pain may often say that they have a history of trauma, as they attribute pain to injury even when there is no clear history of trauma. If injury reported, ascertain the exact mechanism of injury and length of time since reported injury.
- If a patient reports a history of trauma the exact mechanism of injury should be ascertained together with the time that has elapsed since the reported injury.
- Determine if they have been able to carry on activities immediately post-injury; e.g. was the patient able to weight-bear on the injured side, and have they been able to continue to do so?

Do they have an inflammatory overuse problem?

If on direct questioning the patient reports a history of musculoskeletal-type pain with no actual history of trauma it is important to establish the cause. It is likely that this is an acute inflammatory condition which has occurred as a result of overuse—consider whether there is evidence to suggest
- ↑ exercise patterns or repetitive exercise movements.

▶ Take into account the potential impact on function, e.g. hand dominance in upper limb and hand problems may affect:
- Work or personal ADL or
- Impair leisure and sporting pursuits.

Features attributed to a LTC?

Patients may not naturally attribute the presenting problems to their condition, e.g. a recently diagnosed patient with RA may fail to realize that a hot swollen ankle is related to their RA if their clinical features of RA to date have only affected their hands.
- Ask about other medical conditions—they may require specialist advice on musculoskeletal-related complications.
- Explore any acquiescent problems that may relate to the current condition, e.g. a prior history of gout or pseudogout.
- Review any patient-held records or blood monitoring cards.
- If a LTC can be excluded from diagnosis continue with diagnostic assessment.

Primary care: musculoskeletal physical assessment

A clear, accurate history and a thorough physical examination will determine the nature of the patient's presenting problem. The examination sequence outlined should be used particularly for those with limited experience in musculoskeletal examination.

▶ **Specific tests**

These are confined to those that have practical application and can be relatively easily interpreted in a non-specialist setting.

General inspection

Begins as soon as you meet and greet the patient, before they realize that they are being clinically observed, e.g.:
• How does the patient get up from their chair? Do they need help?
• What is their gait like?
• Do they appear in any distress? Immediate distress *may* give an indication of the severity of the presenting problem.
• Can they weight-bear unaided? If there is lower limb musculoskeletal pain patients may report inability to weight bear but unobtrusive inspection may reveal reported 'unable to weight-bear' as meaning 'unable to weight-bear without pain'.

▶ A key observation: in patients with a clear history of a recent leg/ankle/foot injury an observed inability to weight-bear indicates a high index of suspicion for a possible bony injury.

Specific inspection

Specific inspection of the musculoskeletal dysfunction (e.g. painful joint or restricted movement) should always include comparisons with the unaffected side.

▶ Ensure adequate exposure of the affected area and comparative sites, e.g.:
• The shoulder—the patient should remove their upper body clothing to underwear.
• The knee—the patient should remove their trousers/skirt to underwear.

Observe the affected area for:
• Skin redness/swelling/lumps/previous surgical/wound scars.
• Muscle wasting/ anatomical deformity/overlying skin lesions/rashes (e.g. a dermatome distribution of vesicles, would indicate herpes zoster as the cause of pain).
• The integrity of the skin and any associated wounds post-trauma.
• Compare of observations with the unaffected side.

Palpation

Palpation of the affected area include examining any areas for tenderness, overlying skin temperature—e.g. hot to touch, unusual lumps or swelling, loss of muscle bulk, and any bone or tendon crepitus (a palpable vibration).

▶ In a person presenting with a musculoskeletal injury a key concept to understand and detect in palpation is the difference between bony/point tenderness and diffuse tenderness (Box 6.4).

After a musculoskeletal injury the presence of bony/point tenderness may indicate a possible bone fracture requiring x-ray investigation, whilst diffuse tenderness typically indicates soft tissue inflammation such as a ligament sprain or muscle strain.

▶ **Box 6.4 Discriminating bony/point vs. diffuse tenderness**

- Bony tenderness refers to an exquisite, sharp pain elicited on palpating on an area of bony injury. Point tenderness refers to a similar pain, but one occurring only in a discreet part of the affected area.
- In contrast diffuse tenderness refers to a generalized tenderness of the affected area on palpation, without the exquisite pain seen in bony/point tenderness.

Movement

Include range of active movement (ROAM) of the affected joint compared against the unaffected side. Examine to assess:
- Is the ROAM normal? E.g. smooth, pain-free, and equal on both sides.
- Observe for the perceived degree of pain occurring on joint movement.
- Note anatomical location of any pain on movement, and any restriction of movement in comparison with the unaffected side.
- If discrepancies identified in active movement between the affected and unaffected sides, check passive movements of the affected side to identify any loss of function and compare with the normal ROAM.
- Resistance movements may also be checked to assess the quality and strength of muscles between the affected and unaffected sides and any signs of weakness.

▶ Remember that:
- A definitive diagnosis does not need to be established at an initial consultation; instead aim for a more general impression of the problem.
- Focus on an assessment of the severity of the patient's problem, and consider the practical implications of what you can do with the patient in your consulting room, such as:
  - Can they be discharged from the clinic or is there is a clinical indication for onward referral, such as a possible fracture?
  - Remember, vital signs may be required in some instances to help exclude other presenting problems—e.g. temperature recording in patients with neck pain to exclude an infective illness as the cause of the neck pain.

▶ Key features of 1° healthcare musculoskeletal physical assessment:
- Inspection of the patient and the affected area(s).
- Compare against the unaffected limb/joint.
- Absence /presence of warmth, tenderness, or swelling in the joint.
- Palpation of the affected area(s).
- Check range of movement of the affected area, including active, passive, and resistance movements as required.
- Selected special tests of affected joints to assess musculoskeletal function.

Primary care: assessment of neck problems

Introduction

Neck pain is a common non-specific symptom which can be attributed to a wide range of possible differential diagnoses, many of which are not musculoskeletal. The patient may find difficulty in specifically locating neck pain and hence may report that they have neck pain when in fact they have shoulder pain and vice versa; the exact location of the pain can be verified on examination.

Neck history

Neck pain history should include questions that exclude other conditions that require immediate assessment in Accident and Emergency (A&E), e.g.:
- Has there been any recent history of neck or head trauma?
- Do they have any symptoms suggestive of meningitis, e.g. neck stiffness and/or by photophobia?
- Do they have any cardiac symptoms e.g. chest pain?

More general questions to explore the nature of the problem include:
- How does the person feel otherwise?
- Have they had any recent viral illness-type symptoms?
- Do they have any ENT symptoms?
- Have they had a recent fever?
- Do they have a headache?
- Do they have any persisting neck stiffness in association with the above symptoms?

⚠ *Neck injury:* in patients with any history of significant neck trauma or associated cervical spine tenderness (on palpation) the neck should be immobilized with a stiff neck collar (if available) and transferred by ambulance to A&E to exclude a possible cervical spine fracture.

Neck examination

- Inspection:
  - Ensure adequate exposure of the neck and upper back.
  - The head should be held erect and the neck straight.
  - Inspect the neck from all aspects—anterior, posterior, and lateral.
  - Note any obvious swellings, surgical scars, skin lesions, or rashes.
  - Ask patient to indicate area of pain.
- Palpation:
  - Palpate individual spinous processes of cervical spine to C7/T1 junction.
  - Palpate paravertebral muscles on both sides, and trapezius, and sternomastoid muscles, noting any areas of tenderness, muscle spasm, asymmetry, or swelling.
- Movement:
  - Observe active range of movement of cervical spine.
  - Flexion—bending forward.

- Extension—bending backwards.
- Lateral bending/flexion—bending to each side.
- Rotation—looking over each shoulder.
- Also check resistance movement strength controlled by cranial nerve XI—spinal accessory.
- Turning face against resistance—sternomastoid.
- Shrug against resistance—trapezius.
- Neurological:
  - Check upper limb muscle strengths.
  - Test arm reflexes—triceps, biceps, and supinator.
  - Check the integrity of the distal sensations.

Presenting problems of neck pain

Torticollis

This is a common neck problem. Typically:
- The patient wakes with a stiff, painful neck, due to spasm on one side of the neck of the trapezius or sternomastoid muscles.
- May be precipitated by poor body posture or carrying heavy loads on one side of the body.
- Examination reveals the neck held in either right or left lateral flexion, diffuse tenderness and muscle spasm on the affected side, and painful restricted neck movements.
- Neurological examination is typically normal.

Treatment

Simple analgesia (ideally NSAIDs if not contraindicated) and temporary rest from strenuous activities affecting the neck. Encourage maintenance of normal everyday activities. Persistent or recurrent episodes of torticollis may benefit from a referral to a PT assessment and treatment.

Whiplash neck injury

The common presentation typically follows a RTA where:
- Sudden hyperextension of the neck muscles and ligaments has occurred.
- Within 1–2 days of an accident patient complains of neck pain, muscle stiffness, and tenderness.
- Examination of the neck should include the neurological issues as outlined in torticollis or factors that might indicate a need for radiological assessment in A&E.

Where there is no cervical spine bony tenderness or associated neurological impairment, treatment should be as for torticullis plus referral for PT assessment (dependent on local referral guidelines).

Also see Neck and spine, Chapter 6, p.212, 214; Assessing the patient, Chapter 8, p.271; Symptom control: pharmacological and non-pharmacological, Chapter 9, p.289.

Primary care: assessment of common presenting problems—the back

Back problems

Back pain is a common presenting problem in 1° healthcare, both as an acute and a long-term problem. Acute low back pain is often due to:
- Indirect trauma, such as lifting heavy loads.
- Awkward body movements or
- Exercise activities.

▶ In cases of potential direct trauma to the back such as falls or blows to the body any vertebral bony tenderness necessitates referral to A&E.

▶ In cases of thoracic back pain, remember that this may be posterior chest pain and not back pain. Potential organ involvement presenting with posterior chest pain include cardiac, pulmonary, or respiratory conditions must be excluded before focusing the assessment on musculoskeletal back pain. Consider contributing factors that may exacerbate or predicate/prolong back symptoms such as anxiety and depression; these psychological factors should be considered in assessment of patients with back pain.

Back history

Start the clinical questioning and history taking to exclude other causes of back pain such as:
- Genito-urinary, abdominal or chest pathology.
- In patients aged >55 years consider an abdominal aortic aneurysm as a possible cause of back pain; typically this pain is constant and unaffected by movement. A suspected aneurysm requires immediate assessment in A&E.
- Unintended weight loss in patients with back pain of a duration >4 weeks may indicate an underlying oncological cause.
- Sharp nerve-like pains radiating from the lower back down one or both legs as this may indicate nerve root pain or sciatic nerve irritation.

⚠ Spinal cord compression: this is a red flag not to be missed in patients with back pain accompanied by one or more of the following symptoms:
- Disturbance or loss of urinary or stool continence.
- Perineal numbness (saddle anaesthesia).
- Lower limb weakness and/or numbness.

Differential diagnoses should consider those with solid cancer tumours or metastatic spread to the bones—a frequent cause of cord compression.

▶ Consider the high risks related to cancer history + back pain.
▶▶ Back pain + symptoms of cord compression = immediate referral to orthopaedics/neurosurgery or oncology as indicated by their history.

Back examination
- Inspection:
  - Observe the patient's gait.
  - Ensure adequate exposure—view back from all aspects.
  - Look for rashes, lesions, curvature, deformity, and asymmetry.

- Observe the spine bending forward, normal observation is a 'c'-shaped spinal curvature.
- Observe iliac crest height, asymmetry may indicate pelvic tilt or unequal leg lengths.
- Note any obvious swellings, surgical scars, skin lesions, or rashes.
- Ask the patient to indicate area of pain.
- Palpation:
  - Palpate spinous processes from T1 to S2 and paravertebral muscles on each side.
  - Note areas and levels of tenderness.
  - Check for kidney/costo-vertebral angle tenderness on indirect percussion to exclude renal parenchyma inflammation.
- Movement:
  - Observe active range of movement of back.
  - May need to stabilize pelvis by grasping the hips from behind the patient.
  - Flexion—bending forward; extension—bending backwards.
  - Lateral bending/flexion—bending to each side.
  - Rotation—looking over each shoulder.
- Neurological:
  - Check lower limb and ankle muscle strengths.
  - Test lower limb reflexes—knee, ankle, and plantar.
  - Check the integrity of the distal sensations.
- Clinic investigations:
  - Dipstick urine analysis should be considered in order to exclude genito-urinary problems as a cause of back pain.
  - Back x-rays, whilst often requested by patients with back pain, are unnecessary in the majority of patients.

▶ **Back special test—straight leg raising (SLR) test:**

This is a test for nerve root irritation caused by a herniated vertebral disc. This test is especially important in low back pain with accompanying pain radiating down the leg.

- Patient in supine position.
- Examiner *passively* raises patient's straight leg up in the air to the point at which low back pain occurs.
- With the leg still raised, dorsiflex the foot.
- Repeat and compare sides.

▶ It is normal for slight lower back pain and stretching of hamtrings to occur during this test. A positive SLR test occurs with reproduction of sharp back pain extending down the leg. With the affected leg lowered beyond the point of pain, passive dorsiflexion of the foot normally reinforces the pain.

📖 Also see Neck and spine, Chapter 6, pp.212, 214; 📖 Assessing the patient, Chapter 8, p.271; 📖 Symptom control: pharmacological and non-pharmacological, Chapter 9, p.289.

Primary care: assessment of common presenting problems—treatment plans for the back

Back pain presenting problems

Low back pain (simple backache)

This the most common cause of lumbar back pain. The patient presents with a history of low back pain, sometimes associated with heavy lifting or exercise, which worsens on movement.

Examination reveals:

On palpation: localized lumbar spine tenderness with painful, restricted back movements. Neurological examination is typically normal.

Treatment plan

Low back pain can normally be adequately treated with information, reassurance, simple analgesia (NSAIDs may be considered if not contraindicated), and temporary abstinence from strenuous activities affecting the back, whilst attempting to maintain normal everyday activities.

If persistent or recurrent episodes of simple low back pain, consider referral for PT assessment and treatment.

Back pain with associated nerve root pain

This commonly presents as 'sciatica' where the patient complains of a sharp pain radiating from the low back or buttock and down the posterior aspect of the leg of the affected side (often sharp leg pain is perceived as more severe than the accompanying back pain).

Examination reveals:

Commonly the same as for low back pain + SLR test may reproduce the sharp leg pain.

Treatment plan: as for low back pain + urgent referral to PT (dependent on local referral guidelines).

▶ If lower limb neurological examination reveals accompanying paraesthesia, and/or muscle weakness, or altered reflexes on the affected side, further assessment in A&E should be considered

📖 Also see Neck and spine, Chapter 6, p.212, 214; 📖 Assessing the patient, Chapter 8, p.271; 📖 Symptom control: pharmacological and non-pharmacological, Chapter 9, p.289.

Further reading

Hakım A, Clunie G, Haq I (eds) (2006). *Oxford Handbook of Rheumatology*, 2nd edn. Oxford University Press, Oxford.

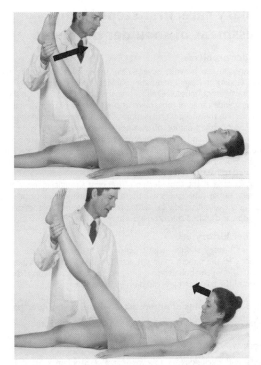

Fig. 6.5 Back examination. Reproduced with permission from Hutson M, Ellis R (2005). *Textbook of Musculoskeletal Medicine*. Oxford University Press, Oxford.

Primary care: first steps in the assessment of shoulder problems

Shoulder problems

Shoulder pain can provoke severe pain, in many cases with limitations in ADL leading to heightened patient anxiety. Shoulder pain may be as a result of other non-musculoskeletal presentations (Box 6.5). The shoulder joint has a wide range of movement at the expense of relative stability, as can be seen in the shallow articulation of the humeral head in the glenoid cavity. The complex nature of the shoulder joint anatomy is dependent upon the integrity and stability of the joint including tendons and muscles of the surrounding rotator cuff (supraspinatus, infraspinatus, teres minor, and subscapularis); hence many shoulder problems seen in 1° healthcare are related to rotator cuff pathology.

Another area at the shoulder tip of frequent shoulder complaints is at the region of the subacromium. If there is inflammation, injury, or swelling rapidly at this site it rapidly presents problems due the anatomical design of the joint and limited subacromium space.

Shoulder history

A precise history should include potential causes of the pain and any limitations to the patient's current activities. They may be unable to differentiate between shoulder pain and neck pain and vice versa; the exact location of the pain can be verified on examination.

Box 6.5 Examples of non-musculoskeletal shoulder pain

Include: ischaemia, pulmonary, and abdominal or pelvic pathologies (e.g. cardiac pain, gallbladder diseases, pulmonary embolism, and ectopic pregnancy).

Assess and exclude/refer following careful problem-focused history taking in patients presenting with non-traumatic shoulder pain.

Shoulder examination

- Inspection:
  - Both shoulders and the upper chest should be exposed.
  - Inspect neck and compare both shoulders.
  - Ask patient to point to the area of pain.
  - Observe the shoulders for shape, symmetry, swelling, deformity, angulations (commonly occurs with shoulder dislocation), skin redness, muscle wasting, scars, and any skin lesions such as vesicles (occur in herpes zoster).
- Palpation: the surface anatomy of the shoulder can be used to provide a systematic approach to shoulder palpation. Carefully palpate the following bony anatomical areas:
  - Cervical spine—if indicated by the history.
  - Suprasternal notch.
  - Sternoclavicular joint/clavicle.

- Coracoid process.
- Acromion/acromioclavicular joint.
- Tuberosities of humerus/humerus.
- Bicipital groove.
- Scapula.

This bony palpation should then be followed by palpation of the following muscular areas:
- Sternomastoid (neck) and trapezius (neck).
- Pectoralis major (anterior chest).
- Biceps (anterior humerus) and deltoid (lateral humerus).
- Triceps (posterior humerus).
- Coracobrachialis (axilla/medial humerus).
- Lattissimus dorsi (posterior chest).
- *Rotator cuff muscles:* supraspinatus, infraspinatus, teres minor, and subscapularis.

Examination must also include assessment of the distal neurological status of the arms and hands. This is achieved by checking the integrity of the axillary nerve at the lateral mid-humerus (badge sign) and the ulnar, median, and radial nerves in their distal distribution of the hand.
- Movement: check neck movements first (if indicated from the history), followed by these active shoulder movements:
  - Flexion (forward movement) and extension (backward movement).
  - Abduction (away from midline) and lateral (external) rotation (arm tucked into chest with elbow flexed, rotating movement away from midline).
  - Medial (internal) rotation (arm tucked into chest with elbow flexed, rotating movement towards midline).
- The following compound shoulder movements can also be checked:
  - Hand touched to back of head (external rotation with abduction).
  - Hand touched to middle of back (internal rotation with adduction).

These first steps can be supported by some simple performed tests for the non-specialist (📕 see Primary care: specific tests for shoulder problems, Chapter 6, p.220).

📕 Also see 📕 Chronic non-inflammatory pain, Chapter 6, p.172; 📕 Assessing the patient, Chapter 8, p.271; 📕 Symptom control: pharmacological and non-pharmacological, Chapter 9, p.289.

Further reading

Hakim A, Clunie G, Haq I (eds) (2006). *Oxford Handbook of Rheumatology*, 2nd edn. Oxford University Press, Oxford.

Primary care: specific tests for shoulder problems

There are a wide range of tests for shoulder function and associated anatomical structures. In many cases these tests are for the specialist assessment of shoulder problems. The following tests are simple to perform and interpret, and are usually sufficient to assess shoulder function and the associated anatomical structures. Referral may be necessary for more complex shoulder problems.

• *Anterior and posterior drawer test.* Stabilize shoulder from behind, applying a downward pressure, and then move glenohumeral joint backwards and forwards to assess anterior or posterior instability. Compare with unaffected side looking for joint laxity in comparison with unaffected side, which would indicate anterior or posterior instability.

• *Sulcus sign.* Stabilize shoulder from the front and pull down on the patient's arm to assess inferior instability. Compare with the unaffected side, looking for a dip (sulcus) appearing below the lateral acromion, which would indicate inferior instability.

• *Active abduction test (painful arc).* Ask the patient to abduct their shoulder. Pain occuring between 70–140° may indicate a subacromial space problem. Pain occuring between 140–180° may indicate an acromioclavicular joint problem (Fig. 6.6).

• *Passive abduction test.* Passively abduct the patient's shoulder. Pain occurring around the acromium may indicate subacromial bursitis.

• *Resisted abduction test.* Ask the patient to abduct their arm whilst you apply an opposing force. Compare with unaffected side. Pain occuring in the superior aspect of the shoulder may indicate supraspinatus tendinitis. Weakness on resistance may indicate a possible rotator cuff tear (supraspinatus).

• *Resisted lateral rotation test.* Ask patient to flex their elbow and press their upper arm into their lateral chest wall, and to move their forearm laterally. Apply an opposing medial force. Pain in the posterior aspect of the shoulder may indicate infraspinatus or teres minor tendinitis. Weakness on resistance may indicate a possible rotator cuff tear (infraspinatus or teres minor).

• *Resisted medial rotation test.* Ask patient to flex their elbow and press their upper arm into their lateral chest wall, and to move their forearm medially. Apply an opposing lateral force. Compare with the unaffected side. Pain in the anterior aspect of the shoulder may indicate subscapularis tendinitis. Weakness on resistance may indicate a possible rotator cuff tear (subscapularis).

📖 Also see Chronic non-inflammatory pain, Chapter 6, p.172.

Further reading

Hakim A, Clunie G, Haq I (eds) (2006). *Oxford Handbook of Rheumatology*, 2nd edn. Oxford University Press, Oxford.

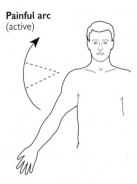

Painful arc
(active)

Action: Patient standing.
Slow arm abduction
(scapular plane).

Positive test: Pain onset (maximal)
at (variable) angular
range.

Fig. 6.6 Painful arc. Reproduced with permission from Hakim A, Clunie G, Haq I (eds) (2006). *Oxford Handbook of Rheumatology*, 2nd edn. Oxford University Press, Oxford.

Primary care: shoulder pain

The most common shoulder problems presenting in 1° care are outlined in this section.

The comprehensive assessment of shoulder problems

- **Supraspinatus tendonitis:** a common problem related to over use, particularly over arm movements (e.g. tasks undertaken by a painter/decorator). Examination reveals localized tenderness over superior aspect of shoulder, painful active abduction 70–140° and painful resisted abduction. Usually resolves after a few days; supportive measures include simple analgesia (NSAIDs if not contraindicated), and temporary rest from the strenuous activity affecting the shoulder.

- **Subacromial bursitis:** history as for supraspinatus, but no pain on resisted abduction, as no muscle or tendon involvement; instead pain occurs on passive abduction as the subacromial space becomes compressed. Tenderness and a soft swelling may be noted at the humeral head. May be related to an inflammatory component (e.g. RA). Supportive measures include simple analgesia (NSAIDs if not contraindicated), and temporary rest from the strenuous activity affecting the shoulder. Some patients with a persisting inflammatory component may benefit from IA corticosteroid injection if not contraindicated.

- **Biceps tendonitis:** often caused by repeated lifting movements, presents with anterior humeral and shoulder pain, tenderness over biceps tendon, and resisted elbow flexion is painful. Rupture of the long head of the biceps may also occur, and presents with pain on lifting and sensation of 'something going' accompanied by palpable lump within the tendon. *Treatment:* temporary rest from lifting and simple analgesia (NSAIDs if not contraindicated).

- **Rotator cuff tear (non-traumatic):** this may be due to fibrosis, tendonitis, or bone spurs. Often >50 years old, presenting with pain and weakness on abduction, may not be able to actively abduct or hold abduction at 90°. Orthopaedic assessment required.

- **Joint instability:** in patients <40 years glenohumeral instability may be seen with a history of recurrent subluxations or dislocations. Older patients (>40 years) may have feelings of shoulder joint instability, accompanied by shoulder pains and clicks; this is often related to long-term rotator cuff problems. Orthopaedic assessment required.

- **Frozen shoulder (adhesive capsulitis):** this long-term condition is more common in ♀, diabetics, and people aged 40–60 years old. Presents with shoulder pain (occasionally debilitating) and limitation in movement, accompanied by diffuse joint tenderness. Compound external/internal rotation movements are painful and restricted which causes difficulty with everyday activities such as dressing and grooming. Initial treatment includes simple analgesia (NSAIDs if not contraindicated), PT, and sometimes local steroid injection. Natural course of the condition is usually about 18 months when it usually resolves spontaneously.

Shoulder injury presenting problems

- *Acromioclavicular joint (ACJ) injury:* fall onto shoulder, elbow, outstretched hand, or a blow to the shoulder tip may cause ACJ injury, ranging from a sprain of the ACJ ligament to disruption of joint. The patient presents with superior shoulder pain and painful decreased shoulder movements, particularly noted on abduction. A bulge or step may be noted in the ACJ articulation. Refer to A&E or Minor Injures Unit for x-ray and further management.
- *Rotator cuff tear:* severe blow or fall on outstretched hand, tenderness may be noted around acromium, active and resistance abduction will be reduced or absent. A complete rotator cuff tear may not be painful, though a lack of active shoulder movement will be evident. Orthopaedic assessment needed.
- *Traumatic effusion:* typically occurs in patients >50 years old, falling onto arm/shoulder, which leads to bleeding/effusion in glenohumeral joint. This is often a delayed presentation with pain and restricted shoulder movement affecting everyday activities such as dressing. Proximal humeral tenderness is noted on palpation due to accompanying humeral fracture. Refer to A&E or Minor Injuries Unit for x-ray and further management.
- *Shoulder dislocation:* this is a relatively common shoulder injury, which normally occurs after falling on the arm or shoulder, or if the arm is pulled sharply. Anterior dislocation of the humeral head is more common than posterior dislocation. The patient appears in discomfort, clasping the affected arm against the body, with a flattening of the anterior outer edge of the shoulder evident. Make the patient comfortable and arrange for immediate transfer to A&E for x-ray and reduction of the dislocation.
- *Clavicular fracture:* this typically occurs after a fall on the outstretched hand. The patient complains of pain and swelling of the injured clavicle, and examination reveals a bony step in the fractured clavicle with associated tenderness and sometimes bony crepitus. X-ray in A&E or Minor Injuries Unit is required to confirm the clinical diagnosis and for fracture clinic review. Most fractures of the clavicle can be successfully managed with a broad arm sling and simple analgesia.

Note: LTCs such as IJDs may present with shoulder problems such as subacromium bursitis as a result of: juvenile arthritis, gout or pseudo-gout, RA, PsA, and AS.

📖 Also see Chronic non-inflammatory pain, Chapter 6, p.172.

Further reading

Hakim A, Clunie G, Haq I (eds) (2006). *Oxford Handbook of Rheumatology*, 2nd edn. Oxford University Press, Oxford.

Primary care: musculoskeletal chest pain

Common causes of musculoskeletal chest wall pain are intercostal muscle sprain caused by minor chest wall trauma; intercostal muscle inflammation caused by repeated coughing; and pain at the sternal junctions caused by inflammation of the costal cartilages.

Chest history

Patients with musculoskeletal chest wall pain typically complain of an intermittent sharp pain which worsens on coughing or sneezing, inspiration, and movement. It is important to ask about the use of simple analgesia as many will have taken minimal analgesia believing such treatment will produce little benefit and are anxious that the pain is cardiac in nature even when they are young and have no risk factors for cardiac chest pain. Careful reassurance, once cardiac problems have been excluded, will help alleviate this anxiety.

⚠ Chest pain of musculoskeletal origin should only be considered as a differential diagnosis when other, more serious causes of chest pain have been excluded, such as cardiac and respiratory or pulmonary problems, with careful problem-focused history taking, including potential red flags, such as: cardiac-type pain, haemoptysis, dysponea, and fever.

⚠ In patients presenting shortly after a potentially significant history of chest trauma, the risk of associated hepatic and splenic trauma should be considered.

Chest examination

- Inspection:
  - Ask the patient to indicate the area of their perceived pain.
  - Note shape of chest and tracheal alignment in the midline.
  - Observe for any deformities or asymmetry of the chest wall.
  - Respiratory pattern—rate, rhythm, depth, effort.
  - Use of neck and chest accessory muscles or intercostal muscle space retraction.
  - Impaired or unequal respiratory movements.
  - Bruising or other traumatic marks on the chest wall.
  - A dermatome distribution of vesicles would indicate herpes zoster as the cause of the chest wall pain.
- Palpation:
  - Palpate ribs, sternal junctions, and intercostal spaces.
  - Palpate anterior and posterior in turn—remember lateral chest walls.
  - Identify areas of tenderness, particularly noting any areas of bony tenderness or bone crepitus, which could indicate a potential rib fracture.

- The sternum can be compressed with 1 hand on the sternum and the other on the spine; in cases of musculoskeletal chest wall pain, particularly rib fractures, a sharp pain will noted at the point of inflammation or injury.

▶ *Respiratory and cardiac examination*
- In patients presenting with musculoskeletal chest wall pain, vital signs (blood pressure, pulse, respiratory rate, temperature, oxygen saturations) should always be recorded and interpreted.
- A chest respiratory examination should be undertaken to exclude respiratory pathology, such as a pleural rub or a respiratory tract infection
- The precordium should be auscultated to exclude abnormal heart sounds such as a pericardial friction rub.
- *Abdominal examination* should also be considered in patients presenting with chest injuries, in order to exclude any associated liver and spleen trauma.

Treatment for musculoskeletal chest wall pain

- Chest x-rays are usually unhelpful in minor chest wall trauma and would not significantly alter treatment plans even if a rib fracture is identified on x-ray. However, the decision must be made based upon the individual assessment of need and whether clinical signs may warrant a chest x-ray.
- Regular simple analgesia (NSAIDs if not contraindicated) is the mainstay of treatment; patients may be reluctant to take such analgesia, but should be gently encouraged to do so, as an effective reduction in pain symptom severity is often seen.
- The patient should be warned that the chest pain may persist, to some degree, for 4–6 weeks after its initial occurrence. Accordingly, strenuous activities affecting the chest, such as lifting, should be avoided during this time period.
- Respiratory movement may be reduced when the patient is in pain, so daily deep breathing exercises should also be recommended, in order to reduce the risk of a respiratory tract infection occurring.

📖 Also see Respiratory investigations, Chapter 17, p.476 and Chapter 13, p.388; 📖 Respiratory complications, Chapter 17, pp.476, 478 and Chapter 12, p.388.

Primary care: elbow problems

The synovial hinge joint of the elbow is a common site of musculoskeletal inflammation. In relation to injuries, the elbow joint is prone to subluxation, dislocation, and fracture due to its relatively superficial overlying soft tissues.

Elbow history

In adults with inflammatory-type problems any history of elbow joint overuse should be elicited. Elbow fractures/dislocations may occur after a fall on the outstretched hand or with direct injury to the elbow. In young children traction force on the elbow can displace the radial head.

Elbow examination

Inspection

- Observe the elbows for shape, symmetry, swelling, deformity, skin redness, muscle wasting, scars, skin lesions, bruising and any wounds post-trauma.
- A fractured elbow is typically held in a degree of flexion supported by the arm of the unaffected side.

Palpation

- As the overlying soft tissues of the elbow are superficial, most of the joint can be easily palpated.
- Start palpation at the lateral edge of the distal humerus, followed by the lateral epicondyle, the recess between the lateral epicondyle and radial head, the radial head, the medial epicondyle, the ulnar nerve behind the medial epicondyle, the medial edge of the distal humerus, and finally the olecranon process.

Movement

- Flexion and extension.
- Forearm rotation (elbows flexed to 90° and held against the lateral chest walls, patient then supinates and pronates their forearms).
- These movements may also be checked on resistance.

Elbow pain presenting problems

Olecranon bursitis

Inflammation of the burse overlying the olecranon may occur spontaneously or as result of repeated pressure over the olecranon. Presents as an egg-shaped swelling over the elbow tip, which is red, hot, and tender. Pain occurs on elbow movement.

Examine the overlying skin carefully to exclude a potential entry site for bacteria such as an insect bite or a small break in the skin, and any corresponding tiredness or fever; such signs of infection would require oral antibiotics in addition to simple analgesia. Otherwise most simple cases of bursitis can be treated with rest of the affected elbow and regular simple analgesia (ideally an NSAID if not contraindicated). Aspiration of the fluid may introduce infection, and should be reserved for cases of traumatic bursitis, where signs of bleeding are evident. This aspiration should be undertaken in A&E.

Epicondylitis

Describes inflammation of the tendons of the lateral or medial aspects of the elbow as a result of overuse or repeated movements. *Lateral epicondylitis (tennis elbow)* presents with pain and tenderness over the lateral epicondyle and pain over the lateral epicondyle on resisted wrist extension. *Medial epicondylitis (golfer's elbow)* presents with pain and tenderness over the medial epicondyle and pain over the medial epicondyle on resisted wrist flexion. Both problems respond to rest from the causative activity and simple analgesia (NSAIDs if not contraindicated). Persistent or recurrent episodes of epicondylitis benefit from PT assessment and treatment. Advice on reviewing grip size of racquet or golf clubs may be helpful as condition may be exacerbated by the wrong grip size.

Elbow injury presenting problems

- *Fractured radial head:* this is caused by a fall on the outstretched hand or direct injury to the elbow. The patient presents with the affected elbow held in flexion, bony tenderness of the radial head, and painfully reduced elbow extension. Requires referral to A&E or Minor Injuries Unit for x-ray and further management.
- *Fractured olecranon process:* this is typically caused by a fall onto the elbow tip. The patient present with pain, bony tenderness, and swelling over the olecranon process and an inability to straighten the elbow. Requires referral to A&E or Minor Injuries Unit for x-ray and further management.
- *Dislocated elbow:* this painful injury normally occurs after a fall on the outstretched hand. The patient presents in discomfort with a swollen and fixed elbow, most commonly caused by dislocation of the radial head and fracture of the proximal ulna. Requires urgent assessment in A&E.

Primary care: wrist and hand problems

The complexity of the wrist and hands joints must be carefully considered when assessing patients with wrist and hand problems. It is important to have a low threshold for onward referral for expert advice.

Wrist and hand history

The wrist and hand are prone to inflammation or trauma. Consider:
- Any history of overuse or repeated movements should be elicited.
- The patient's occupation may have an impact on the presenting problem.
- Finger, wrist, or hand fractures. Hand fractures typically occur after a punch-type injury, which the patient may initially be reluctant to reveal. Finger fractures usually occur after crush injuries or from forced flexion or extension of the interphalangeal joints. Remember that accompanying wounds in hand and finger injuries may have associated tendon and/or nerve injuries.

Wrist and hand examination

Inspection
- Observe the wrists, hands, and fingers for shape, symmetry, swelling, deformity, skin redness, scars, skin lesions, bruising, and any wounds post-trauma.

Palpation
- *Wrist:* palpate the distal radius, ulna, radial and ulnar styloids, and carpal bones. Pay particular attention to tenderness in the anatomical snuffbox (scaphoid bone). Note any crepitus of the wrist extensor tendons.
- *Hand and fingers:* palpate the metacarpals, the metacarpophalangeal (MCP) joints, the proximal phalanx, interphalengeal joint (IP), and distal phalanx of the thumb and the proximal phalanges, proximal interphalangeal joints (PIPs) middle phalanges, distal interphalangeal joints (DIP), and distal phalanges of the fingers. Palpate the thenar and hypothenar eminence at the base of hands for swelling and tenderness.

Movement
- *Wrist:* check the active range of wrist flexion, extension and radial and ulnar deviation.
- *Hand:* check the active range of thumb abduction, adduction, extension, flexion and opposition. Flexion and extension of the MCP and IP joints should also be checked. Comparative resistance movements of the IPs can be checked to assess extensor and flexor tendon function. Resistance movement testing is particularly important to assess with finger lacerations and forced extension/flexion finger injuries.
- *Neurological:* check the integrity of the ulnar, median, and radial nerves in their distal distribution of the hand.

Wrist and hand pain presenting problems

- **Tenosynovistis (tendonitis):** is relatively common at the wrist in the extensor and flexor tendons. Patients present with wrist pain on movement and slight swelling over the affected tendon, tenderness and crepitus is noted on palpation. This responds well to rest from the causative activity and regular simple analgesia (NSAID if not contraindicated).

Wrist and hand injury presenting problems

- **Colles' fracture:** most often occurs in older people, falling on their outstretched hand. The injury sustained is a displaced fracture of the distal radius and ulnar styloid. The patient presents with pain, swelling and reduced movement of the wrist. Requires urgent further assessment in A&E for x-ray and reduction of the fracture.
- **Scaphoid fracture:** a fracture of this small carpal bone is normally sustained from a fall on the outstretched hand. The patient presents with a painful wrist and ↓ movement. Examination reveals slight swelling and bony tenderness in the anatomical snuffbox (located inferiorly to the distal radius). Requires referral to A&E or Minor Injuries Unit for x-ray, immobilization, and review. Fracture may not be detectable on initial x-ray—repeat x-ray or bone scan 2–3 weeks later. Clinical signs of fracture are sufficient for a diagnosis.
- **Metacarpal fractures:** are associated with a punch injury of the hand, the 5th metacarpal is particularly prone to fracture. The patient presents with swelling, pain, and bony tenderness of the affected metacarpal(s). Requires referral to A&E or Minor Injuries Unit for x-ray, immobilization, and review. If injury is a punch injury, human tooth wounds are sometimes also present; local guidelines on infection prophylaxis and immunization should be consulted.
- **Finger sprains and strains:** the collateral ligaments and muscles of the thumb and finger can be sprained or strained presenting with a swollen finger, pain on movement, and diffuse tenderness. The collateral ligaments should be stressed to identify any excess comparative laxity, which would require hand clinic assessment. Otherwise treat using the neighbouring finger as a support to strap together and use simple analgesia (NSAID if not contraindicated).
- **Finger fractures:** avulsion fractures of the phalanges can occur with either forced hyperextension or forced flexion of an IP joint. The fracture occurs as result of a hyperextended flexor tendon avulsing a small piece of bone on the flexor surface (volar plate injury) or an hyperflexed extensor tendon avulsing a small piece of bone on the extensor surface (mallet finger injury). Fractures of the proximal and middle phalanges can also occur from direct trauma, such as fall (presents with swelling and tenderness of the affected area). Mallet finger injury—a visible droop of the distal phalanx is evident. All injuries require referral to A&E/Minor Injuries Unit for x-ray, immobilization, and fracture or hand clinic review.

Primary care: hip problems

The ball and socket joint of the hip is stable particularly when compared against the shoulder. This is due to the deeper articulation of the head of femur in the acetabulum, the rigid bones of the pelvic girdle, and the stabilizing strong femoral ligaments. In the 1° healthcare clinics, acute inflammation and injuries of the hip are less common presentations. In older people fractures of the neck of femur are common after simple falls.

Hip history

⚠ Non-traumatic acute hip pain should be approached with caution in certain groups of adult patients as it may indicate:
- Hip infection (📖 pp.196, 252, 379).
- Metastatic spread in patients with cancer (solid tumours).
- Avascular necrosis in patients with risk factors such as SLE.
- Abdominal or pelvic pathologies.

Hip examination

Inspection
- The patient should be undressed to underwear.
- Observe the patient standing, noting any leg length discrepancy or asymmetry of the iliac crest heights.
- If possible, observe the patient's gait.
- Note any overlying bruising, wounds, scars, skin lesions, or redness.
- Observe for muscle wasting.
- If a fractured neck of femur is suspected observe the affected leg for shortening and external rotation

Palpation
- Palpate the bony landmarks—iliac crest, iliac tubercules, anterior iliac spines, pubic tubercules, and the greater trochanters.
- Palpate the femoral triangle and inguinal ligament—with the hip externally rotated and abducted.
- The ischial tuberosity may also be palpated with the patient lying on their side or prone.

Movement
- Flexion—bend hip and knee toward chest.
- Extension—returning leg to straight position.
- Abduction—move leg from midline.
- Adduction—move leg back to midline.
- Lateral (external) rotation—roll the extended leg outward.
- Medial (internal) rotation—roll the extended leg inward.

Hip presenting problems
- **Hip muscle strains:** can commonly occur at the adductor longus and magnus (groin tenderness and pain on resisted adduction); gluteus medius (iliac tubercle tenderness and pain on resisted abduction); (iliopsoas (anterior tenderness and pain on resisted flexion); gluteal and biceps femoris (posterior tenderness and pain on resisted extension when prone). These muscle strains respond to rest and simple analgesia (ideally an NSAID if not contraindicated).

- *Hip bursitis:* can occur with overuse in greater trochanter bursa (pain on adduction in lateral hip); iliopsoas bursa (pain on flexion in anterior hip); and the ischial bursa (posterior pain, pain on sitting). Hip bursitis normally responds to rest and simple analgesia (NSAID if not contraindicated). In patients with significant pain soft tissue corticosteroid injection may be considered.
- *Fractured neck of femur:* typically occurs in an older person after a fall. The patient complains of a painful thigh and hip and is unable to weight-bear. With the patient supine shortening and external rotation of the affected leg is evident. Requires immediate ambulance transfer to A&E.

📖 Also see Osteoarthritis of hip and knee, p.14; 📖 Chronic non-inflammatory pain, p.171; 📖 Assessing the patient, p.271; 📖 Symptom control: pharmacological and non-pharmacological, p.289.

Further reading

Hakim A, Clunie G, Haq I (eds) (2006). *Oxford Handbook of Rheumatology*, 2nd edn. Oxford University Press, Oxford.

Primary care: knee problems

The condylar joint of the knee, despite being a significant weight-bearing joint is dependent on its cruciate and collateral ligaments for its stability; hence problems with these ligaments give rise to many knee presenting problems.

Knee history

⚠ If any of the post-knee injury problems noted here or in the examination refer to A&E for further assessment: dislocated patella, inability to weight-bear, inability to flex/extend the knee, a grossly swol-len knee (large effusion), inability to raise leg (SLR), bony tenderness of the patella or head of fibula, any distal neuro-vascular deficit, and any knee injuries in people >55 years old.

Knee examination

Inspection
- Exposure—knees, pelvis, lower legs.
- Inspect and compare.
- Walking, standing, sitting, supine.
- Standing—is pelvis level? Knees symmetrical, anterior/posterior, leg lengths.
- Swelling, erythema, scars/wounds.

Palpation
- Patella/patellar ligament/prepatellar bursae.
- Quadriceps.
- Check for effusion with patellar tap.
- Medial/lateral femoral epicondyles.
- Medial/lateral menisci.
- Medial and collateral ligaments.
- Gastrocnemius area (posterior).

Movement
- Active SLR.
- Flexion.
- Extension.

▶ Knee special tests

As with the shoulder there is a wide array of special tests for assessing knee dysfunction and instability. The following selected special tests are simple to perform and interpret, and are usually sufficient to diagnose specific knee problems.

- **Valgus stress test**: for assessing the integrity of the MCL. Patient supine and test knee in extension and flexed to 15–20°. Push knee medially with 1 hand whilst applying an opposing lateral force at ankle with other hand. Laxity in extension indicates MCL disruption as feel separation of tibia and femur. Flexion stress—isolates MCL, looking for ↑ laxity in comparison with unaffected side.
- **Varus stress test**: this assesses integrity of LCL. Opposite manoeuvre to valgus stress test. Push knee laterally with 1 hand whilst applying an

opposing medial force at ankle with other hand. Again looking for ↑ laxity in comparison with unffected side.

- *Anterior/posterior drawer test*: for ACL, anterior drawer test, where patient is supine with knee flexed to 90°. Grasp tibia just below joint line and pull forward with both hands. Intact ACL will move forward a few mm and then stop abruptly/hard end point. Injured ACL will have more forward movement and a 'soft' end point. With the knee in the same position a reverse posterior movement can be applied to assess the PCL.

- *Apley/grinding test*: to assess the menisci. Is joint line pain meniscal or ligamentous? Patient prone, affected knee flexed 90°, apply external/internal rotation, with downward force—pain indicates meniscal damage. Repeat external/internal rotation, with upward force, pain indicates collateral ligament injury.

- *McMurray's test*: an alternative to the Apley test. Patient supine and the knee fully flexed. Fingers placed on the medial or lateral joint line, and the knee is slowly extended with the tibia externally rotated for medial meniscus or internally rotated for lateral meniscus. Look for a painful clicking at medial or lateral joint line.

Knee presenting problems

- MCL injury: the MCL is the most commonly injured knee ligament. Valgus (lateral) stress, or external rotational stress with leg firmly planted. If force great, ACL also often damaged. History findings— effusion <12 hours after injury, localized swelling and tenderness over injured area, typically at the superior origin of the MCL. If there is no excessive ligament laxity: rest and simple analgesia (NSAID if not contraindicated) is normally sufficient. Excessive laxity on stress testing A&E/orthopaedic referral is required.

- ACL injury: 2nd most commonly injured knee ligament. Non-contact pivoting/twisting with foot planted, non-contact hyperextension, sudden deceleration, forced internal rotation, sudden valgus (lateral) impact. There is often an accompanying meniscal injury. The patient is normally unable to continue activity, has extreme pain at time of injury, feels a 'pop' in knee or a tearing sensation, swelling 1–2 hours after injury, knee tense and painful, and has episodes of 'giving way'. Requires further assessment in A&E.

- Meniscal injuries: medial more common as the lateral is more fixed. Normally occurs as a result of rotational force to flexed knee. Often with ACL injury. Typically can continue activity, 'popping' sound at time of injury, effusion >12 hours after injury, painful locking or 'giving way' of knee, followed by stiffness. A clicking sensation often accompanies meniscal problems. Requires orthopaedic referral.

📖 Also see Anterior knee pain (Patellofemoral syndrome), pp.198, 202, 286; 📖 Baker's cyst, pp.198, 202, 286; 📖 Osteoarthritis, p.7; 📖 Septic arthritis, p.384; 📖 Gout, pp.102, 104.

Primary care: lower leg and ankle problems

Ankle and foot pain/swelling are frequent presenting complaints in 1° healthcare. Pain is often due to musculoskeletal causes, whether this be injury, acute inflammation, RA, gout, or vasculitis. However wider systemic causes of ankle and foot pain/swelling such as endocrine, cardiac, hepatic, or renal pathologies must also be considered.

Lower leg/ankle/foot history

⚠ Until definitively proven otherwise patients presenting with non-traumatic calf pain should be presumed to have a DVT and referred to A&E for further assessment.

⚠ In patients presenting with ankle or foot injuries with accompanying malleolar pain or midfoot pain, the following clinical findings are suggestive of a possible fracture requiring referral for x-ray: bony tenderness at the posterior edge or tip of the lateral malleoleus or the navicular or the base of the 5th metatarsal or alternatively an observed inability to weight-bear on the injured ankle/foot.

Ankle/foot examination

Inspection
- Observe lower leg, ankle, and foot for any bruising, swelling, wounds, scars, skin lesions, redness, or anatomical deformity.
- Remember to inspect the plantar surface of the foot and the toe web spaces.
- Observe the gait; can the patient weight-bear on the affected side?

Palpation
- Palpate from below the knee, including the fibular head, calf muscles, the Achilles tendon, the calcaneum, the medial and lateral malleoli, the navicular, and 5th metatarsal.
- If a foot injury is suspected also palpate the other tarsal bones and the toe phalanges.

Movement
- Ankle dorsiflexion, plantarflexion, eversion, and inversion.
- Remember that resistance movements of the ankle will always be painful and reduced in a recently sprained ankle; so initially this may not be of clinical significance.
- Toe flexion and extension.

Lower leg, ankle, and knee presenting problems
- **Calf strain (gastrocnemius tear):** presenting as a sudden onset of calf pain with a forceful forward leg movement such as running and stopping suddenly. Presents with tenderness and swelling over the calf muscles and pain to weight bear fully. Dorsiflexion ↑ the

calf pain. Responds well to rest, ice, simple analgesia (NSAID if not contraindicated). Physiotherapy referral may also be useful (dependent on local guidelines).

- *Tenosynovitis (tendonitis)*: inflammation of either the Achilles tendon or extensor hallicus longus due to excessive walking or running is relatively common. Presents with pain on movement and crepitus of the affected tendon. Responds well to rest from the causative activity and regular simple analgesia (NSAID if not contraindicated). Physiotherapy assessment may be required for persisting Achilles tendonitis.

- *Ankle sprain*: occur as a result of an inversion or eversion injury. Presents with malleolar pain, swelling, ↓ movement, and sometimes bruising. Diffuse tenderness and warmth of the affected ligaments is noted. Patients may need to be encouraged to attempt to weight-bear during their examination; but this is an important observation in order to exclude a potential fracture. Treatment includes rest, elevation, and simple analgesia (NSAID if not contraindicated).

- *Plantar fasciitis*: typically presents with unilateral calcaneum pain which worsens on standing and walking. Examination is often unrevealing; with only slight tenderness of the affected plantar surface sometimes being noted. Treatment comprises raised heel pads and simple analgesia (NSAID if not contraindicated). May take some time to settle. Local steroid injection may be required in refractory cases.

- *Toe bruising/fracture*: a common injury, which normally occurs after 'stubbing' the end of a toe. The toes are important for foot balance when walking, so this relatively small injury can have a large impact on everyday activities. Both fractures and bruising are very painful and can be difficult to differentiate clinically. X-ray is not needed unless a dislocated toe is suspected or if there is an accompanying crush injury and subungual haematoma. Treatment includes neighbour strapping of toe and sufficient analgesia (co-dydramol may be required in some cases). The patient should be advised that pain may continue for 2–3 weeks post-injury even with regular analgesia.

Primary care: skin and wound infections

Introduction

In patients presenting with musculoskeletal injuries, there can often be accompanying skin or wound infections. In patients with possible musculoskeletal acute inflammation, local infection should always be considered as an additional differential diagnosis, because the cardinal symptoms of skin redness, pain, and swelling are key features of both infection and inflammation. The commonest pathogens in skin or wound infections are *Staphylococcus aureus* and *Streptococcus pyogenes*. Fungi, yeast, and the herpes group of viruses may also cause local skin infections and should therefore be considered in clinical decision making.

⚠ *The following types of traumatic wounds carry a high risk of infection and should be considered with caution:* delayed presentation (>12 hours) of wounds requiring closure; dirty wounds, e.g. those contaminated with soil, grit, or grease/oil-like substances; penetrating and/or puncture wounds; wounds with areas of non-vascularized tissue; wounds overlying potential bony injuries, which should be treated as compound fractures; and animal or human bites. These types of wounds are ideally treated in A&E or Minor Injuries Unit.

⚠ It should also be remembered that patients with possible immune compromise, by virture of their medical and/or drug history, are at higher risk of devloping skin or wound infections, and there should be a lower threshold for diagnosis and treatment of skin/wound infection in at-risk immune compromise patients.

Cellulitis

Cellulitis typically describes an acute bacterial infection of the skin, which may present in isolation or else in conjunction with a traumatic wound. Symptoms include a defined area of redness, swelling, and pain of the affected skin area, often accompanied by general malaise and sometimes associated regional lymphadenopathy. On examination the affected erythematous skin is hot and tender on palpation, most often with a well-defined border.

⚠ The patient should be examined for signs of spreading cellulitis, which may require hospital assessment: fever, tachycardia, red tracking marks/ascending lymphangitis, and a worsening malaise.

If signs of spreading cellulitis are not present most patients can be successfully treated with oral flucloxacillin, or co-amoxiclav, or erythromycin (if penicillin allergic) as per *BNF* dosage schedules and local guidelines, in conjunction with simple analgesia, rest, and advice regarding worsening and persisting signs of infection. The area of skin redness can be marked with a pen to monitor the progression/regression of local infection.

Wound care in musculoskeletal injuries

Musculoskeletal injuries with accompanying wounds require careful inspection and thorough cleansing, so as to ↓ the chances of cellulitis occurring or developing further, if already present.

- Any visible contaminants, such as grit or soil, should be removed from a wound. This may require wound irrigation in conjunction with wiping with saline-soaked gauze, applied with a sufficient pressure to remove wound debris. If required, topical anaesthetic gel can be applied prior to wound cleansing.
- Wound debris removal is particularly important in skin abrasions, otherwise, retained pieces of grit/soil ↑ the chances of infection occurring or being prolonged, and also of causing permanent skin marking.
- If an acute wound is >2–3mm deep, some form of wound closure will need to be used, whether this is adhesive skin strips, skin glue, or suturing.
- Once cleaned the wound should be covered an appropriate non-adherent, absorbent dressing, and reviewed at regular intervals. Bacteriological wound swabs may need to be considered in discharging wounds.

⚠ Tetanus immunization status should also be determined. Adult patients who give a clear history of 5 or more tetanus vaccines (3 pre-school, 1 at secondary school, and 1 as a young adult), most probably have lifetime immunity and so do not require any further booster dosages. If there is not a clear history of 5 vaccines, and the last booster dose was >10 years ago, a tetanus booster dose should be given as per BNF recommendations and local guidance.

- In patients with no clear history of any prior tetanus immunization, a full tetanus immunization course and tetanus immunoglobulin will need to be considered. This is particularly the case in tetanus prone wounds:
  - Wounds with devitalized skin.
  - Puncture wounds.
  - Soil/manure contaminated wounds.
  - Wounds with signs of infection.

📖 Also see Infections in musculoskeletal conditions, p.379; 📖 Septic arthritis, p.384.

Orthopaedic surgery

Orthopaedic surgery: overview

Advances in orthopaedic surgery have substantially improved the overall function and quality of life for individuals with arthritic conditions. Arthroplasties (joint replacements) are now available for almost every joint, with hip and knee arthroplasty being the most commonly performed orthopaedic operation in the UK.

Individuals who fail to gain satisfactory results from conservative management of their MSC, or have a progressive disease may benefit from a surgical procedure. Assessment by a surgeon for suitability for surgery is best carried out before the patient develops joint deformity or instability, muscle contractures, or advanced muscle atrophy. Delaying surgery until these problems develop can compromise the results and ↑ the risk of surgical complications occurring.

Planning surgery involves consideration of:

- The degree of pain and functional limitation perceived by the patient.
- The joints involved, as no joint can be considered in isolation.
- Possible surgical and conservative treatments, including the expected short- and long-term outcomes.
- Potential risks of surgery/anaesthetic.
- The patient's individual circumstances including an understanding of their social and occupational needs.
- An understanding of the patient's goals and expectations. Clarification of whether these goals are attainable and their expectations realistic should be confirmed from the surgeon's perspective; unrealistic expectations of surgery can ↓ patient satisfaction with surgical outcome.
- An assessment of motivation. Some surgical procedures require patients to undergo intensive physiotherapy/rehabilitation programmes to attain the best surgical outcome.

Aims of surgical intervention.

The 1° aims of any surgical procedure are to:
- Relieve pain.
- Prevent and correct deformity.
- Prevent destruction of cartilage or tendons.
- Maintain or improve function of joints by ↑ or ↓ motion.
- Enable individuals to maintain their independence.

Relief of pain and loss of function are the 1° reason for consideration of any type of surgical intervention. If the pain cannot be controlled by conservative means and the patient's life, in particular his/her sleep is affected, surgery should be considered. Cosmesis is not a prime consideration, but for patients with RA this can bring benefits in the form of improved self-image so should not be overlooked.

Integrated care pathways (ICPs)

ICPs are now a common approach to care planning. These are locally agreed multidisciplinary documents that embed guidelines, protocols, evidence-based practice and patient-centred best practice into individual patient care. In addition they record deviations from planned care in the form of variances. ICPs work well in orthopaedic units as a patient's care is expected to follow a set pattern, for a defined procedure, within a given time frame.

An ICP aims to have:
- The right people.
- Doing the right things.
- At the right time.
- In the right place.
- With the right outcome.
- Give attention to the patient's experience.
- Comparisons of planned care with the actual care given.

The additional benefits of ICPs are:
- A reduction in the amount of documentation health professionals need to complete.
- The fostering of multidisciplinary working.
- The ability to free practitioner's time so that individual problems can be dealt with when they occur, rather than focusing on potential problems.
- Quality outcomes and costs can be balanced

The use of ICPs also allows different healthcare units to make comparisons between the care they provide in each area.

Further reading

National Electronic Library for Health (2003). Integrated Care Pathways. Available online at: ⁀ www.nehl.nhs.uk/carepathways/intro

de Luc K (2001). *Developing Care Pathways*. The Handbook. Oxford. Radcliffe Medical Press, Oxford.

Orthopaedic surgery: preoperative assessment

Preoperative assessment begins as soon as the decision referral for possible orthopaedic surgery is made. Early health screening should take place in the 1° care setting and is often coordinated before referral for consideration of surgery. The aim of screening is to detect and treat any underlying health or social problems that could affect the outcome of surgery or necessitate a planned operation being cancelled (see Box 7.1). It is important to begin the process of discharge planning at this point to ensure everything is in place to facilitate a smooth discharge postoperatively (📖 see Discharge planning, p.254).

NICE[1] have issued guidance on the use of routine preoperative tests for all grades of elective surgery. These take into account the planned procedure and comorbidities and suggests a preoperative testing regimen that determines the patient's fitness to undergo surgery.

> ### Box 7.1 Anaesthetic high-risk patients
>
> - Past history of anaesthetic problems.
> - Unstable diabetes/hypertension.
> - Severe obesity.
> - Symptomatic emphysema.
> - Difficult airway.
> - Abnormal U&Es.
> - Unstable ischaemic heart disease.
> - Previously unidentified heart murmurs/aortic stenosis.

Smoking cessation

This needs to be initiated at least 2 months before surgery for optimal effect. Smoking cessation can reduce the risk of cardiac ischaemia and postoperative chest infection. Heavy smoking can ↓ the oxygen carrying capacity of the blood equivalent to the loss of 2g/dL of Hb, ∴ giving up smoking can give a benefit of a 1–2 unit blood transfusion postoperatively.

Weight reduction

Current evidence supports weight loss if morbidly obese, yet consideration should also be given to potential improvements in quality of life.

Obesity is not a contraindication for surgery but can ↑ the risk of:
- Anaesthetic complications.
- Intraoperative blood loss.
- DVT.

Hospital based pre-admission assessment

It is essential that all preoperative screening is complete and the patient is fit for surgery before the day of admission as patients are routinely admitted to hospital on the day of surgery. Pre admission assessments usually take place 14–21 days preoperatively, although in many cases this may be undertaken at the initial outpatient appointment where the decision for surgery is made. Assessment often involves all members of the MDT.

Aims of pre-admission assessment clinics
- To identify and treat any previously unrecognized medical/social conditions which could affect outcome of surgery. This should include:
  - Screening for the presence of methicillin-resistant *Staphylococcus aureus* (MRSA) colonization.
  - Checking for any breech of the skin which could be infected.
  - Checking for fungal infections under the patient's nails.
  - Vascular assessment.
- To assess fitness to undergo an anesthetic.
- To establish baseline measures of health outcomes, and allow the healthcare team to anticipate and prepare a care plan unique to the individual patient's problems.
- To ensure the patient has an understanding of the surgical procedure and rehabilitation to be able to give informed consent to proceed.
- To continue to the process of discharge planning.

Patient education and consent

The UK Department of Health requires patients to have access to sufficient information to be able to make an informed decision about whether to consent to surgery.[2] Information should be provided on:
- The planned procedure.
- The risks and common complications.
- The type and extent of postoperative rehabilitation.
- Expectations for postoperative pain relief.
- Expectations for function.
- Alternative treatments.

Verbal information should be supported by additional written or visual information (e.g. DVD) to refer to after the consultation to reinforce the information provided and act as a formal record.

The provision of such information has been shown to:
- ↓ anxiety.
- ↑ patient satisfaction.
- ↑ patient outcomes.
- ↓ the use of analgesia

Some voluntary organizations such as NRAS and Arthritis Care may also provide patients with the opportunity to discuss issues with patients who have successfully undergone proposed procedures. This can be facilitated by the hospital team or by contacting the organizations directly.

References

1. National Institute of Clinical Excellence (2003). *Pre operative tests. The use of routine preoperative tests for elective surgery.* NICE, London.

2. Department of Health (2002). *Good practice in consent implementation guide: consent to examination and treatment.* Department of Heath, London.

Orthopaedic surgery: postoperative care

A named professional should be responsible for the coordination of care between all members of the MDT. It is important that the patient and their carers are able to identify the key persons concerned and they should be actively involved in continuously negotiating and influencing their care.

Track and trigger

An early warning system in acute surgical areas was recommended in 2003. The system was devised in order to detect if a patient's condition is deteriorating and allows a prompt and potentially appropriate response to the occurrence of life-threatening situations. The recommendations from this early warning system state:

- A clear physiological monitoring plan detailing the parameters to be monitored and the frequency of observations should be made for each patient.
- There are explicit statements of parameters that should prompt a request for review by medical staff or expert MDT members.
- Respiratory rates should be monitored at any point when other observations are made.
- Staff require education and training in the interpretation and understanding of pulse oximetry readings.

Such schemes should be backed up by 'outreach' services to support ward staff in managing patients who are 'at risk'.

Prevention and treatment of potential postoperative complications

Any major surgical procedures that require a general anesthetic and have the potential for complications are discussed in the following sections. Specific complications, nursing instructions, and patient education requirements are discussed in the relevant section relating to individual surgical procedure. For detailed information see Kneale and Davis.[1]

Haemorrhage and shock

Significant blood loss can occur with major orthopaedic procedures. Consideration needs to be made to ensure a balance is made between anticoagulation to prevent DVT and pulmonary thrombosis and the risk of haemorrhage.

Signs and symptoms of haemorrhage/shock

- Patient complains of ↑ anxiety, fatigue, ↑ pain over wound site.
- Blood loss apparent from drain or wound site.
- Tachycardia or irregular pulse, hypotension, ↑ respiration rate, ↓ urinary output.
- FBC shows ↓ in RBC, Hb, and heamatocrit values; however, if patient is hypovolemic, the heamatocrit may not be ↓ as it is a ratio of blood cells to serum.
- If blood loss is severe—coagulation studies to detect clotting abnormalities.

Nursing management

- Stop or minimize blood loss. Apply pressure dressing to area of bleeding.
- Blood and fluid replacement—if Hb is <9g/dL consider treatment with blood transfusion or autologous transfusion.
- Depending on the result of coagulation screen and the amount of blood loss, fresh frozen plasma and platelets may be administered in addition to whole blood.

Reference

1. Kneale J, Davis P (eds) (2005). *Orthopaedic and Trauma Nursing. Churchill Livingstone*, Harlow.

Orthopaedic surgery: pain management

Acute postoperative pain has been identified as an important factor influencing the patient's perceptions of progress and recovery. Analgesia is the mainstay of postoperative pain control and should be provided according to the patient's perceived pain level and response to medication. Pain relief should be sufficient to allow mobilization; rest and pain free sleep, but avoid drug side effects.

Signs and symptoms of pain
- Patient appears pale and clammy, restless.
- Tachycardia, hypertension.

Management of pain: regional anaesthesia

An injection of local anaesthetic agent at some point along the distribution of a nerve to block the sensation of pain. Regional anesthesia, particularly spinal and epidural techniques, are often used for patients who have to undergo surgery, but who may not be medically fit enough to receive a general anaesthetic.

Spinal block

Local anaesthetic is injected into the sub-arachnoid space, where it mixes with the cerebrospinal fluid (CSF). A spinal needle is inserted below the termination of the spinal cord, usually at the level of the 3rd or 4th lumbar space. The local anaesthetic diffuses through the CSF and blocks the cord and nerve roots. It can diffuse both up or down therefore there is a risk of respiratory muscle paralysis if the needle is inserted too high in the column.

Epidural block

Injection or infusion of a small volume of local anesthetic into the epidural space usually recommended for use during major lower limb surgery. Epidural analgesia is usually prescribed as a low concentration local anaesthetic and opiate agent, to achieve minimum motor block and good analgesic effect. Pre printed prescriptions are generally used with standard mixtures in pre-filled syringes to ↓ risk of calculation errors.

Monitoring and record keeping during spinal or epidural block

Throughout the procedure observations are taken and documented more frequently (usually every 30min/determined by local policy) during the first 6 –12 hours of the infusion, and for the first hour following a top up injection or change of infusion rate.

Observations include:
- The effectiveness of pain relief achieved at rest and on movement.
- Level of sedation.
- Level of sensory and motor blockade so that potentially serious complications can be detected early.

For epidural infusions, records must also be kept of the epidural infusion rate, inspection of epidural insertion site, patency of IV access and integrity of pressure areas. Contemporaneous records must be kept during the infusion including consent, insertion of the catheter, prescription, monitoring, additional doses, and notes about any complications or adverse events.

It is advised that patients who have undergone orthopaedic surgery must be observed for possible development of compartment syndromes (□ see Compartment syndrome, p.249).

Advantages of epidural analgesia
- Patient experience ↓ pain and sedation ∴ can participate in their nursing care and rehabilitation.

Disadvantages relating to potential complications of the epidural
- Nerve damage.
- A dural tap.
- Epidural abscess.
- Headache, backache.
- Urinary retention.
- Nausea and vomiting.

Systemic side effects of local anesthesia include:
- Cardiovascular effects such as hypotension, bradycardia, heart block, cardiac arrest (ventricular tachycardia or fibrillation).
- CNS effects such as agitation, euphoria, respiratory depression, twitching, convulsions, and sensory disturbances.

Peripheral nerve block
Topical application or injection of local anaesthetic to infiltrate peripheral tissues. Used for minor procedures. Complications are rare and usually related to overdose or accidental intra-vascular injection.

Nursing care during regional anaesthesia
Preoperative preparation is the same as for general anaesthesia, including careful monitoring of vital signs. Additional support is required for psychological needs of the patient who remains conscious during the procedure.

Pressure areas and superficial nerves are vulnerable to pressure damage while the patient's limbs are numb.

Further reading

Carr E, Mann E (eds) (2000). *Pain: Creative approaches to effective management.* Palgrave Macmillan, Hampshire.

Royal College of Anaesthetists (2004). *Good practice in the management of continuous epidural analgesia in the hospital setting.* RCoA, London.

Patient-controlled analgesia

PCA is an electronic device that is used to enable the infusion of analgesia (morphine) intravenously, on demand. An initial loading dose is administered, and when able, the patient is instructed in the use of the device. A preset dose is administered at the push of a button, with a lock out period between doses of usually 5min.

Advantages of PCA

- Analgesia is tailored to patient's specific needs.
- Avoids delays from waiting for oral or IM analgesia to be given.
- Can be used if oral fluids are restricted.
- Gives control of pain relief to the patient.

Monitoring

General principles of monitoring PCA analgesia are similar to epidural analgesia.

The administration of regular oral/IM analgesia following the discontinuation of any form of spinal, epidural, or PCA analgesia is essential to enable mobilization/rehabilitation to progress.

Acute compartment syndrome

A complication of trauma, caused by muscle ischaemia and necrosis and has a serious sequlae. Irreversible, can lead to amputation, renal failure, and loss of life. Early detection of ACS through careful monitoring of clinical signs and symptoms and the evaluation of the neurovascular status of the extremities is vital.

Signs and symptoms: the 6 Ps

Pain
- Out of proportion to the injury.
- Unrelieved by narcotics.
- Excessive use of analgesia devices (PCA).
- ↑ by movement of distal digits.
- Described as deep or throbbing.
- ↑ with elevation of the extremity.
- May not be present if central/peripheral sensory deficits are present.

Paresthesia
- Subtle first symptom.
- Best elicited by direct stimulation.
- Patients complain of a burning sensation.
- Can lead to hypoesthesia (numbness) pain.

Pressure
- Involved compartment or limb will feel tense and warm on palpation.
- Skin will be tight and shiny.
- Skin occasionally appears cellulitic.

Pallor
- Late sign.
- Pale/whitish tone to the skin.
- Prolonged capillary refill >3sec.
- Cool feel to skin due to lack of capillary reperfusion.

Paralysis
- Late sign.
- May start as weakness in active movement of involved or distal joints.
- Leads to inability to move joints or digits actively.
- No response to direct neural stimulation due to damage of myoneural junction.

Pulselessness
- Late sign.
- Very weak or lack of palpable or Doppler audible pulse.

Diagnostic tools have been developed to provide an objective measurement of compartment pressures as an adjunct to signs and symptoms in detecting ACS; these include continuous compartmental pressure monitoring. Treatment of ACS is fasciotomy of the affected compartments; this may require additional procedures such as skin grafting.

Postoperative complications: deep vein thrombosis/pulmonary embolism

The development of DVT and PE are significant complications of major orthopaedic surgery (Box 7.2). The risk of DVT is ~40%, most of these are minor, asymptomatic, and do not require treatment. The risk of fatal PE is <0.1%.

> **Box 7.2 Patient-related risk factors for venous thromboembolism**
>
> - Active cancer or cancer treatment.
> - Active heart disese or respiratory failure.
> - Acute medical Illness, including recent MI or stroke.
> - Age >60 years.
> - Antiphospholipid syndrome.
> - Behçet disease.
> - Central venous catheter in situ.
> - Continuous travel of >3 hours ~4 weeks before or after surgery.
> - Immobility (prolonged) i.e. bed rest, limb in plaster.
> - Inflammatory bowel disease.
> - Myeloproliferative diseases.
> - Nephrotic syndrome.
> - Obesity (BMI >30kg/m^2).
> - Personal or family history of DVT.
> - Pregnancy or puerperium.
> - Severe infection.
> - Use of oral contraceptives or HRT.
> - Varicose veins with associated phlebitis.
> - Inherited thrombophillias.

Signs and symptoms of DVT

- Pain, tenderness swelling, redness at or below the site of thrombosis.
- Pyrexia.
- Mild-to-severe pitting oedema may occur.
- Homan's sign (forced dorsiflexion of the foot causing pain in the calf) is not sensitive or specific for DVT.

Venous US is an accurate, sensitive, and noninvasive examination for locating thrombus within deep and superficial veins.

PE

If part of a thrombus breaks away it may lodge in the pulmonary arteries and cause a PE. PE is the commonest cause of sudden death in hospital. PE results in:

- ↓ cardiac output.
- Hypertension.
- Impaired oxygenation.
- Bronchospasm.

Management

Prophylaxis

To reduce venous stasis:
- Elevate limb.
- Regular dorsiflexion of the ankle when resting.
- Early ambulation.
- Anti-embolism stockings or mechanical pumps.

To reduce hypercoagulability:
- Adequate hydration.
- Anticoagulant therapy. Clinical guidelines have been developed based on the determination of risk of PE and major bleeding, with prophylaxis being prescribed as a result of the risk assessment.
- Patients can be trained to self-administer subcutaneous low molecular weight heparin injections at home (usually delivered for up to 10 days postoperatively).

Assessment of risk

Risk calculations for DVT can be assessed using scales such as the Autar scale.[1]

Risk categories

- Patients who are at standard risk for PE and bleeding.
- Patients who are at elevated (above standard) risk for PE but standard risk of major bleeding.
- Patients who are at standard risk for PE and at elevated (above standard) risk of major bleeding.
- Patients who are at elevated (above standard) risk for both PE and major bleeding.

Mechanical prophylaxis is advised in all patients. The suggestion for additional prophylaxis differs in each of the other 4 categories and involves the options of aspirin, warfarin and low molecular weight heparin.

👉 Local guidelines exist in units in the UK.

Reference

1. Autar R (2004). Venous thromboembolism prevention: an update. *Journal of Orthopaedic Surgery*, **8**, 50–6.

Further reading

The American Association of Orthopaedic Surgeons (2007). Clinical guidelines on the prevention of symptomatic PE in patients undergoing total joint replacement. Available at: 🖰 www.aaos.org/research/guidelines/guide.asp

Postoperative complications: infection, delayed wound healing, and pressure ulcers

Infection

Wound infection is a potentially serious complication of surgery and is associated with poor outcome (Box 7.3). Infection following joint replacement surgery can lead to an infected joint and can be a major cause of joint failure. If this occurs the patient will have to undergo a prolonged stay in hospital and an extensive course of antibiotic therapy.

> **Box 7.3 Risk factors that contribute to delayed wound healing**
>
> - Patient's age, older persons are at ↑ risk.
> - Poor skin condition.
> - Poor nutritional status.
> - Comorbid conditions such as diabetes, malignancies, respiratory and cardiovascular disease.
> - Use of long-term corticosteroids.

Wound dressings

To provide optimum protection a dressing must be able to:
- Absorb excess exudates.
- Prevent contamination of the wound and surrounding tissues.
- Not adhere to the healing tissues.

Multi-resistant infections

MRSA is carried on 30–50% of the general population, causing a high risk of transmission to patients following orthopaedic surgery as the natural barrier of the skin has been breached. Preoperative screening for the colonization of MRSA organisms is performed during the pre-assessment visit. High-risk factors for colonization are:
- ♂.
- >70 years old.
- Previous hospital admission.
- Nursing home residents.

The main precautions in preventing the spread of MRSA are:
- Good hand hygiene, for all staff that come into contact with patients, including the use of alcohol hand gel after each contact.
- Isolation of known carriers of MRSA.
- The use of protective clothing such as gloves, disposable aprons etc.
- Safe disposal of linen.
- High standards of hospital cleanliness.

Drug treatment of infections

- MRSA is treated by the use of vancomycin or teicoplanin.
- Other resistant organisms include vancomycin-resistant *enterococcus*, penicillin-resistant *pneumococcus*, multi-resistant *pseudomonas aeruginosa* and muli-resistant *mycobacterium tuberculosis*. Refer to *BNF* and local policies for prescribing guidance for infections.

Prevention of pressure ulcers

A constant pressure of 60mmHg can cause irreversible tissue damage within 1–2 hours. Pressures of 4–100mmHg have been documented over the ischial, posterior trochanter, and thigh areas when clients are sitting in a wheelchair, even when using wheelchair cushions. Bony prominences such as the sacrum, heels, spine, hips, costal margins, and occiput are especially at risk when in a lying position. Shearing and friction forces contribute to the development of pressure ulcers.

All patients undergoing surgery should be assessed by the use of a recognized assessment tool i.e. Waterlow Score, to determine their risk of developing a pressure ulcer (Box 7.4). A plan of care to prevent the development of pressure ulcers should be determined by the MDT, in agreement with the patient. The plan should be documented, implemented, and evaluated along with evidence of ongoing reassessment as the patient's condition changes, throughout the pre-, peri- and postoperative period.

> ### Box 7.4 Pressure ulcers: additional risk factors for development
>
> - The individual's health and nutritional status.
> - Ability to change position unaided.
> - Incontinence.
> - Medication such as corticosteroids which alter the quality of skin.

Grades of pressure ulcers

- Grade 1: non-blanchable erythema of intact skin. In individuals with darker skin, discoloration of the skin, warmth, oedema, or hardness may also be indicators.
- Grade 2: partial thickness skin loss involving epidermis, dermis, or both. The ulcer is superficial, and appears clinically as an abrasion, blister, or shallow crater.
- Grade 3: full thickness skin loss involving damage to, or necrosis of, subcutaneous tissue that may extend down to, but not through, underlying fascia. The ulcer appears clinically as a deep crater with or without undermining of adjacent tissues.
- Grade 4: full thickness skin loss with extensive destruction, tissue necrosis, or damage to muscle, bone, or supporting structures. Undermining and sinus tracts may also be associated with a grade 4 ulcer.

Pressure ulcer prevention and care of immobilized patients

- Regular turning/repositioning schedule (at least every 2 hours).
- Toileting regimens for incontinent patients.
- Use of positioning/pressure relieving devices including mattresses and cushions, positioning devices etc.

Further reading

National Institute of Clinical Excellence (2003). *Pressure ulcer prevention.* NICE, London.

Discharge planning following orthopaedic surgery

The way certain ADL are carried out may have to be adjusted depending on how surgery affects an individual. Such adjustments should be anticipated preoperatively and form part of the discharge process. Planning for discharge should begin at the point the patient is listed for surgery and the plan should be constantly updated throughout the current episode of care.

Patients and their relatives should be informed of the anticipated length of stay in hospital for the procedure they are undergoing.

Nurse-led discharge

The nurse is often the key coordinator in a patient's discharge, making decisions regarding the patient's fitness to leave hospital and coordinating the activities that facilitate this. This involves communication with other health professionals both in 1° and 2° care settings and the patient's family to ensure that services are in place for a safe discharge.

Discharge plans are multidisciplinary and include:
- An assessment of physical condition including general health, recovery from anaesthetic, pain control, infection screen, and wound healing.
- An occupational therapy assessment. This addresses aspects of personal care, ADL, and work that may have been affected by the surgery. The need for living aids or assistive devices is assessed and these should be provided prior to discharge.
- Physiotherapy includes assessing the patient's mobility, and mobility of any affected limb/joint. General advice on the need to be active and suggestions for sensible activities to ↑ post-discharge fitness is given.
- Social factors. Ensuring any care that may be required from relatives is available such as help with shopping, cleaning and with transport.
- Falls prevention. The risk of falling should be determined based on previous and current medical status, medications taken, the environment, visual acuity, and balance. Tips for accident prevention are given in 📖 p.42.
- Arrangements for transport home.

Patient education

Prior to discharge patients should be advised of:
- Any changes to medications that have been instituted in hospital, and in particular regrading the use of analgesics.
- Details of any follow-up care required, i.e. for removal of sutures, outpatient physiotherapy, and consultant review.
- A point of contact for use if they have any questions regarding their care or in the event of any problems, particularly if these occur out of hours.
- The need to inform dental practitioners of prosthetic joint replacements. Antibiotic cover is required for any dental procedures lasting >30min.

- Details of the implant type and size will be registered, with the patient's consent, on the National Joint Register. This is important should there be any requirement for revision of the implant at any point in the future.

Hospital at home (H@H)/supported discharge schemes

The aim of such schemes is to facilitate early discharge from hospital by providing intensive levels of care and rehabilitation that otherwise would be given in hospital, in the patient's home, for a defined time period.

Detailed admission and discharge criteria for the scheme have to be agreed and patients can then be referred from the scheme to community nursing services if required. All staff working in such schemes require multiple skills as it is not cost effective to duplicate nurses and therapist visits to an individual patient.

There are two organizational models of H@H schemes:

- *Model 1:* nursing and therapists care is coordinated by a team of specialist practitioners from the 2° care sector. The medical responsibility for care remains with the orthopaedic consultant. Advantages of this model are that the practitioners are experts in the care that some patients require, which gives the consultants confidence in utilizing such services. In addition, access to reassessment or admission to hospital if necessary can be easier.
- *Model 2:* a community based generic H@H service for a defined geographical population. This is an extension to existing community nursing services, with community nurses providing the care, and the responsibility of that care being with the GP. For this model of care to succeed specialist training for staff involved is essential.

Postoperative follow-up

Due to changes in healthcare delivery and, in particular, a reduction of outpatient appointments, review of patients following orthopaedic surgery may be carried out by experienced practitioners, either nurses or PTs, who work as part of the surgical team. These may be undertaken in 1° or 2° care settings.

Not all surgical procedures require a follow-up visit; some follow-up consultations may be made by telephone.

Surgery to the spine

Various disorders affect the lower back. The most common causes of low back pain that are considered for surgical intervention include:

Herniated vertebral disc

The nucleus pulposus extrudes through the annulus fibrosis, exerting direct contact on neural structures. The size of the spinal canal, the location of the defect, and size of herniation play a part in the decision to operate or treat conservatively. Pain is the 1° symptom. This can be intermittent in severity and frequency. Sciatica described as numbness, tingling, or burning sensation down the limb, is present if the damage is in the L4 region. Localized epidural steroid injection can offer sustained relief of pain in some patients.

Spondylolysis

Defect or break in the neural arch between the superior and inferior articulating surfaces. May progress to spondylolisthesis

Spondylolisthesis

Forward subluxation of 1 vertebrae on another. Can be congenital or degenerative. Surgical treatment is considered if there is evidence of neurological deficit, persistent pain, a progressive slip, or a slip of >50%.

Spinal stenosis

Narrowing of the spinal canal. Can be congenital or degenerative and can occur at any region in the spine. Significant neurological compromise can occur if a narrowed canal is invaded by disc material. Signs and symptoms include neurogenic claudication, presenting as leg pain after walking, which is relieved by sitting or squatting.

Long-term results of spinal surgery are comparable to conservative treatment, ∴ surgery is only considered in the presence of significant neurological deficit or red flags (Box 7.5).

Conservative management of back pain include:
- Individualized exercise regimens/pain management techniques.
- NSAIDs and regular analgesia/antidepressants.
- Heat/ice./TENs machines.

Box 7.5 Red flags: possible indicators of serious pathology

- Thoracic pain.
- Fever and unexplained weight loss.
- Bladder and bowel dysfunction.
- History of carcinoma.
- Ill health.
- Progressive neurological deficit.
- Disturbed gait, saddle anaesthesia.
- Age of onset <20 years or >55years.

Spinal decompression

The common goal of decompression surgery is to ensure careful freeing of the affected nerves by removal of bone, disc, and facet capsule. A combination of surgical techniques including discectomy, laminectomy, and foramenotomy are used to ensure a proper decompression of the nerve elements.

Spinal fusion

Spinal fusion aims to restore stability and spinal alignment. There are several approaches to spinal fusion including an anterior, posterior, or circumferential fusion, which can be performed with or without instrumentation.

Factors affecting outcome of surgery

Despite initial high success rates for spinal surgery, outcomes for patients can be disappointing over time (Box 7.6).

Box 7.6 Causes for poor outcome from spinal surgery

- Recurrent disc herniation or spinal stenosis.
- Chronic nerve injury.
- Incomplete decompression.
- Infection.
- Failure of fusion to develop or poor postoperative alignment of spine.
- Loosening of instrumentation.
- Nerve irritation from instrumentation and subsequent pain.
- Incomplete diagnosis of problem preoperatively.
- Junctional failure of the spine where there is collapse/instability of a segment of the spine adjacent to a previously operated area.

Principles of postoperative management after spinal surgery

Patients require a period of immobility postoperatively, ∴ prevention of complications such as chest infection, wound infection, ↑ risk of DVT and pressure ulceration are key factors in postoperative management.

- *Assessment of neurological function:* sensory and motor function should be assessed every 2 hours for the first 24 hours postoperatively. Then 4–8-hourly. Cases of neurological damage have been reported up to 36 hours after surgery.
- *Pain control:* use of PCA in the immediate postoperative period (📖 see pp.246, 260). Analgesia needs to be sufficient to allow early mobilization, and tailored to the individual patients requirements.

General principles of body mechanics following spinal surgery

- Sleep on the side with knees bent and a supporting pillow between the legs.
- Avoid sleeping prone.
- Place a pillow under the knees for support when sleeping supine.
- Post-cervical surgery, use a flat pillow only.
- When getting up from the bed, the patient should roll onto their side, use their arms to push up while allowing the legs to swing slowly over the side of the bed.
- Avoid all movements that twist the neck or lower back.
- Avoid lifting weight >~2.5–4.5kg (~5– 10lb) in initial 6 weeks postoperatively.

Surgery to the hip and knee

Arthroplasty

Prosthetic arthroplasty (joint replacement) can relieve pain and improve function for patients with moderate-to-severe destruction of cartilage and subchrondral bone. Arthroplasty of the hip is the most common operation performed in the world closely followed by arthroplasty of the knee.

Total hip arthroplasty/replacement (THR)

The surgeon may choose to use cemented or un-cemented prosthesis or a combination of the two. Selection of prosthesis is dependant on:

- Underlying pathology.
- Associated medical conditions.
- Patient's age.
- Potential postoperative activity.
- Choice of the surgeon.
- Implant availability.

THR has been demonstrated to give excellent function for 15–20 years.

Surface replacement hip arthroplasty

Involves using surface replacement prosthesis (metal on metal) and follows removal of diseased surfaces of the joint. The main advantage of this procedure is that less bone stock is removed, making revision to a conventional THR simpler. This is often the procedure of choice for younger patients, undertaken as a first stage with a view to revision to a full THR at a later date.

Total knee arthroplasty/replacement (TKR)

TKR is the current treatment choice for bi- or tri-compartmental knee arthritis. TKR prosthesis are designed to replace only the joint surface necessitating minimal bone resection, therefore bone stock is preserved which maintains treatment options in the event of joint failure. A major factor in preventing early joint failure is that all TKR prostheses allow some rotation and unlimited flexion. TKR prostheses can be cemented or un-cemented.

Contraindications to TKR

- Relative contraindications: high activity expectations and long life expectancy.
- Absolute contraindications: presence of active infection, including conditions that may produce non-healing ulcers of the ipsilateral lower extremity.

Unicompartmental knee replacement

If OA is limited to the medial or lateral compartment a unicompatmental knee replacement may be considered. The success rate of this procedure is 95% after 5 years. Hemi-arthroplasty does allow conversion to TKR if necessary in the future.

High tibial osteotomy of the knee (HTO)

Osteotomy is undertaken to reduce/alter the loading forces on the most severely affected part of the tibial plateau. The procedure involves resection of a wedge of bone from either the lateral or medial side of the upper tibia. Due to the success rate of knee arthroplasty, HTO is rarely undertaken; however, for younger patients with an isolated cartilage defect this procedure can used to realign and unload a damaged compartment. In the future, the procedure may be undertaken in combination with osteochondral alografting techniques or autograft meniscal transplantation.

Arthrodesis/fusion of the knee

This is the treatment choice for pain control in:
• Young active or heavy patient with end-stage unilateral disease.
• Those with relative or absolute contraindications for arthroplasty.

Surgery involves trimming of the articular surfaces of the distal femur and proximal tibia to provide flat surfaces across which fusion can occur. Postoperatively, the joint is immobilized usually in an Ilizarov external fixator frame for a period of up to 3 months. Partial weight-bearing may be necessary during this time.

Knee fusion results in an immobile joint fixed in extension, with a shortening of the limb by approx 1cm. This procedure is performed rarely and is poorly tolerated by patients.

Arthroscopy and debridement

Arthroscopy involves the visualization of the inside of the joint with the aid of an arthroscope. NICE guidelines indicate this procedure for continued locking and giving way of the knee joint.[1]

Autologous cartilage transplant

This is a 2-stage procedure, involving taking cartilage cells form a non-weight-bearing aspect of the patients joint and transplanting these cells 4–6 weeks later onto the defective area of the joint. This procedure has the potential to restore damaged joint surfaces.

Reference

1. National Institute for Health and Clinical Excellence (2008). NICE Guidelines for the management of osteoarthritis. NICE, London. Available at: ⌖ www.nice.org.uk

Principles of postoperative care for total hip/knee arthroplasty

ICPs are often used to provide a framework for planning and delivering care during a surgical episode of care[1] (📖 also see Surgery to the hip and knee, p.258).

Nursing management

- Management of pain (📖 see Symptom control, pp.246, 248, Chapter 9).
- Assessment of neurovascular status in both lower limbs.
- Monitoring fluid balance and vital signs.
- Assessment of dressings/drains for excessive output.
- Chest physiotherapy.
- Encouragement of leg exercises to reduce risk of DVT.
- Initiating mobilization and return to independence.

Common postoperative complications of THR/TKR

DVT

Follow locally accepted guidelines for the prevention of DVT/PE

Dislocation of THR prosthesis

Occurs most commonly 2–5 days postoperatively. Signs and symptoms of dislocation include:
- Severe pain.
- Internal rotation of the limb.
- Limb shortening.

Infection

Risk reduced in the immediate postoperative period to ~1% due to modern surgical techniques and the use of prophylactic antibiotics.

Late complications

- Late sepsis around the prosthesis. Can occur 6–24 months postoperatively in 1–4% of THR prosthesis. Delayed infections in TKRs have been reported in 4.1 % of patients, an average of 7 years postoperatively. Treatment of joint infection usually requires a 2-stage operative procedure to remove the infected prosthesis and treatment with IV antibiotics for at least 6 weeks before insertion of a new joint.
- Long-term prosthetic loosening—may necessitate revision surgery. Failure rate of THR revision surgery is 10% at 5 years.
- Leg length discrepancy—may require orthotic shoe raise to correct

Postoperative education for THR and TKR

Discuss the use of prophylactic antibiotics for future surgical dental procedures that can cause transient bacteraemia and ↑ the risk of joint infection.

Patient education post-TKR (Box 7.7)

- Swelling of the leg up to 1 year post peratively is normal.
- Exercise is vital to achieve potential range of movement.

- Surgeons usually suggest patients do not kneel for 6 months following TKR although it is not an absolute contraindication. Numbness of the knee may result in hesitancy to kneel. Patients should be taught to kneel on a soft surface and to rise from kneeling using the unaffected leg.

Box 7.7 Precautions following THR

Avoid extreme positions until surrounding soft tissue is healed—up to 6 weeks postoperatively.
- Avoid bending >90°:
  - Dress operated leg first, and undress last.
  - Do not bend at the waist to tie shoes.
  - Use high chair with supportive arms/raised toilet seat.
  - Use long-handled aids to pick things up from the floor.
  - Lead with un-operated leg when ascending stairs.
  - Lead with operated leg when descending stairs.
  - In the absence of pain, sexual intercourse may be resumed 6 weeks postoperatively, unless advised otherwise by the surgeon.
- Avoid crossing operative leg past the body's midline (adduction):
  - Get out of bed on the operated side.
  - Sleep on your back (6 weeks); may need to use pillow to maintain abduction.
- Avoid twisting the leg in or out (internal/external rotation):
  - Lead with your feet when changing direction, avoid twisting your body.
- Use correct walking aid.

Reference

1. de Luc K (2001). *Developing Care Pathways. The Handbook.* Radcliffe Medical Press. Oxford

Ankle surgery and foot surgery

Ankle surgery

Treatment of end-stage ankle arthritis remains controversial. Treatment options include:

Arthrodesis of the ankle

Normally carried out using internal fixation methods. If performed relatively early in the hindfoot for significant flat foot deformity, a simple subtalar fusion may suffice. With longer established deformities and subluxation of the talonavicular joint, a triple arthrodesis may be required. This involves fusion of the talonavicular, calcaneocuboid, and subtalar joints. The planned outcome of the surgical procedure is ensuring that the foot is plantirgrade or flat to the ground. Postoperative rehabilitation requires a period of non-weight-bearing for up to 6 weeks, often in a short leg cast, followed by a further 6 weeks in an ambulatory cast.

Arthroplasty/replacement of the ankle

The advantage of arthroplasty is that when successful, it maintains motion and reduces strain on adjacent joints. Problems such as wound healing complications and implant subsidence have improved with newer designs of prosthesis in recent years; however, if the joint fails, salvage can be difficult, particularly after deep infection, which if painful and non-responsive to treatment may require a below-knee amputation.

Foot surgery

Excision arthroplasty

Surgical reconstruction of the forefoot is performed to:

Correct hammertoes

The proximal joint is fixed in flexion whist the distal and MTP joints are extended. The pressure of shoes over the deformity causes painful callosities, which if the skin becomes broken, and can be a potential source in infection.

Dorsal dislocation of the lesser MTP joints

Often occurs in patients with RA. Patients complain of callosities under the metatarsal heads and pain is described as 'walking on pebbles' Excision of the metatarsal head is performed to allow realignment of the forefoot

Severe hallux valgus deformity (bunion)

This is a static subluxation of the first MTP joint in which there are 3 features:

- The 1st toe angulates laterally towards the 2nd toe.
- The middle portion of the first metatarsal head enlarges.
- The bursa over the medial aspect of the MTP joint becomes inflamed and thick walled.

This may be asymptomatic or a source of chronic pain and disability. Conservative management includes advice on good footwear and padding of the deformity. Surgery involves metatarsal osteotomy, or excision of the proximal phalanx. Arthrodesis of the MTP joint is also considered an option for advanced hallux valgus deformity.

Nursing management

- Foot surgery can be extremely painful, ∴ adequate pain management is essential.
- Knowledge of the postoperative plan of care is essential to enable patients to take an active part in their recovery. Mobility may require the use of crutches or alternative walking aids. Practice preoperatively may help to allay anxiety.

Wrist and hand surgery

Good hand function is essential for performing most ADL and leisure pursuits. The wrist and hand joints are prone to both forms of arthritis; however, surgical intervention is more commonly performed for patients with inflammatory arthritis. In RA erosive damage to hand joints can occur very early in the disease process.

Common deformities of the hand as a result of RA include:

- Ulnar drift caused by damage at the MCP joint, aggravated by normal activities
- Swan neck deformities: hyperextension of the PIP joint with flexion of the MCP and DIP joint
- Boutonnière deformity: flexion if the PIP joint and hyperextension of the DIP joint
- Z deformity of the thumb: instability of the MCP or IP joint. Fusion of the thumb is usually the procedure of choice, giving the patients a stable thumb and ↑ the strength of the pinch grip.

Surgical interventions to the hand and wrist include:

Carpal tunnel decompression

CTS is the most common compression neuropathy affecting the hand. Pain is caused by compression of the median nerve as it passes with the flexor tendons, through the carpal tunnel at the wrist. Symptoms can vary from a mild tingling on the palmer aspect of the thumb and 1st 3 fingers, to loss of motor function and intense pain that disrupts sleep. There can also be a loss of grip strength and wasting of the thenar muscle.

Surgical decompression is usually carried out as a day case. Normal activities are encouraged as soon as comfortable postoperatively. Grip strength and endurance may take 3–6 months to achieve, and for some may remain incomplete.

Arthrodesis (fusion) of the wrist

Advanced degenerative disease of the IP joints, carpus, and wrist are commonly treated by arthrodesis which affords long-term pain relief and stability.

Synovectomy of the wrist

Synovial proliferation can destroy articular cartilage, causing instability and 2° deformity. When the articular cartilage is intact early synovectomy can be of benefit.

Tendon rupture/transfer

The loss of extension at the MCP joint, due to rupturing of the extensor tendon—particularly of the little finger—requires urgent surgical attention as direct repair of the tendon can only be undertaken in the acute phase.

Prophylactic tenosynovectomy

If it is clinically suspected that the extensor tendons are at risk, prophylactic tenosynovectomy may be performed. This is often undertaken with resection of bony prominences at the distal radio-ulnar joint.

MCP joint arthroplasty

Silicone MCP implants may be used for hands that are painful and have fixed deformities. Patients generally report a subjective functional improvement and improved appearance postoperatively; however, reported rates of fracture of implant can vary between 0–50%.

Nursing management and common postoperative complications

- *Pain relief:* usually managed with oral analgesia (□ see Postoperative care, pp.246, 260).
- *Assistance with self-care and ADL:* the ability to wash and dress and carry out other self-care tasks may be impaired postoperatively. Referral to the OT preoperatively may result in the provision of aids to help in the performance of such activities. Help may be required on discharge and assessment of self-care should form part of the discharge planning process.
- *Splintage:* splintage to help pain control and support the operated area in an acceptable position is common following all types of hand/wrist surgery while healing is taking place.
- *Altered body image:* disfigurement of the hand and wrist can have a profound affect on an individual's body image. Surgery may be corrective; however, limiting a person's ability to self-care and the use of sometimes prolonged splintage can have a negative impact on body image. Good preoperative information and the opportunity to discuss and view the splintage may avoid unnecessary distress.

Elbow surgery

OA of the elbow is usually mild as the elbow joint is a slight weight-bearing joint when compared to the lower limb joints. However, individuals who extensively overuse their upper extremities, i.e. labourers or athletes, can experience disabling pain and loss of movement as a result of OA of the elbow.

Elbow arthroplasty

Total elbow arthroplasty (TEA) is more often carried out as a result of 2° OA following an injury to the humeral, ulnar, or radioulnar joints, or for patients with RA or hemophilia. Results of TEA for 1° OA and those of a younger age group can be poor due to the heavier loading applied on the replaced joint. However, the results for surgery for individuals with RA are comparable to THR/TKR, in that 90% of patients report dramatic pain relief. Functional improvements of 90% ↑ in strength of flexion and 60–70% ↑ in pronation and supination have also been reported. These ranges include the functional arcs of movement required for ADL.

Presenting symptoms

- Pain and stiffness at the elbow.
- Limitations in ADL, i.e. difficulty in:
  - Lifting or receiving an item onto the hand (supination).
  - In writing (pronation).
  - In eating, dressing, or grooming which require flexion at the elbow.

The aim of surgery is to provide a stable painless range of movement during ADL.

2 types of prosthesis are commonly used:

- An unconstrained surface replacement—main problems postoperatively relate to joint instability in 20–50% of cases.
- A linked semi-constrained prosthesis—the ulnar and humeral components are linked to reduce the risk of dislocation, but the linkage allows a degree of laxity that permits the soft tissue to absorb some of the stresses that would normally be applied to the prosthesis–bone interface and reduces the risk of joint loosening.

Nursing management/common postoperative complications

- Pain control.
- Assessment of neurovascular status. Risk of temporary/permanent ulnar nerve injury during surgery. Evaluate motion and sensation of 4th and 5th fingers on operated side. Immediately postoperatively, oedema may minimize the patient's ability to abduct/abduct the fingers. Some numbness may continue for 6–8 weeks post surgery.
- Assessment of dressings/drains. As the skin around the elbow is thin with little subcutaneous tissue, the wound may be prone to complications including infection or wound breakdown. Infection rates have been reported between 2–5%.
- Assistance with aspects of ADL. Post-surgery the joint is protected in 90% flexion with a back- slab or firm padding and crepe bandaging. This may be replaced with a polyurethane splint after 48 hours. This splint may be used for up 6 weeks except when exercising.

Exercise
- Gentle, active, assisted elbow flexion, passive gravity extension, and forearm rotation are commenced 1–3 days postoperatively.
- Gradual strengthening exercises for triceps and biceps are added as healing progresses.
- Avoid extension >30% to prevent subluxation or dislocation.
- Encourage extension after 6 weeks.

Patient education
- Normal activities, such as light housework, can be resumed after 4–6 weeks.
- Light gardening after 6 weeks.
- Driving after 8 weeks.
- Strenuous activities such as carrying heavy shopping and contact sports should be avoided.

Synovectomy and excision of the radial head

More commonly performed in individuals with 2° OA as a result of RA or haemophilia.

Presenting symptoms
- Persistent synovitis around the elbow.
- ↓ ROM, particularly extension.
- Pain particularly on supination and pronation.
- On examination, clinical involvement of the radio humeral or radio-ulnar joint.

Nursing management and patient education

Mild, active assisted motion of the elbow is commenced 4 days postoperatively, progressing to active motion as pain allows. Pain usually improves as strength improves.

Pain can continue to reduce over the initial 3–6 months postoperatively. ROM can continue to improve for 6 months.

Shoulder surgery

The shoulder is the most mobile joint in the body. OA of the shoulder often occurs from either significant trauma, 2° to RA or a chronic tear in the rotator cuff. Shoulder motion is provided by the rotator cuff and deltoid muscles ∴ any tear in the rotator cuff can be associated with significant ↓ in ROMs which can compromise the results of any chosen surgical option.

Surgical repair of torn rotator cuff

The commonest cause of rotator cuff damage is from repetitive injury. Commonly presents in patients >40 years of age. Surgery may not lead to any improvement in pain, compared to exercise. Some large rotator cuff tears may not be repairable. In this instance decompression and debridement may be the treatment of choice.

Presenting symptoms

- Pain.
- Limitation of active abduction beyond 25°. If the arm is passively abducted the patient may then be able to hold it in that position due to the action of the deltoid muscles.
- Limitation of backwards extension and external rotation. This affects activities such as putting the arm into a sleeve.

Surgical repair can be undertaken using an open or arthroscopic approach. Arthroscopic surgery may not lead to any difference in outcome in the long term, compared with open surgery but recovery may be quicker.
Advantages of an arthroscopic approach include:

- Smaller skin incisions.
- No deltoid detachment.
- ↓ soft tissue dissection.
- ↓ pain.
- ↓ hospital stay.

Nursing management

- Immobilization of the affected joint, to promote tissue repair.
- A polysling is worn when not exercising to provide support and pain relief.
- Passive elevation and external rotation exercises are commenced whist in hospital and continued for 6 weeks postoperatively.
- Patients are encouraged to lift the arm with the elbow bent to create a short lever and less stress in the first 3 months post-surgery. The arm must not be lifted above shoulder level.
- Active exercises are commenced after 6 weeks with the aim of mobilizing the shoulder and strengthening muscles when the tendon has healed.

Common postoperative complications

- Deltoid detachment or failure of the repair.
- Deep infection.

Patient education

- Postoperative rehabilitation including the ability to fully self-care can be prolonged. This must be fully understood preoperatively. In some instances support with ADL may need to be organized on discharge.
- Driving can be recommenced after 6 weeks.

Total shoulder arthroplasty (TSA)

Primary OA and RA account for approx 85% of all TSA. The main indication for surgery is relief of pain, particularly night pain. Restoration of movement and strength is dependant on the condition of the rotator cuff. Patients needs to motivated and understand that it can take up to 12 months before the full benefit of surgery is obtained.

3 main types of prosthesis are used:

- Unconstrained—used when the patient has a functioning rotator cuff.
- Constrained—used for patients with severe pain in an unstable shoulder with a poor rotator cuff.
- Semi-constrained—primarily dependant on the rotator cuff mechanism, but does have some constraint built into the design.

Nursing management and common postoperative complications

Pain relief: may necessitate the use of PCA analgesia (see Patient-controlled analgesia, p.248). Step-down analgesia is essential to enable patients to take part in rehabilitation. A polysling is worn when not exercising for support

Neurovascular assessment: risk of damage to axillary nerve and brachial plexus during surgery.

Assessment of nerve function

- Motor function of the radial nerve—assess the patient's ability to abduct the thumb.
- Motor function of the ulnar nerve—abduct or spread the fingers apart against pressure.
- Axillary nerve function—ask the patient to push the elbows out against resistance.

Assistance with ADL: patients require help with most care activities in the initial postoperative period.

Exercise

- 48 hours postoperatively—passive motion exercises. Aim to achieve 140° of forward elevation and 40° degrees of external rotation.
- 10 days post surgery—assisted exercises to gain rotation and isometric exercises to strengthen the rotator cuff and deltoid muscles Followed by active abduction and flexion.
- 3 weeks post-surgery—resisted exercise and passive stretching, commenced, to ↑ muscle power and improve active/passive ROM.
- Exercise to be continued for minimum of 6 months.

Patient education

- Avoid housework for 4 weeks.
- Driving and sedentary work can be recommenced after 6 weeks. Patients with more strenuous jobs may not be able to return to work for up to 12 weeks.

Assessing the patient: clinical examination and history taking

Assessing the patient

History taking and examining the patient are essential to making a diagnosis. An accurate medical history is the key 1st step to making a diagnosis and will help inform the examination and determine appropriate investigations. A good clinical history can guide the practitioner to a diagnosis whereas examination and investigations merely confirm or refute that considered diagnosis.

The essentials of good consultation and history taking

- Put the patient at ease.
- Establish a rapport with the patient.
- Use open questions to allow the patient to tell their story. Explore the problem using open and closed questions to clarify and elicit a full history.
- Use your listening skills to be attentive to the patient and the information they provide.
- Remember non-verbal communication is as important as verbal, e.g. eye contact, facial expression, posture, and position.
- Clarify, reflect back, and summarize to verify your understanding of what the patient is saying.
- Explore the patient's ideas and beliefs, concerns, and expectations.
- Establish a logical sequence of events.
- Show empathy and interest.

History taking consists of a series of topics, which move sequentially to explore the whole of the history (Box 8.1).

> **Box 8.1 A sequence to use for history taking includes:**
>
> - Presenting complaint.
> - History of presenting complaint.
> - Previous medical history.
> - Drug history.
> - Family history.
> - Social history.
> - Systems review—general examination.

Presenting complaint

This is a short statement summarizing the patient's presenting symptoms that have brought the patient to seek advice.

History of presenting complaint

An exploration of the symptoms to elicit the cause and effect and factors that precipitated the problem or specific factors that brought on the symptoms. If the patient is able to recount any specific event consider factors such as trauma, overuse, or infections. Infections prior to onset of symptoms are important in viral or reactive forms of arthritis. When the symptoms are insidious in nature they are less likely to be able to pinpoint any specific event.

Pain

As pain is the most common presenting complaint in musculoskeletal medicine it is important to explore the nature of the pain.

A structured approach to the consultation and examination should be undertaken and mnemonics such as SOCRATES may be helpful (see Box 8.2).

Box 8.2 An example of using SOCRATES for exploring pain

S	Site	Where? Radiation? Numbness? Pattern
O	Onset	When and how it started? Changed factors?
C	Character	E.g. type of pain—shooting, burning, tingling?
R	Radiation	Does the pain go elsewhere?
A	Associated feature	Aggravating/relieving factors.
T	Timing	Is it best or worse at different times of day?
E	Exacerbation	Exacerbating or relieving factors.
S	Severity	Rated on a scale of 1–10, e.g. effect on sleep

Previous medical history

Related to an existing diagnosis/longstanding disease? Relevance of past medical history, e.g. associated diagnostic criteria. Previous blood tests, investigations, or presenting features, e.g. an asthmatic using long-term steroids leading to osteoporosis.

Drug history

Past and present if prescribed.

Family history

Predisposing or genetic factors to aid diagnosis, e.g. a family history of IJD.

Social history

Explore the context of the symptoms and how they are affecting the patient.

Systems review

Examination of all health systems to identify all factors that might confirm or reveal signs aiding diagnostic decisions

📖 History taking and clinical examination, Chapter 8, pp.271, 274.

History taking and examination: practical points

There are three key screening questions to ask the patient:
- Do you have any pain or stiffness in your muscles, joints, or spine?
- Are you able to dress or undress yourself without any difficulty?
- Are you able to walk up and downstairs without any difficulty?

In addition to the routine clinical history taking and full examination some specific factors should be considered:
- *Stiffness*: present in both inflammatory and degenerative joint disease. Ask the patient if there is any particular time of day when symptoms are present or worse:
  - Presence of EMS is a classic finding in IJD. Duration of stiffness is an indicator to the severity of the problem, e.g. in poorly controlled inflammatory arthritis (e.g. RA) stiffness can last all day.
  - In contrast, mechanical or degenerative joint disease (e.g. OA) stiffness is usually associated with inactivity or at the end of the day.
- *Swelling*: in the absence of trauma it may be indicative of an inflammatory process:
  - Is the swelling localized or diffuse swelling?
  - Site of swelling, e.g. on the joint line or in the periarticular structures such as tendons (tenosynovitis) or bursae (bursitis)?
  - Patterns of joint involvement aid diagnosis, e.g. distribution of joint involvement in seronegative spondyloarthropathies.
- *Tingling, numbness or parasthesia*: may indicate nerve entrapment, e.g.:
  - Tingling in the thumb, index, middle and half of the ring finger seen in CTS.
  - Numbness and tingling down the leg below the knee—consider sciatica nerve entrapment.
- *Muscle weakness*: is this localized or generalized weakness?
  - Localized weakness indicates a focal problem, e.g. peripheral nerve lesion.
  - Generalized weaknesses—consider a systemic cause such as a myopathy.
- *Deformity*: may be associated with pain but can cause concern to the patient even if symptoms are absent.
  - E.g. Heberden's nodes, on the DIP joints caused by OA, can be quite disfiguring, but are not always painful.
- *Systemic symptoms*: may indicate a more serious inflammatory process or sinister pathology:
  - Weight loss.
  - Anorexia.
  - Fatigue.
  - Malaise.
  - Night sweats.
  - Fever.

- *Sleep disturbance*: several factors may interfere with normal sleep patterns including anxiety and depression. Poor sleep pattern is also a feature of fibromyalgia.

Previous medical history

Are symptoms related to an existing diagnosis/longstanding disease? Explore past medical history for causal factors that may put patient at risk, e.g. an asthmatic using long-term steroids without bone protection leading to osteoporosis.

Drug history

Detailed drug history (past and present):

- Consider a drug side effect (e.g. statins causing myalgias) or precipitating problems (e.g. drug-induced lupus or diuretics precipitating an acute flare of gout).
- Review prescribed medications and benefits of treatment were achieved. May also provide an indication of an existing diagnosis the patient has failed to mention.

Family history

Some rheumatic conditions have a familial predisposition (e.g. family history of psoriasis, uveitis, or inflammatory bowel disease may point to a diagnosis of a spondyloarthropathy).

Social history

Provides an insight into how the condition affects the patient's life. Considerations should include:

- Marital status and dependants.
- Home environment (bathroom facilities, stairs etc.).
- Occupation and ability to maintain work with current symptoms.
- Infrastructures the maintain independence e.g. car owner or ability to access public transport.
- ADL restrictions or problems as a result of current problem, including hobbies and participation in social interaction.
- Psychological status including perceptions related to the presenting complaint, expectations, needs and health beliefs/behaviours will have an effect on the individual's ability to cope with symptoms and possible treatment options. Managing expectations of the patient may need to be negotiated.

Review of systems

This is a methodical approach to examine all health systems to identify any key indicators that may lead to or confirm a diagnosis.

History taking: assessing the patient, p.272.

History taking and clinical examination: systems review

The clinical examination is part of a comprehensive process necessary to identify clinical findings in relation to a patient's presenting complaint. Combined with history taking the clinical examination should enable the practitioner to define abnormalities or indicators that build a diagnostic picture (📖 see Assessing the patient, p.272; 📖 Primary care walk-in clinics, p.208).

Systems review

A full clinical examination should always include a review of all body systems to ensure an accurate diagnostic picture. There are many common characteristics or links in MSC, yet there are also areas where a differential diagnosis is sought between 1 musculoskeletal condition and another (e.g. scleroderma or SLE). Take note of:

- General: weight loss, anorexia, night sweats are all common systemic features of IJD.
- Cardiovascular or respiratory: episode of pleuritic or pericardial pain (SLE); breathlessness may be associated with anaemia of chronic disease (RA) or pulmonary fibrosis (seropositive arthritis); absence of peripheral pulses (vasculitis); haemoptysis (WG).
- GI/abdominal GI symptoms such as diarrhoea (ReA or a seronegative arthritis associated with inflammatory bowel disease if chronic); oesophageal reflux and dysphagia (systemic sclerosis).
- Genitourinary/gynaecological symptoms: urethral discharge (ReA); genital ulceration (Behçet disease); dysparuenia due to vaginal dryness (SS); late miscarriages (APS).
- Skin and mucous membranes: psoriasis, photosensitive rash (SLE or another CTD); oral ulceration (SLE); xerostomia, i.e dry mouth (SS); symptoms of Raynaud's phenomenon worsening in later life or new-onset Raynaud's is associated with CTDs or exacerbated by medications, e.g. beta blockers.
- Eye symptoms, particularly episodes of acute red eyes: conjunctivitis (ReA); uveitis (spondlyoarthropathies); episcleritis (painless); scleritis (painful); keratoconjuctivitis (RA) or xerophthalmia i.e dry eyes (SS); visual disturbance and blindness (temporal arteritis).

General examination including joint examination

Routine checks

All patients with musculoskeletal disease, whether being admitted to a ward or being seen in clinic should have regular assessments that include:

- Urinalysis checked for blood, protein, and glucose:
  - Blood and protein are indicative of renal involvement; particularly important if the patient has a CTD.
  - Blood and protein may indicate an infection in a patient on immunosuppressive therapy, indicating a need for further investigation (e.g. MSU).

- Some drugs require monitoring of the urine for side effects, e.g. ciclosporin, cyclophosphamide.
  - Glycosuria may be present and may indicate the development of diabetes (key in those treated with long-term corticosteroid therapy).
- Blood pressure:
  - ↑ blood pressure may again indicate renal involvement in CTD or hypertension requiring further treatment.
  - Regular monitoring is required for some medications of the blood pressure, e.g. ciclosporin and leflunomide.
- Weight and height should be recorded for baseline measurements:
  - Weight may be required to calculate drug dosages.
  - Height is also useful for assessing if there is a loss of height as a result of osteoporosis.

General principles of joint examination

A good musculoskeletal examination relies on patient cooperation in order for them to relax their muscles so that important clinical signs are not missed:

- Always introduce yourself before undertaking any joint examination.
- Explain what you are going to do and gain the consent of the patient.
- Ask the patient to let you know if they experience any pain or discomfort at any time during the examination.
- Musculoskeletal examination should compare both sides of the body to assess for asymmetry in colour, deformity, swelling, function, and muscle wasting (Figs. 8.1, 8.2).

Gait, arms, legs, spine (GALS)

GALS is a brief and sensitive way of assessing the whole of the musculoskeletal system for any signs of early disease and to identify areas where there is a problem that needs to be examined in more details. It looks at the first movements affected in any musculoskeletal disease or pathology.

Box 8.3 shows the recording of a normal GALS where gait is normal and appearance and movement of arms, legs and spine are all normal. The findings of the GALS can be tabulated in a short hand form where A stands for appearance and M stands for movement.

> **Box 8.3 A normal GALS**
>
> | | A | M |
> |-------|---|---|
> | Gait | A | M |
> | Arms | ✓ | ✓ |
> | Legs | ✓ | ✓ |
> | Spine | ✓ | ✓ |

📖 Also see Musculoskeletal physical examination, pp.186, 271; 📖 Primary care walk-in clinics, p.208.

If an inflammatory arthritis is suspected

Patients may present and there may be a strong index of suspicion based upon the clinical assessment that the presenting signs and symptoms identify a possible inflammatory arthritis.

An important assessment tool for on-going management of RA is the 28-joint Disease Assessment Score (DAS28). Tender and swollen joints commonly affected are examined and scored, together with bloods for ESR or CRP and a patient global assessment of their general well-being using a VAS. The DAS28 has been validated for use with either ESR or CRP. However, whichever blood test is used the subsequent assessments should use the same blood test for calculating DAS28. The calculation (using a DAS calculator) provides a composite score, e.g. 5.15, the DAS28 score. The DAS28 score for eligibility criteria for treatment with biologic drugs is under review but currently set at 5.15.

📖 Also see Rheumatoid arthritis: assessing and managing the disease, p.62.

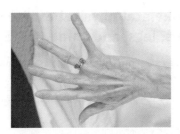

Fig. 8.1 Examination of hands. Reproduced with permission from Castledine G, Close A (2009). *Oxford Handbook of General and Adult Nursing.* Oxford University Press, Oxford.

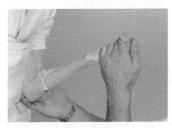

Fig. 8.2 Examination of arms. Reproduced with permission from Castledine G, Close A (2009). *Oxford Handbook of General and Adult Nursing.* Oxford University Press, Oxford.

Musculoskeletal physical examination: gait, arms, legs, and spine (GALS)

There are 3 key screening questions to ask the patient:
- Do you have any pain or stiffness in your muscles, joints, or spine?
- Are you able to dress or undress yourself without any difficulty?
- Are you able to walk up and downstairs without any difficulty?

Gait
Observe the patient walking, turning, and walking back.
- Look for symmetry of movement in the arms, legs, and pelvic movements, normal stride length, and the ability to turn quickly.
- Observe for an asymmetric antalgic gait where pain and deformity causes the patient to hurry from 1 leg onto the other.

Inspection of the patient in standing anatomical position
- Observe from posterior, anterior, and lateral views.
- Inspect for normal muscle bulk and symmetry of shoulder girdles, spine, arms, buttocks, thighs and calves.
- Observe for any obvious signs of swollen or deformed joints, including knees and toes or signs of flexion deformity, e.g. at the elbows.
- Inspect for normal spinal curves—cervical lordosis, thoracic kyphosis, lumbar lordosis, or signs of scoliosis in the spine.
- Look at symmetry of level iliac crests, gluteal folds.
- Signs of valgus or varus deformities in the knees or ankles, hip or knee flexion deformities, or signs of hyperextension of the knee (known as genu recurvatum).
- Signs of rheumatoid nodules of extensors surfaces of elbows and Achilles tendons.
- Signs of olecranon bursitis (at the elbow) or Achilles bursitis.
- Normal alignment and thickness of the Achilles tendon.
- Popliteal swelling, indicating a Baker's cyst.
- Loss of the medial arches of the foot.
- Ask patient to open their jaw and move it from side to side (temperomandibular joint).
- Ask the patient to try and put their ear to their shoulder on each side (lateral flexion of cervical spine).
- Press over midpoint of supraspinatus muscle, and roll the skin over the trapezius muscle. A wince and withdraw indicates the hyperalgesic response of fibromyalgia.
- Ask the patient to bend forward from the waist to touch the toes, place a couple of fingers over the spinous processes and see if they move together on standing upright (if they do not this may be a sign of inflammatory spine disease).
- Place the patient's hands behind their head and push their elbows back (this tests abduction and external rotation of the shoulders as well as flexion at the elbows).

- Keeping their elbows tucked in ask the patient to bring their hands up to in front:
  - Inspect the palms of the hands for swelling, wasting or other deformity
  - Turn hands over keeping elbows tucked in to side (this test pronation and supination of both elbows and wrist).
  - Inspect dorsum of hands for muscle wasting, swelling, and deformity.
  - Inspect the nails for any signs of pitting or onycholysis (seen in psoriatis), nailfold infarct, or splinter haemorrhages (possible vasculitis activity).
  - Ask the patient to make a fist, test power grip.
  - Touch the pulp of each of the fingers to the thumb (opposition).
  - Squeeze across the MCP joints—pain indicate signs of inflammatory synovitis.

Examination of the patient lying on the couch

- Ask the patient to bend their knee and bring their heel as close in to their buttock as they can, 1 leg at a time.
- Place your hand over the knee to feel for any crepitus.
- Whilst the knee is flexed, take the hip up to 90° and internally rotate the hip:
  - Achieved by holding the lower part of the leg and pushing the foot outwards.
  - Note how far the hip moves—in ♀ this ROM is >♂.
  - Early disease in the hip will elicit pain radiating into the groin.
- Return the leg to the neutral straight position and test for any signs of swelling using:
  - A balloon and bulge sign.
  - A patellar tap.
- Inspect the feet for any signs of deformity.
- Inspect the toe nails (as for the finger nails).
- Inspect the soles of the feet for any signs of callus formation due to subluxation of the metatarsal heads.
- Squeeze across the metatarsals—pain on doing this is indicative of signs of synovitis in the metatarsals.

📖 See Box 8.3 for an example of a normal GALS chart, p.278.

📖 Also see Regional examination of the musculoskeletal system, p.186; 📖 Primary care walk-in clinics, p.208; 📖 History taking and clinical examination, p.272.

Regional examination of the musculoskeletal system

Regional examination of the musculoskeletal system (REMS) is a system of examination developed to ensure that examinations are conducted in a standardized way.

The key steps in any musculoskeletal examination are:
- Look.
- Feel.
- Move.
- Function.

Look

- Always start with a visual inspection of the patient at rest.
- Compare both sides for symmetry.
- Look for skin changes, scars, muscle bulk, and swelling in and around the joint and the periarticular structures.
- Also look for any signs of deformity in alignment and posture of the joint.

Feel

- Feel the skin for temperature using the back of the hand, in particular across the joint line and at other relevant sites.
- Any swellings should be assessed for fluctuance and mobility.
- Hard, bony swellings of OA can be distinguished from the soft, boggy swelling of synovitis in IJD.
- Tenderness is an important clinical sign to elicit both in and around the joint.
- Synovitis is detected by the triad of warmth, swelling, and tenderness around the joint line.

Move

- The full ROM of the joint should be assessed.
- Both sides need to be compared.
- As a general rule both active and then passive movement should be assessed. (Active is where the patient moves, passive where the examiner moves the joint.)
- When examining the joint, loss of full flexion or extension should be detected and that restriction recorded as mild, moderate, or severe restriction in ROM.
- The quality of the movement should also be noted with reference to abnormalities such as crepitus being recorded.
- In some instance the joint may move beyond the normal range—this is called hypermobility.

Function

It is important as part of a musculoskeletal examination to relate findings to function, e.g. .limited elbow flexion—can the patient still feed themselves?

📖 Also see Musculoskeletal physical examination, p.280; 📖 Regional examination of the musculoskeletal system, p.186; 📖 Primary care walk-in clinics, p.208; 📖 History taking and clinical examination, p.272.

Examination of the upper limbs

Examination of the hand and wrist

Look

- With hands palm down look for obvious swelling, deformity, posture, muscle wasting particularly of the interossius muscles of the back of the hand, and scarring.
- Look at the skin for thinning and bruising (steroid use) or rashes.
- Look for nail changes of psoriasis (pitting and onycholysis), splinter haemorrhages, ands nail-fold infarct (vasculitis).
- Which joints are affected, are the changes symmetrical or asymmetrical?
- Ask the patient to turn their hands over.
- Inspect the palmar aspect of the hands, look for the same things as palms down, in particular wasting of the thenar and hypothenar eminences, signs of palmar erythema.

📖 Also see Connective tissue disease, p.115.

Feel

- Assess for temperature over the joint lines of wrist, MCP, PIP, and DIP joints using the back of the hand.
- Feel for radial pulses.
- Gently squeeze across the MCP joints to assess for tenderness.
- Feel for swelling and tenderness over each of the joint lines and over the tendon sheaths.
- Test for median and ulnar nerve sensation by stroking over the thenar and hypothenar eminences.
- Assess radial sensation over the web space of the thumb and index finger.
- Palpate the patients' wrists.
- Feel up the arm to the elbow to look and feel for rheumatoid nodules or psoriatic plaques over the extensor surface.

Move

- Ask the patient to straighten their fingers fully.
- Get the patient to make a fist (power grip).
- Assess wrist flexion and extension, with patient actively doing, then passively.
- Touch finger pulp of each finger to thumb (pincer grip).
- Move each joint passively feeling for crepitus.

Function

- Ask the patient to grip your 2 fingers to assess power grip.
- Ask the patient to pinch your finger to assess pincer grip.
- Ask the patient to pick up a small object such as a coin or paper clip from your hand. This is to assess pincer grip and function.

📖 Also see Primary care walk-in clinics, p.208; 📖 Regional musculoskeletal conditions, p.186.

Examination of the elbow

Look
- Skin changes (scars, psoriatic plaques).
- Swelling (synovitis, bursitis over the olecranon process, rheumatoid nodules).
- Deformity or muscle wasting.

Feel
- Temperature.
- Joint line for:
  - Swelling.
  - Tenderness.
  - Crepitus on movement.
- Medial and lateral epicondyles for tenderness.
- Olecranon bursa for swelling and tenderness.

Move
- Active and passive flexion and extension, pronation and supination.
- Compare 1 side to the other.

Function
- Being able to get hand to mouth is an important function of the elbow.

Shoulder examination

Look
- From the front (skin changes, scars, swelling, attitude).
- From behind (wasting, deformity).
- Compare both sides, are they symmetrical?
- Is posture normal?

Feel
Palpate in turn the sternoclavicular joint, acromioclavicular joint, and glenohumeral joint for:
- Temperature.
- Joint line tenderness.
- Swelling or crepitus.
- Palpate the muscle bulk of supraspinatus, infraspinatus, and deltoid.
- Identify any muscle tenderness.

Move
Active ROM:
- Ask the patient to put their hands behind their head and then behind their back.
- Abduction (assessing for scapular movement and painful arc).
- Flexion and extension.
- Internal and external rotation with the elbow flexed at 90° and held by the patient's side.

Passive range of movement, if active movement is restricted.

Function
- Includes getting the hands behind the head and behind the back as these movements are needed for washing and grooming.

Examination of the lower limbs

Hip examination

Look

Inspection of the patient when standing:
- From the front for a pelvic tilt or rotational deformity.
- From the side for flexion deformity or scars overlying the hip
- From behind for muscle wasting (gluteal muscle bulk in particular).
- Is there any suggestion of leg length inequality?
- Measure real leg length with a tape measure.

Feel
- Palpate over the greater trochanter.

Move
- Assess full hip flexion with the knee flexed at 90°; observe the patient's face for signs of pain.
- Assess for fixed flexion deformity of the hip by performing Thomas' test. To do this, fully flex hip whilst the opposite hip is observed to see if it lifts off the couch, if it does this confirms a fixed flexion deformity in that hip.
- Assess internal and external rotation with the knee in 90° flexion, passively—often limited particularly in internal rotation in hip disease.
- A Trendelenburg test involves the patient standing on 1 leg., if there is any hip disease the pelvis dips on the non-weight-bearing side when the patient stands on the affected hip.

Function

Inspection of the walking patient:
- Do they have an antalgic gait which is a painful gait resulting in a limp?
- A Trendelenburg gait seen when proximal muscle weakness results in and as a result the patient walks with a waddling gait.

Knee

Look
- Inspection of the patient on the couch.
- Attitude.
- Skin changes, scars, psoriasis.
- Swelling.
- Valgus or varus deformity.
- Quadriceps wasting.

Feel
- For temperature ↑ using the back of the hand.
- Palpate the borders of the patella for tenderness.
- With the knee flexed palpate for joint line tenderness.
- Feel in the popliteal fossa for swelling (Baker's cyst).
- Insertion of the collateral ligaments.
- Effusion—include bulge sign, patellar tap, and balloon sign.

Move
- Assess full flexion and extension actively and passively.

- Assess stability of the collateral ligaments of the knee by placing the leg in 15° of flexion and alternately stressing the joint line on each side, by placing 1 hand on the opposite side of the joint line to that which you are testing.
- Anterior drawer test for anterior cruciate ligaments is performed by placing both hands around the upper tibia, with thumbs over the tibial tuberosity and index fingers tucked under the hamstrings to make sure they are relaxed. Stabilize the lower tibia with the upper forearm and gently pull the upper tibia forward. If there is any laxity of the anterior cruciate ligaments there will be a significant degree of movement.

Function
Inspection of the patient in standing
- From the front for genu varus, genu valgus.
- From the side for flexion deformity, posterior tibial subluxation, genu recurvertum.
- Inspection of the walking patient.

Foot and ankle
Look
With the patient sitting on the bed:
- Observe the feet, comparing both side for symmetry.
- Inspect the dorsal surface for skin changes, nail changes, and scars.
- Look for alignment of the toes and evidence of hallux valgus of the big toe.
- Look for joint clawing of the toes, swelling, and callus formation.
- Soles of the feet for callus formation, adventitious bursae.
- Inspect the patient's footwear for any abnormal wearing or evidence of poor fit. Also look at any orthoses.

With the patient weight-bearing:
- Look at the forefoot for toe alignment and the midfoot for foot arch position.
- From behind look at the Achilles tendon for thickening or swelling.
- Observe for normal alignment of the hindfoot; in disease of the ankle there may be varus or valgus deformity at the ankle.

Feel
- Temperature over the foot and ankle and check for peripheral pulses.
- Metatarsal squeeze for MTP joint tenderness.
- Palpate the midfoot, ankle, and sub-talar joint for tenderness.

Move
- Move actively and passively assessing for pain, crepitus, ↓ ROM.
- True ankle joint—dorsiflexion and plantar flexion.
- Subtalar joint—abduction and adduction.
- Midtarsal joints—inversion and eversion.
- 1st MTP joint—flexion and extension.

Function
- If not already done, assess the patient's gait for the normal cycle of heel strike, stance, toe off, and swing.

Examination of the spine

Look

At the patient when standing:
- From the back for any signs of scoliosis, muscle spasm, pelvic tilt, skin changes.
- From the side for normal cervical lordosis, thoracic kyphosis, and lumbar lordosis (see Fig. 8.3).

Feel

Palpate the spine starting at the occiput to the sacrum and sacroiliac joints feeling for:
- Temperature.
- Swelling.
- Paraspinal muscles for spasm or tenderness.
- Spinous processes for alignment or local tenderness.

Move

With patient standing:
- Lumbar spine flexion and extension (assess using fingers on a couple of spinous processes).
- Lateral flexion of lumbar spine, by asking the patient to run each hand in turn down the outside of the adjacent leg.

With the patient sitting:
- Thoracic spine rotation.
- Cervical spine movements of flexion, extension, lateral flexion, and rotation.
- With the patient lying as flat as possible perform a SLR.
- Assess limb reflexes (upper and lower) and dorsiflexion of the big toe.

📖 Also see Neck and spine, pp.212, 214.

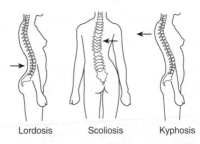

Lordosis   Scoliosis   Kyphosis

Fig. 8.3 Abnormal spine curvature. Reproduced with permission from Castledine G, Close A (2009). *Oxford Handbook of General and Adult Nursing*. Oxford University Press, Oxford.

Symptom control: using pharmacological and non-pharmacological methods

Overview

The most common presenting symptom for MSC is that of pain. Pain is a complex phenomenon and a number of contributing factors can ease or exacerbate the perceived pain. Pain may be as a result of new trauma or a progressive deterioration of condition. These conditions may be mild, self-limiting, or progressive. Reported symptoms other than pain may include fatigue, depression, poor sleep patterns, or deterioration in functional ability.

The essential components of achieving symptom control require a comprehensive assessment. Good clinical history taking and a thorough physical examination need to be considered in the context of symptom control and clinical assessment tools Pain can be experienced by the individual in the joint itself, surrounding tissues, or as referred pain.

Assessment

All management must focus on identifying effective methods to evaluate symptoms such as pain, stiffness, and fatigue.

Assessment of the overall condition

- How active (acute) is the condition or disease presenting?
- Can the presenting symptoms be attributed to a chronic condition previously diagnosed?
- If presenting symptoms are related to an underlying condition is the disease well controlled? Are medications being taken appropriately?
- Are the presenting symptoms debilitating/self-limiting or do they indicate a medical emergency such as a septic arthritis?

Factors that influence levels of perceived pain/functional changes

Following a full physical examination to elicit physical changes, other factors should be considered including key indicators that might influence the individual perceptions of pain. Consider social and psychological assessments that include:

- The level of social support and social need that may have an impact on perceptions of pain and achieving symptom control.
- Cultural and religious beliefs. In some communities pain is to be borne and accepted as natural phenomenon or a form of retribution.

Assessing disease activity

Some MSC have global objective measures to assist in assessing disease activity. A 1st approach should include:

- Examination of joint or joints affected (comparing against unaffected joint):
  - Are they tender, swollen, hot or red?
  - Able to function normally and weight-bear? With or without pain?
- Are there any indicators from blood tests such as inflammatory markers that might guide the clinical picture? E.g. CRP, ESR, uric acid, or changes in complement levels (C3 and C4).
- How do these markers compare to recent or last investigations?
- Are there other factors that may exacerbate the condition, e.g. intercurrent infections or other comorbidities, poorly controlled (e.g. control of diabetes, chronic obstructive pulmonary disease (COPD))?

Management

On completion of the comprehensive assessment a decision needs to be made as to whether the perceived changes in symptom control are as a result of changes in disease/poor understanding of the condition or are non-disease-related factors (e.g. for medication concordance, stress of social/psychological issues which impact on the individual) which may be improved by non-pharmacological options. E.g. non-pharmacological options include:

- Information on the conditions and understanding symptoms. Empowering the individual to self-manage is an important component of achieving symptom control.
- Non-pharmacological options include walking aids, appropriate footwear to manage load bearing and impact, muscle strengthening exercises, and joint protection.
- Additional non-pharmacological strategies that individuals can readily use in the home include cold and warm packs, rest and relaxation, and the use of assistive devices or splinting to protect joints.

If the assessment indicates an ↑ in the level of disease control or disease activity consider:

- Concordance of current medication regimens—dose and frequency.
- Drug interactions that may have an effect on medication regimens— e.g. an episode of diarrhoea and vomiting will effect absorption.

If the global picture supports a change in disease control/activity with patient reported changes, review with prescribing clinician to review treatment options. Patients may require:

- Change in drug therapy.
- ↑ dose of current treatment or change in route of administration, e.g. subcutaneous injection for those failing to tolerate oral therapy (e.g. MTX).
- The addition of another drug therapy (combination therapy).
- Treatment to manage side effects altering bio-availability or a review of blood picture to consider any toxicities.
- Exclusion of a new disease process or exacerbation of a comorbidity (e.g. diabetes or GI disorders).

In some cases the picture can be mixed with evidence of some aspects of disease exacerbation and factors that could be considered poor symptom control. Specialist nursing advice may be to guide management.

📖 Also see Assessing the patient, p.272; 📖 Assessment tools p.539; 📖 Rapid access and emergency issues p.379; 📖 Blood tests and investigations p.461; 📖 Pharmacological management p.419.

Assessing pain

MSCs in the UK cause a significant burden to the individual and society with high levels of incapacity claims and loss of work. The relief of pain is a basic human right yet there is still much to be done to improve symptom control for those with debilitating musculoskeletal pain. The interpretation of pain is an individual unique experience based upon perceptions of altered bodily sensations. It is a subjective, multi-faceted phenomenon affecting sensory and emotional experiences that influence the perception and experience of pain. Pain can be classified in a number of ways.

• Acute or chronic.
• Chronic malignant or nonmalignant pain (benign).
• Inflammatory or non-inflammatory.

Not all pain will require medications to relieve it but a thorough assessment of the issues involved in the patient's experience of pain together with any underlying disease process that may require modification to reduce the sensation of pain is required. Factors that must be considered include physical, social, spiritual, and emotional aspects of the patient experience related to the pain.

Factors that affect pain include:

Pathophysiology

• Tissue damage, e.g. neurological damage or injury to soft tissues.
• A review of underlying disease activity, e.g. inflammatory component for IJDs such as ReA or gout.

The nature of the pain

• The patient-reported symptoms of pain including evaluation of the level of pain experienced by the individual (quality and quantity):
  • E.g. the use of VASs to assess the level of pain.
• Relieving or exacerbating factors.
• Distribution of pain, e.g. distribution represents neurological pathways.
• Type of pain experience:
  • Intermittent or constant.
  • Trauma (sudden/acute episode) or insidious onset (relapsing and remitting).
  • Description of the pain sensation (shooting, pins and needles).
  • Affect on bodily functions/functional ability.

⚠ Night pain waking a patient at night is an indicator of inflammation.

Personal interpretation of sensations

• Prior experiences of pain.
• Cultural and ethnic beliefs and interpretations of pain.
• Social and psychological factors that influence the individual's ability to interpret painful symptoms.

Consider the consultation in the context of practitioner and patient-centred models of consultation. A mnemonic to aid recall—PQRST:

• P = provoked by.
• Q = quality and quantity.
• R = region and where does it radiate to.

- S = severity.
- T = timing.

The nursing process

- Recognition that the pain is 'real'. Providing empathy and support.
- Listening to the patient and their experience/sensations of pain.
- Identify factors that exacerbate or relieve symptoms.
- Explore the context of the pain experience:
  - Sudden or insidious onset.
  - Interpretation of pain (attitudes, beliefs, cultural factors).
  - Exacerbating psychological factors (e.g. fear and anxiety).
- Current symptom relieving strategies (pharmacological and non-pharmacological) and the efficacy.
- Interpreting the level of pain using tools that aid in the nurse/patient therapeutic relationship—informed and shared decision making.
- Negotiate a goal setting approach to optimize pain control using a range of pharmacological and non-pharmacological options.
- Set agreed review process to evaluate changes in pain sensations following planned pain relieving strategies.

Measuring pain and its effects

The VAS is a recognized simple clinical tool consisting of a horizontal 10cm line (Fig. 9.1). The patient is asked to mark along the 10cm line the point which reflects their perceived pain at that time. The mark is then measured using a ruler to attribute the number along the line (e.g. 8 out of total score of 10).

Other examples of pain assessment tools include:
- Body maps (pictorial) or verbal rating scales (the use of word to describe pain).
- Faces pain scales (pictorial – may be useful with language/communication barriers).
- Pain questionnaires such as the McGill Pain Questionnaire.
- Scales to assess for the older person with cognitive impairment/communication problems (e.g. the DOLOPLUS 2 scale).
- Other tools to assess mood, function, cognition, health beliefs.

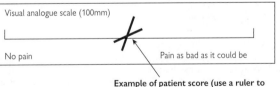

Fig. 9.1 Example of a VAS scale (note not to scale). The cross indicates the patient's measure of their pain over the last week.

Assessment of pain: red and yellow flags

Introduction

The principle of using an assessment approach that refers to 'red' or 'yellow' flags has been used for some 30 years. The red and yellow flag system allows clinicians to have a rapid system of identifying high-risk indicators when undertaking a clinical examination.

Red flags—medical

A red flag approach enables treatments/assessments to be undertaken by non-medical teams provided they were able to identify those requiring rapid referral for medical examination (red flag). They are often used in a pathway approach or protocol where most of the common pathology is identified and guidance is included in the pathway—depending upon the expertise and facilities available to investigate.

The use of red flags works as a teaching aid, enhancing the need to identify key diagnostic criteria that prompt rapid screening, investigation, and treatment. There are different red flags according to the bodily system being reviewed. Red flags usually identify relatively rare but important diagnostic factors that may indicate serious disease requiring further medical examination.

Signs of symptoms that indicate serious underlying pathology might include features that indicate:
- Neurological disease.
- Malignancy.
- Infections.
- Fractures.

An example of red flags for back pain can be seen in Box 9.1.

Box 9.1 Example of red flags for back pain

- Night pain.
- Pyrexia + sweats.
- Weight loss.
- High ESR.
- History of malignancy.
- Altered sphincter disturbances + neurological deficit/impairment.

Yellow flags—psychological

The other important indicators that need to be identified in care are those that indicate underlying psychological issues that may require further specialist or medical support. Yellow flags are used to identify prognostic indicators that may require further assessment and will affect outcomes or indicate an additional psychological component to the presenting condition. These factors may require further investigation/referral or require additional consideration during the consultation (Box 9.2).

Box 9.2 Example of yellow flags for pain

- Family history.
- Previous pain syndrome.
- Pain-related work problems.
- Poor coping skills/difficult life challenges.
- Previous history of depression/anxiety.
- Unresolved post-viral symptoms.
- Poor sleep patterns.
- Significant emotional distress.

Symptom control: pain relief

Pharmacological and non-pharmacological treatments

Achieving symptom control for those presenting with a wide range of MSCs requires:

- A patient-centred consultation that includes thorough musculoskeletal examination and history taking and exploration of the patient's perspective on the condition, personal impact, expectations, anxieties, and fears.
- Information should be provided about the condition, prognosis, and treatment choices (written and verbal).
- Recognition of the value of practical aspects of symptom control that enhance self-management.
- Access or signposting to voluntary or community support that can complement healthcare support.

In some circumstances additional support may be required, such as:

- Prompt referral to specialist expertise for those with long-term systemic inflammatory conditions—such as SLE, CTDs, IJDs (e.g. RA, AS, and PsA).
- Cognitive behavioural therapy (CBT).
- Referral or specific guidance on occupational health advice related to work-related functional issues.
- Advice may be required on welfare/financial issues such as those provided by the Citizen's Advice Bureau or how to claim incapacity benefit.

📖 Also see Chronic non-inflammatory pain, p.171.

Pharmacological options

Patients should be advised when effective pain relief is sought that medications should be taken at regular intervals and treatment should not be delayed until the pain becomes unbearable. Pharmacological options should be complemented by non-pharmacological options to achieve maximum treatment effect. Nurses should consider using the WHO analgesic pain ladder if it is an appropriate choice, taking into account the degree of pain experienced and previous pharmacological approach. For example, a person experiencing severe pain from septic arthritis may not achieve effective pain control using paracetamol, rest, and cold packs. Advice on dose and frequency of administration are essential for effective pain control (see Box 9.3).

Non-pharmacological options

The use of non-pharmacological options should be encouraged. A wide range of options can be offered to suit to presenting problems, preferences of the patient, and ability to carry out procedures/treatment plans. (Box 9.1) In some circumstances CBT may also be helpful, particularly if higher levels of psychological support are required to aid rehabilitation.

📖 Also see Chronic non-inflammatory pain, p.171.

Box 9.3 Pharmacological and non-pharmacological options

Therapeutic options
- Simple analgesia (non-opioid): paracetamol—advise on dose and frequency.
- Compound analgesia (simple analgesia with opioid component):
  - Co-codamol—different dose regimens.
  - Nefopam hydrochloride.
- Topical anti-inflammatory, rubefacients, or capsaicin:
  - Topical NSAIDS—diclofenac sodium, ibuprofen, ketoprofen.
  - Rubefacients—create a deep heat sensation.
  - Capsaicin creams—chilli pepper inhibits substance P.
- NSAIDs (which includes COX-2 inhibitors).
- Opiod (short- or long-acting)
  - Tramadol hydrochloride—short acting.
  - Transdermal fentanyl patches—long acting.

Supporting therapies
- Amitriptyline for neuropathic pain—given at a lower dose than used to treat depression.
- Pregabalin, an anti-epileptic therapy, may also be effective in neuropathic pain.
- Corticosteroids can aid pain relief in inflammatory condition—taken orally for systemic effect, or IA, or soft tissue injections (local benefit to swollen joint).
- Hyaluronic acid courses may provide relief to those with knee OA.
  - ◈ Further evidence required for cost-effectiveness/benefit

Non-pharmacological options
- Information, advice, and support (patient support groups) advice lines.
- Guidance on condition, prognosis, and treatment choices.
- Joint protective devices—splints, kettle tippers, walking sticks, orthotics.
- Exercise (improves mood) and muscle strength.
- Pacing, rest, relaxation, distraction techniques.
- Self-management programme—e.g. EPPs.
- Goal setting, problem solving approach/stress management.

Options with limited evidence base include:
- Thermotherapy—use of hot or cold.
- TENS.
- Complementary therapies:
  - Glucosamine sulfate.
  - Fish oils for OA. RA patients have an ↑ risk of cardiovascular disease so may warrant offering this as a choice for patients to consider.
  - Acupuncture—some evidence in OA.
- Swimming programme.

NB the limited level of risk/harm related to some of these options warrant consideration particularly when enhancing patient-perceived self-efficacy.

Symptom control: depression and fatigue

Fatigue and depression are strongly associated with pain. For those with a MSC, the pivotal factor that drives them to seek medical advice is that of relieving their pain. The pain itself, the fear of pain, and what pain 'means' causes a severe burden on the individual. Unrelieved pain, changes to functional ability (such as ↓ ROM), and disturbed sleep can build up a picture of negative attitudes and beliefs resulting in:

- Fatigue.
- A sense of vulnerability.
- Poor self-esteem and threats perceived.
- Self-efficacy related to positive health behaviours.
- Depression/anger/apathy.
- Loss of motivation.

Patients require early and effective support to prevent a downward spiral of ↑ disability, fatigue, depression, and potential loss of their role in society (work, independence). Depression and fatigue are complex phenomenon with a number of causes and contributing factors. Depression, fatigue, and pain are strongly linked with poor healthcare outcomes. These factors are also important to consider in the context of functional ability in MSCs.

Definition of depression

Depression is a general term to describe a negative change in mood. This change can be seen as a normal process, e.g. a short-lived low mood might be as a result of a temporary response to an event. Depression is commonly reported for those with LTCs. Social isolation and economic distress are linked to depression. Clinical depression is defined as symptoms lasting >2 weeks, and are so severe they affect ADL.

People with depression may report:

- Negative emotions—feeling of unhappiness, everything is a problem.
- Apathy—loss of interest in previous hobbies, activities, food.
- Poor self-esteem and loss of expressions of emotions.
- Sleep disturbances—insomnia, early wakening.
- Poor concentration and irritability.
- Feelings of being 'changed'.
- May have 'real' physical symptoms, unrelieved by treatment.

Definition of fatigue

Fatigue is characterized by feelings of exhaustion or weariness which may be directly attributed to the use of excessive energy. Fatigue related to long-term MSCs can also be as a result of coping with unrelieved pain and stiffness in combination with active disease and/or an anaemia of chronic disease. Functional ability and the additional energy required to undertake normal ADL when there is functional impairment should also be considered when assessing fatigue. The interpretation of fatigue is also a subjective state related to an awareness of ↓ capacity for physical or mental activity.

Depression and fatigue

Depression and fatigue are symptoms that can be subject to an underlying pathology but also affected by psychosocial issues. It can sometimes be difficult to unravel the social and psychological factors when a patient with a chronic non-inflammatory condition (such as fibromyalgia) reports depression and fatigue, particularly as the diagnosis of the condition itself results chiefly upon a group of self-reported symptoms.

A nursing assessment in the context of depression and fatigue

To understand and support patients with depression and fatigue good practice should ensure:

- Ensure early access to a healthcare professional.
- Provide a patient-centred and holistic assessment.
- Use validated tools to measure depression (e.g. Hospital Anxiety and Depression Scale) and fatigue (SF36 vitality subscale).
- Identify contributing factors that may precipitate depression/fatigue.
- Build a framework of support that is based upon encouraging active coping styles and self-management principles.
- Avoid reliance on medication and 'quick fixes' for those conditions/patients that may have strong psychosocial issues:
  - Identify social vulnerabilities/needs.
  - Psychological factors and any prior treatments offered.
- Identify physical factors that may lead to depression or fatigue:
  - Poor disease control of inflammatory conditions—anaemia, weight loss, ↑ inflammatory markers.
  - Prior history of depression or poor mental health.
  - Functional limitations ↑ burden on ADL.
  - Unrelieved pain which disturb sleep.
  - Adverse side effects to medications.

Useful advice

Depression and fatigue combined with poor pain control may require referral to specialist support for:

- Diagnosis and treatment of any underlying condition (e.g. RA) or management of depression.
- Prompt referral to pain management teams.
- If a long-term MSC—review of disease control.

Practical support to give the patient

- Exercise—goal setting-approach graded appropriate exercise programme.
- Review diet.
- Pacing, rest, and relaxation.
- Manage contributing factors to fatigue:
  - Poor sleep patterns.
  - Inflammatory disease or poor disease control.
  - Anaemias or anaemias related to chronic disease.
  - Psychosocial factors—consider CBT.

Further reading

Callaghan P, Waldock H (2006). *Oxford Handbook of Mental Health Nursing*. Oxford University Press, Oxford.

Supporting patients with pain

Patients who experience pain need recognition that their pain is real and that support and guidance is available to help them achieve symptom control.

The impact of unrelieved pain

- Poor self-esteem.
- Depression.
- Fatigue.
- Disturbed sleep.
- Reduction in functional ability.
- Poor perceived self-efficacy and self-esteem.
- Negative health behaviours.
- Inability to carry out normal ADL e.g. changes to career progression/redundancy.

Interpretation of pain

The unpleasant sensations associated with pain will differ from person to person based upon a range of factors including:

- Underlying disease pathology.
- Social and psychological factors related to prior experiences of pain and cultural beliefs related to pain.
- Interpretation of what the pain 'means' to the individual (fear of malignancy), level of incapacity as a result of the pain.
- Nature of the pain—relapsing, unremitting.

Patients will need information and guidance on why they are experiencing pain and what options there are to relieve the symptoms. The nursing assessment process should be used to encourage the patient to be an active participant in their management and review of how effective pain relieving strategies have worked. Assessment tools must be used to allow a level of objective review of pain scores and treatment effect (e.g. VAS)

Common mistakes

In many cases patients are not advised about the basic principles of how pain works. As a result there are common mistakes that patients make in managing their symptoms. These include:

- Only taking pain relief when the pain gets really 'bad'.
- Not taking regular doses over a 24-hour period, choosing to take a large dose infrequently.
  - This may result in discarding simple analgesia given regularly (e.g. paracetamol for OA).
- Failure to advise on the non-pharmacological options, e.g.:
  - Rest and relaxation, cold packs.
  - Use of aids (walking sticks) e.g. functional problems related to knee pain.

Also see Assessing pain, p.292; Chronic non-inflammatory pain, p.171.

Further reading

Arthritis Research Campaign. Information leaflets on pain: ⌐ www.arc.org.uk

Beckwith S, Franklin P (2006). *Oxford Handbook of Nurse Prescribing*. Oxford University Press, Oxford.

Hakim A, Clunie G, Haq I (eds) (2006). *Oxford Handbook of Rheumatology*, 2nd edn. Oxford University Press, Oxford.

The British Pain Society. Pain scales in multiple languages: ⌐ www.britishpainsociety.org

The National Rheumatoid Arthritis Society. Information on how pain works: ⌐ www.rheumatoid.org.uk

Frequently asked questions

Is a goal setting approach helpful in trying to improve symptom control?

Patient-centred goals can be set in a structured and formal way that includes regular reviews and revision of goals. In other cases a more informal approach may be sufficient. (A goal may be simply by the next appointment the patient will have stepped down their paracetamol dose to 500mg a day at lunchtime from 1g.)

Goal setting can be effective if used as part of a patient-centred assessment. Goals should be small and achievable and may help to dispel anxieties or prior learnt health behaviours that reinforce negative thoughts about symptom control. Once positive results are achieved it is easier to build upon these goals and increase self-efficacy (belief that they have some control over their condition and how to manage symptoms).

All treatment options can then be refined and reduced/changed according to the assessment and review following goal setting.

How do I decide which treatment options (pharmacological and non-pharmacological) are most appropriate for each patient?

Pharmacological and non-pharmacological options should be offered as an overall package. The nurse should offer the patient a range of approaches/practical tools they can use themselves to improve control and importantly enhance self-management principles. Important factors to consider include:

- The patient's health assessment and underlying risk factors (e.g. if high cardiovascular risk NSAIDs/COX-2 therapies may be contraindicated) (🕮 See Pharmacological management pain relief, p.403).
- Decisions should consider the patient's informed decision following education about their condition and potential risks and benefits of treatment options.
- All symptom control should consider treatments that provide the maximum benefit but most importantly with the least possible risk acceptable to the patient and the clinician. Consider advising on how to manage the side effect of medications, e.g. the use of bulking agents when patients start pain relieving medications that may result in constipation.
- Treatment should consider the degree to which symptoms are distressing/affecting the patient and how they rate their symptoms (e.g. high VAS score for pain).
- The healthcare professionals' knowledge of the condition and guidelines/evidence related to best treatment options in the context of a disease assessment.
- Prior treatments tried and prior side effects or benefits of that treatment.
- Treatment benefits should be reviewed in the context of symptoms and benefits. Patients should be educated on how to step up or step down treatment wherever possible.

Practical advice for self-limiting conditions

Musculoskeletal disorders cover a wide range of conditions. It is no surprise ∴ that from time to time individuals may present with a wide range of problems related to joint or soft tissue disorders. Many of these are general short-term problems that require appropriate treatment and advice with resolution over a short time frame (treatment, surgery, or spontaneous resolution).

Conditions that require specialist support

Patients who have systemic, life-threatening or long-term inflammatory conditions that require on going specialist management. These include:
- CTDs, e.g. SLE, scleroderma, WG.
- IJDs, e.g. RA, PsA, AS.
- Metabolic bone diseases, e.g. osteoporosis.
- Infections, e.g. septic arthritis.
- Orthopaedic trauma.

These problems outlined next may be confined to pain or functional limitations related to a joint or the soft tissues surrounding the joint.

Examples of self-limiting conditions include:
- Back pain—early access to advice is essential for the best outcome.
- Injuries related to falls or trauma.
- Soft tissue disorders affecting tendon, ligaments, bursae, muscles, fascia or joint capsule—occupational or sports injuries (e.g. tennis elbow).
- Musculoskeletal pain.
- Early functional limitations related to 1 joint such as seen in OA of the knee.

Evidence supports prompt access to:
- Symptom relief.
- Information about the problem, prognosis, and how to self-manage the condition.
- Provision of aids or devices to aid the management of functional problems.
- Regimens to return to full normal functional ability.

Practical advice on managing self-limiting conditions
- Immediate soft tissue injury (Box 9.4).
- Outline the long-term prognosis of the condition.
- Identify aspects of bone healthy lifestyle—exercise, diet, risk reduction in sports injuries by using appropriate equipment. Occupational factors such as reducing risks related to back pain.
- Encourage self-management options, including:
  - Use of walking aids, appropriate footwear or devices, e.g. insoles for plantar fasciitis.
  - Educate on appropriate use of joints and equipment, e.g. occupational issues such as equipment that exacerbate the pain and functional difficulties, such as poor posture, lack of wrist support for a typist.

- Describe pharmacological pain relief options and how pain works to ensure concordance.
- Identify non-pharmacological options that can support pain relief—thermotherapy, exercise, rehabilitation use of goal setting.

▶ Most importantly, encourage a healthy positive perspective on long-term outcome and return of normal functional ability.

Box 9.4 Acute phase management of soft tissue injury

- Protect.
- Rest the injured area.
- Ice (10–20min every 2–4 hours).
- Compress.
- Elevate.
- Support.

Pain relief may also be required in the short term (e.g oral or topical NSAID where not contraindicated).

Work-related issues in musculoskeletal conditions

There are >2.2 million people receiving incapacity benefits as a result of a MSC (the highest group after mental health conditions). MSCs account for 9.5 million lost working days in 2005/6 and the impact of work-related illness in MSC is 2 × higher than in those suffering from 'stress'. The introduction of biologic therapies may significantly improve these figures but rely on early pro-active management if patients are to remain in employment. The cost to society has been estimated to be >£7 billion (based upon analysis from 1995/6 costs). Some statistics include:

• >2.5 million people in the UK visit their GP with back pain every year. >80% of adults will suffer significant back pain at some time in their life.
• Almost 400,000 people have RA with 12, 000 new cases each year, a quarter of who will stop work within 5 years of diagnosis. This can significantly rise if effects of related conditions (depression cardiac and respiratory complaints) are taken into account.
• >200,000 patients with AS visit their GP each year. Unemployment rates are 3 × higher in those with AS compared to the general population.

These facts are disappointing because evidence suggests significant benefits can be achieved if patients receive prompt support. Pilot studies have shown a 6-fold ↑ in those actively wishing to return to work after early proactive support.

Surveys have also revealed that patients generally rate their quality of life, mood, and social factors (relationships, independences, role in society, satisfaction with care and self-esteem) more highly if they are actively employed.[1]

The role of the nurse

• Early intervention is essential—ensure prompt support and advice including access to multi-professional teams (especially OTs) for advice on functional and occupational issues.
• Focus on positive issues related to capacity not incapacity of the patient. Encourage positive messages that reinforce the individual's belief that they will be able to maintain some form of employment with the right support—provide early practical guidance and information. Early referral to occupational therapy and information such as patient information leaflets on maintaining work.[2]
• Encourage flexible working and review of work stations or other functional limitations to maintaining work.
• Flag the need to think beyond the biomedical model and highlight the psychosocial benefits of participation in society and work.
• Consider more than just direct costs (use of health resources) but consider indirect costs e.g. costs to the patient, loss of social interaction, independence, financial burden, role in society.
• Be proactive in reviewing and supporting those with MSCs.

References

1. The National Rheumatoid Arthritis Society Surveys (2004, 2005, 2007). Available at: ✋ www.rheumatoid.org.uk

2. Available at: ✋ www.rheumatoid.org.uk.

Further reading

The Work Foundation (2007). Fit for Work? *Musculoskeletal disorders and labour market participation.* The Work Foundation, London.

Nursing care issues in management of pain

The prevalence of pain varies considerably in published literature but ranges from 7–16 million people reporting musculoskeletal pain in the UK.

Patients who experience pain will require empathetic and knowledgeable support. Pain evokes fear and anxiety particularly if the cause of the pain is poorly understood. The experience of pain is debilitating, affects self-esteem, and can negatively impact on the patient's ability to use positive health behaviours.

Acute or chronic pain

Although there are important factors to consider in the different management approaches for acute or chronic pain, the relief of pain for the patient is the aim of both.

Acute pain

In acute pain the painful sensations are related to a condition that endangers other bodily functions, requiring prompt intervention of the underlying disorder causing pain (e.g. acute prolapsed interveterbral disc).

Chronic pain

The considerable heterogeneity in definitions of chronic pain means that estimates of chronic pain range from 7–55% of the population in the UK. Chronic malignant pain is generally well managed with patient pathways of care and expertise readily accessible to most patients with malignancy. Chronic non-malignant pain tends to have more negative connotations with healthcare professionals and as a result is often less well managed.

Chronic pain is a complex mix of issues that are often referred to as the biopsychosocial model of care:
• Nociception—nerve fibre impulses.
• Behavioural responses.
• Cognitive factors.

Acute on chronic pain

A classic example of acute on chronic pain is that of a patient with a LTC with an underlying pathology (e.g. IJDs such as RA). The underlying, ongoing low-grade inflammation is exacerbated by acute episodes of 'flares' of the condition ↑ the pain sensations.

Although there are different experiences and responses to acute or chronic pain, perceived views of pain will be developed over time and prior illness experiences/health beliefs and coping styles, e.g.:

Physical
• The underlying pathology causing pain.
• Recognition of the condition.
• Ability to comprehend the diagnosis/acceptance of diagnosis.

Psychological factors
• Cognitive abilities.
• Health seeking behaviours, beliefs.

- Coping styles whether they have a preference for:
  - Active—gentle exercise, distraction techniques.
  - Passive—bed rest, avoidance strategies.

Social factors
- Cultural or religious beliefs related to pain and treatments.
- Language barriers may add to social issues/anxieties.
- Partner/family support related to the pain/condition.
- Level of financial support and ability to manage factors associated with pain (e.g. able to purchase aids, home environment, work flexibility).
- Work-related issues.
- Additional factors that affect the emotional response to the pain at that time:
  - Death of a family member/divorce/financial worries.

Nursing issues in pain management
Prompt and empathetic approach to those experiencing pain is important:
- Undertake a holistic and patient centred assessment:
  - Scope the patient's interpretation of pain and treatments.
  - Review medications (dosing and frequency) and efficacy of previous treatments.
- If appropriate, provide pharmacological and non-pharmacological options:
  - A review of medications may need to be discussed with prescribing/diagnosing clinician.
- Evaluate pain using a tool such as a VAS which encourages patient–practitioner communication with shared goals (reducing pain score).
- Ensure the patient understands the cause of pain (and/or diagnosis) and prognosis:
  - Try to reduce emotional distress related to pain/condition.
- Provide strategies that encourage self-management using a goal setting approach:
  - Exercise, pacing, rest, relaxation, distraction techniques.
- Consider CBT or pain management programme for those who require psychological treatment of pain.

Useful resources
- *The Pharmacist* is an excellent resource in medicine reviews for pain management.
- Pain Management teams or Psychological team (CBT).
- Specialist team dealing with underlying pathology (e.g. rheumatologist for RA).
- Consider volunteer and support groups /community health/well being programmes.
- The British Pain Society website: ⌐ www.britishpainsociety.org

Further reading
Hakim A, Clunie G, Haq I (eds) (2006). *Oxford Handbook of Rheumatology*, 2nd edn. Oxford University Press, Oxford.

Holistic and patient-centred care

Holistic assessment

Introduction

Holistic care is that of considering the 'whole' person in the context of the physical, social, psychological, and spiritual needs. The essence of nursing is that of ensuring a holistic approach is considered for all aspects of care. Early and proactive support should focus on encouraging individuals to be informed about their condition and the treatment options. For the individual with a MSC this approach is imperative, irrespective of condition.

A nursing consultation

If a truly holistic assessment encompassing a patient-centred approach is to be achieved, the nurse must allow adequate time in an environment conducive to exploring the factors outlined in the introduction. In a similar way to qualitative interview techniques a framework to the consultation needs to be borne in mind. It should not be so prescriptive that it fails to enable the patient to build a therapeutic alliance with the nurse.

Holistic assessments should include:

- Social circumstances—age, sex, work-related issues, functional ability, and level of social support.
- Ethnicity or cultural needs.
- Family and clinical history.
- Health and lifestyle issues—smoking, diet.
- Psychological or educational issues/needs.
- Any impairment—visual or hearing.
- Health and illness beliefs (see Fig. 10.1 for a holistic framework to care).

Once a detailed assessment has been undertaken the care planned and treatment required should be negotiated taking into account:

- Their condition in the context of the present symptoms and needs.
- The wider social and psychological aspects of the patient and their perceived additional needs.
- The strategy required to optimize their quality of life in the context of their perceived needs and independent state.

It is widely recognized that patient outcomes for those with LTCs can be improved if actively encouraged to participate in their healthcare decisions.

Further reading

Beckwith S, Franklin P (2006). *Oxford Handbook of Nurse Prescribing*. Oxford University Press, Oxford.

Drennan V, Goodman C (2007). *Oxford Handbook of Primary Care and Community Nursing*. Oxford University Press, Oxford.

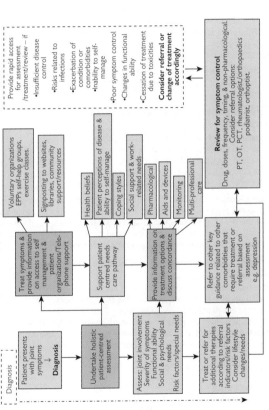

Fig. 10.1 Holistic approach to care.

Patient-centred care

Introduction

The term 'patient-centred care' appears to be attributed to work undertaken by the Picker Institute in 1991. Patient-centred care theories encompass a number of domains in the consultation process. These include:
- Exploring the experience and expectations of disease and illness.
- Understand the 'whole' person—holistic view of care.
- Identifying common ground or a partnership in treatment plans.
- Health promotion.
- Enhancing the therapeutic relationship.

This approach can present challenges for HCPs particularly in 1° care where consultations may have insufficient time allocated to exploring the patient needs.

Achieving a patient-centred approach to care must have patients who are:
- In an environment conducive to exploring their health beliefs.
- Empowered and informed about their treatment.
- Understand the potential risks/benefits of the planned treatment.
- Actively involved in their care in the context of their holistic assessment and integral to discussions about their care.

The patient-centred approach tailors the management plans more appropriately to the priorities and needs of the patient (Fig. 10.2). Evidence has outlined the benefits of this approach and increasingly this type of consultation fits with important aspects of informed decision making in relation to treatments or surgical interventions in line with clinical governance.

Benefits of a patient-centred and holistic consultation

This approach ↑ the potential for patients to:
- Enable health beliefs to be explored and discussed.
- Develop positive health-seeking attitudes and behaviours.
- Encourage active participation in managing their condition.
- Promote awareness of other positive health-seeking opportunities.
- Improve the quality of healthcare communication. Poor professional patient communication is linked to poor patient outcomes.
- Support the needs of the vulnerable patient (either from a psychosocial perspective or for those who are generally unwell).

Further reading

Mitchie S, Miles J, Weiman J (2003). Patient centredness in chronic illness: what is it and does it matter? *Patient Education and Counseling*, **51**, 197–206.

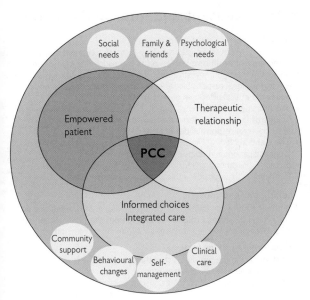

Fig. 10.2 Patient-centred care.

Patient consent and informed consent

Introduction

Before any physical investigation or any form of treatment can be given it is the duty of healthcare professionals to ensure that the patient consents to the treatment/investigation proposed. The duty of care is part of the statutory legal responsibilities of healthcare professionals and as such includes the ethical principles of valid consent:

- The Nursing and Midwifery Council (NMC) Code of Conduct, Standards for conduct, performance and ethics (2004) state the essential legal responsibilities of protecting the patient.
- The General Medical Council Consent document (2007) outlines Consent; patient and doctors making decision together.
- Employing organization, Healthcare Trust will have governance frameworks that consider ethical and professional responsibilities.

Seeking patient consent

If in doubt about your abilities to adequately inform the patient and document decisions, guidance should be sought from the NMC or an experienced colleague. In seeking consent it is important to remember:

The responsibility of the nurse

- That you act in the best interest of the patient.
- Consent is obtained before treatment.
- That the process of establishing consent is rigorous, transparent, and demonstrates a clear level of professional accountability.
- The process of consent and decisions are accurately recorded.

Consent must be valid

- Consent must be given voluntarily.
- The patient must be an adult.
- The patient must be presumed to be mentally competent to provide consent (or have a legally nominated guardian).
- The decision to provide consent is based upon accurate and valid information to enable a decision that reflects the risks/benefits of the treatment.
- The patient should be informed if the treatment is unlicensed or part of a research trial.

Consent-specific patient issues

- The HCP providing the treatment or undertaking the investigation should seek consent from the patient.
- It is an ongoing and continuing pre-requisite of all treatment/investigations provided throughout the patient's healthcare journey. It is not a one-off decision.
- Patient decisions must be respected.
- Consent may be implied, verbal, or written.
- The patient should be aware of their right to seek a 2nd opinion if required.

Consent—the young or those do not have the mental capacity to provide consent

- Young people >16 years of age are presumed competent to make decisions about their care and treatments.
- Children of younger age may also provide consent if they are seen as competent and able to comprehend the information in relation to the decision, the Gillick competent ruling (otherwise the legal parent or guardian can make the decision).
- Mental capacity—requires:
  - Ability to understand simple language and purpose of treatment.
  - Understand risks and benefits or other treatment options.
  - Recognize the consequences if treatment were not administered.
  - Ability to retain information long enough to make a decision.

Documentation of consent should include:
- The treatment or procedure.
- The date and time that consent was given.
- The name and title of the practitioner seeking consent.
- An outline of key factors related to risks related to the treatment and the information provided.
- Any specific instructions that the patient outlines in giving consent.

Informed decision making

The validity of any consent provided rests with the ability of the patient to make a truly informed decision about their care based upon the information that the HCP provides.

There is an ↑ interest in providing tools to aid patient decisions about treatment benefits and risks. These aids vary but some provide the detailed facts and then interpret the risk based upon visual images of risks and benefits (Fig. 10.3).

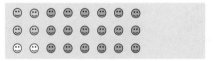

Fig. 10.3 Decision aids. An example of a visual aid to improve decision making. No treatment—e.g. 4 people will improve by 75% without any treatment, 2 patients will stay get worse without treatment, and 18 people will achieve a 75% improve with the suggested treatment. Adapted with permission from Tugwell, P. et al. (2003). *Evidence based rheumatology.* Copyright John Wiley and Sons Limited.

Further reading

O'Conner AM, et al. (2006). Decision aids for people facing health treatment or screening decisions. *Cochrane Collaboration.* Issue 3. John Wiley and Sons Ltd., Chichester.

Education

Education is a core component of the support nurses provide to patients and may vary from a one-off information-sharing approach to a clearly defined treatment to an ongoing planned educational component for a patient-centred consultation for someone with a LTC.

In the past, delivering education was considered part of a structured training package frequently delivered in a group setting over a clearly defined time frame (for example a 2-hourly weekly programme delivered by a multi-professional team delivered over 6 weeks). Increasingly, there is recognition that this approach may not be effective as tailoring education/information giving with an emphasis on tailoring information to the patient's specific needs and expectations with the aim of achieving behavioural changes.

Group education programmes delivered using cognitive behavioural approaches (i.e. ↑ motivation, self-efficacy, and promoting health behaviour change) are significantly more effective than providing a series of short weekly lectures with brief practice from members of the MDT.

However, current models of one-to-one educational approaches have had surprisingly little evaluation. Education should be tailored to meet people's information needs and enable making treatment decisions. To help make health behaviour changes, it should be structured, use goal-setting, and be supported with printed materials. Increasingly there is a focus on developing various lay-led models to deliver self-management programmes within a community setting, these include the EPPs.

Patient education is strongly associated with other aspects of healthcare and should aim to:
- Endorse and empower patient self-management principles.
- Enhance patient satisfaction and perceived self-efficacy.
- Strengthen governance and reduction of risks.
- Professional responsibility in seeking informed consent for treatment/examination.
- Reduce litigation.
- Adoption of health behaviours and beliefs conducive to optimal patient outcomes.
- Improve concordance to treatment and monitoring.

The scope and depth of information/education provided may vary according to the nature of the condition and treatment offered, e.g.:
- The personal preferences of the individual in relation to informational/educational needs, e.g.:
  - Active or passive coping style.
  - Health beliefs and behaviours.
  - Cognitive abilities.
- Acute or chronic condition (one-stop rather than ongoing).
- Medical intervention (high or low risk treatment).
- Complexities related to treatments (e.g. risks and benefits of drug therapies).

- The mediating factors that improve outcomes (e.g. prompt treatment of infections).
- The level of distress of anxiety experienced by the patient (and their family).
- The rehabilitation or recovery phase.

Further reading

Iorik K, Fries JF (2006). *The Arthritis Helpbook*. Da Capo Press, Cambridge, MA. A tested self-management programme for coping with arthritis and fibromyalgia.

Social and psychological aspects of a new diagnosis

When a person receives a diagnosis it may be perceived as a threat to health and well-being. The ability to adapt to a diagnosis and the consequences vary significantly. This ability to adjust to a diagnosis is often independent of disease severity and correlates more closely to levels of perceived control (self-efficacy) and active coping styles.

For some the diagnosis can result in a perceived change from (healthy) person to (sick) patient. The level of threat may rest upon:

• The perceived (or actual) threat (or actual) of the diagnosis and treatment.
• Prior experiences of ill health or knowledge of condition, e.g. family history.
• The adaptation to health and lifestyle as a result of new diagnosis.
• The stigma attached to the continued illness, e.g. OA is a considered a disease of the elderly.
• The effects the diagnosis has upon their perceived role in society and within the family infrastructure/community.
• The patient's psychological status and coping styles.
• Acute or chronic status of condition.
• Predictable nature of symptoms/disease changes.

Adjustment phase

The practitioner–patient relationship is frequently cited in research as an important factor in aiding the patient's ability to adjust to their diagnosis. However, individuals differ in many ways to their diagnosis and in the length of time taken to 'come to terms' or 'adjust' to their condition.

Patients may be aware of changes in their mobility or limitation in ADL. These losses can impact on independence, self-esteem, and relationships. In acute conditions these losses may be short lived. In LTCs the loss can be compounded by the unpredictable yet deteriorating nature of the disease. The effects can be profound in psychological and social terms (e.g. poor self-esteem, denial, financial losses due to work-related issues). Self-reported pain and depression in MSC is high. Deterioration in physical ability is a contributing factor to poor outcomes in MSC.

During the adjustment phase patients may be in 'denial' and fail to actively participate in healthcare decisions or recall important information. This phase may also result in numerous stressors that may be social or psychologically driven. These factors may mean patient ability to retain or recall information may be sub-optimal

Key message

Educational opportunities must be taken whenever the patient appears responsive to receiving information. Education should be an ongoing aspect of nursing care and should not be considered a 'one-stop shop'.

Educating the patient and the family

Educating the patient about their condition and treatment options is a perquisite of all nursing support. Education should be delivered using a patient-centred and holistic approach, enabling a strong therapeutic relationship to develop. Patient education is the precursor to self-management.

MSCs are poorly understood and there are many lay perceptions about the conditions, treatment efficacy, and long-term outcomes—the common quoted term (even by some HCPs) is that 'nothing can be done to treat arthritis', for instance.

Dispelling lay perceptions and building a positive and informed approach to practical aspects of managing conditions such as 'arthritis' will start the patient on the right pathway through their healthcare journey, and will enhance the patient's perceived control over their disease.

Key points and tips to educating the patient and their family

- Encourage the patient to bring a partner or family member along to the consultation.
- If the partner attends clinic (and the patient consents to their participation) recognize the partner's role in supporting the patient and include them in the consultation where appropriate.
- Always ensure that information provided at the consultation is supported by written information for the patient to take home with them.
- For those who do not have English as their first language a partner or family member can be very helpful in interpreting but also advising on lifestyle issues (e.g. fasting times, pain beliefs).
- A partner may provide additional importance advice about family responsibilities or functional difficulties that the patient is reticent about reporting.
- Patient support groups or volunteer activities can be mentioned which include the patient and the partner involvement, e.g. the National Rheumatoid Arthritis Society has a volunteer network training programme that includes patients and their partners.
- Partners may aid recall and questioning of issues.
- The HCP is seen by the partner to give full recognition to the patient's condition and symptoms.
- Partners may become integral to the patients' care over time and active involvement helps to build a relationship with the multi-professional team, e.g. poor hand function may mean a partner will offer to administer subcutaneous injections

Challenges in educating the patient and family

- The patient may decline to have the partner involved in care.
- Anxieties of a partner can be higher than those of the patient.
- Managing the consultation may be more complex.
- In some cases there may be tensions between patient and partner.

Self-efficacy and concordance

Self-efficacy (SE)

SE is the perception or belief that a person has the ability to undertake important activities that benefit their lives. SE focuses on the person's perception of their ability rather than the actual ability of undertaking the task. Believing someone has control over their life and the ability to undertake certain tasks in their life can improve health outcomes. This perceived ability is called SE, originally defined by Bandura in 1977.

SE related to health behaviour is predictive of future health status and is amenable to change through education (unlike other psychological traits that are resistant or prove difficult to change). SE is an important outcome to focus on because:

• Beliefs can powerfully determine the level of commitment a person applies to achieve defined outcomes.
• Evidence supports timely targeted patient education interventions improving SE.
• SE can be used as a patient-centred outcome measure.
• Assessment tools can provide evidence on baseline SE for pain and other symptoms.

There are specific SE tools for arthritis:
• The Arthritis SE Scale (ASES).
• The Rheumatoid Arthritis SE scale (RASE).
• Self-Efficacy Scales (SES).

📖 Also see Assessment tools, p.539

Concordance

The extent to which patients take prescribed treatments is an area of extensive research. Concordance is a term used to describe an interactional decision process that creates a therapeutic partnership. Developing concordance with a patient is an important and effective approach to treating a patient with therapies that they wish to be prescribed and feel able to take. Healthcare resources can be used more effectively and patient satisfaction and outcomes are likely to benefit from this approach. Concordance is an important component of:

• A holistic patient-centred consultation.
• Patient empowerment and self-management.
• Clinical governance and risk management.
• Responsible prescribing.

📖 Also see Holistic assessment, p.312; 📖 Patient-centred care, p.314.

Further reading

Katz PP (ed) (2003). Patient outcomes in rheumatology A review of the measures. *Arthritis Care and Research*, **49** (Special Issue), S1–S233.

Oliver S (ed) (2004). *Chronic Disease Nursing: A Rheumatology Example*. John Wiley & Sons Ltd: Chichester.

Self-management: what is it?

Introduction

The term self-management describes the ability of an individual to effectively manage their condition on a day-to-day basis. The ability for a person to self-manage is the aim of all patient education and these 2 concepts go hand-in-hand. These are different models for delivering EPPs. Educational aspects also need to be considered in the context of the bio-psychosocial model of health and illness (🕮 see Patient education, p.318, 321).

Following on from patient education, the patient should recognize the scope and potential benefit of undertaking some level of self-management of their condition. This usually comes once the patient has made an initial adjustment to their diagnosis and received sufficient education to enable them to feel confident in their ability to self-manage and to effectively cope with some aspects of their condition.

Self-management principles include:

- Taking responsibility for their lives, health, and disease states.
- Recognizing the importance of making informed decisions about their treatment
- How to manage exacerbations of their condition using pharmacological and non-pharmacological treatments.
- Monitoring aspects of their treatment and potential side effects/toxicity.
- Knowing when to seek medical advice and who to go to.
- Recognizing additional health behaviours that are beneficial to general well-being.

It is important to remember that MSCs are:

- Chronic—treatable but rarely curable.
- Have a very variable course—characterized by episodic exacerbations of symptoms.
- Have a variable outcome—symptoms may deteriorate slowly, a few have infrequent, mild exacerbations, a minority suffer constant, severe symptoms.
- Access to help is not available 24 hours a day, 7 days a week, so people must learn to self-manage non-life threatening fluctuating symptoms and problems.

The biopsychosocial model of health and illness

The biopsychosocial model of health and illness recognizes the influence of people's perspective on their physical, psychological, emotional, and social well-being. These perspectives include the individual's:

- Attitudes.
- Health beliefs.
- Understandings.
- Experiences.
- Emotions.
- Personal relationships.
- Social environment.
- Social networks.

The biopsychosocial model advocates a holistic approach to management of chronic conditions. The individual's experiences of living with the consequences of ill health (physical, social, and psychological) must be recognized to ensure appropriate strategies are provided to aid the individual adjust and learn to self-manage and enhance self-efficacy. The biopsychosocial model identifies the importance of:

- Positive experiences enhance appropriate health beliefs and behaviours and negative experiences are detrimental to self-efficacy.
- Psychosocial traits as key determinants of poor health behaviours ('catastrophizing' or 'fear-avoidance').
- Health behaviours (or traits) may not be easy to change. Factors that will affect the individual's ability to modify or change health behaviours include:
  - Prior health behaviours and beliefs.
  - Perceived threat to the individual's health and health beliefs.
  - Anxieties and needs of the individual.
  - Prior experiences in achieving self-efficacy.
  - The predictable or unpredictable aspects of their condition.
  - Beliefs in the ability to access support and advice when self-management principles have been exhausted.

Self-management strategies

- Challenge erroneous ill-health beliefs.
- Teaches coping skills.
- Enhances self-efficacy.
- Reduces helplessness.
- Reduces social isolation.

Achieved by:

- Information and knowledge about the condition.
- Endorsing and empowering self-management principles.
- Encouraging alternative supportive 'non-medicalized' infrastructures (voluntary or support groups).
- Demonstrating self-efficacy principles.

Simple self-management strategies for symptom control

Non-pharmacological self-management strategies include a range of options. The strategies work on reducing the heightened awareness to pain sensations by distraction or changing mood. Perceived self-efficacy is enhanced reducing anxieties. A number of tools can be considered.

Heat and cold (thermotherapy)

- Some people find warming a joint relieves pain, others find cooling more effective.
- Commercial heat/cold packs are available, but can be made by wrapping a hot water bottle, ice cubes, or frozen peas in a towel; a warm bath or thermal clothing coolant sprays are also effective. Advise to :
  - Position yourself comfortably so the joint is supported.
  - Place the hot/cold pack over the joint for 10–15min.
  - Remove the pack and gently move the joint.
  - Replace the hot/cold pack on the joint for another 5–10min.
- Gently warming or cooling a joint is very safe. The sensation of heat/cold should not become uncomfortable. People with circulatory problems or ↓ thermal sensation (diabetes) should use it cautiously.

Transcutaneous electrical neuromuscular stimulation (TENS)

TENS produces pulsed electrical stimulation delivered to the skin using electrodes placed on the skin. The current then activates specific nerve fibres which may inhibit pain sensations to the brain. TENS may deliver:

- High frequency.
- Low frequency.
- A pulsed form of TENS that can switch between high and low frequency.

The use of TENS carries very little risk and is non-invasive.

- Safe, non-invasive electrical stimulation.
- Self-applied using relatively cheap readily available machines.

Massage

- Rubbing a pain is an innate reaction to pain.
- Direct human physical contact has a profoundly comforting effect, inducing relaxation and calm.
- The pain relief produced by moisturizers, oils, gels, lotions, and creams is partially due to the massaging action needed to apply these agents.
- Gently massaging painful joints or muscles for 5–10min is a simple, effective, safe, and pleasurable (!) way to relieve pain.

Joint protection

The use of aids and devices to support, protect, or rest the affected or painful joint. Forms of joint protection include:

- Splints particularly used in inflammatory forms of arthritis or where instability or pain is present (📖 see Joint protection, p.530; 📖 Why split joints?, p.532).

- Aids and devices include equipment used to relieve the stressors to the joint, e.g.:
  - Tap turners, chair raisers, vegetable peelers, kettle tippers.
  - Dressing aids, Velcro straps.
  - Walking aids and specific footwear.

📖 Also see Equipment aids and devices, p.344.

Pacing, rest, and relaxation

Rest–activity cycling

'Rest–activity cycling', or pacing, encourages people to intersperse activity with periods of rest. Muscle fatigue causes abnormal movement which can lead to pain and damage. People often do activities (especially chores like gardening, housework, shopping) in spite of ↑ discomfort and pain. Adopting good habits and behaviours can avoid fatigue, pain, and damage (Box 10.1). Initially this may seem be seen an inconvenience, but gradually individuals should find that as the time of activity between rests ↑, the activity becomes easier with much less pain.

Physical activity

- Physiologically physical activity improves joint mobility, strength, endurance, 'normalizes' motor neuron transmission, and biomechanics.
- Psychologically appreciating what they can do makes people feel good, ↓ depression, and ↑ self-confidence, self-esteem, and independence.
- For simple ways of ↑ physical activity see 📖 Exercises, p.350.

Box 10.1 Advice to patients on rest–activity cycle

- Identify activities that cause pain, e.g. gardening, hoovering, etc.
- Think about the way you are doing them—most people begin to experience pain after a relatively short time, but continue the task until it is completed or pain forces them to stop.
- Recognize how long it takes you to begin to feel tired and some mild discomfort (e.g. after 20min); take a break at this point (5–10min), before returning to the task.
- Take another break if pain starts to ↑ again, or finish the task later.

Pacing, rest, and relaxation as an additional option for symptom control

For those with severe or inflammatory pain, they may need to build in a period of total relaxation to enable them to cope with an otherwise full day of activity—particularly during exacerbations of their condition.

- To achieve effective relaxation, a timed period of total muscle relaxation resting on the bed listening to restful music or reading may reduce levels of fatigue and ultimately reduce pain levels.
- The time spent relaxing can be ↓ gradually as the flare settles.

Self-management principles: relaxation and breathing techniques

Perception of pain is heightened by stress, anxiety, worry, and depression, ↑ muscle tension, poor shallow breathing patterns, and feelings of being helplessly controlled by pain. Left unchecked, individuals can start to 'catastrophize' based upon the learnt behaviours and beliefs.

These feelings can be modified and ultimately changed by allowing individuals to recognize the effects of their feelings on signs of stress, tension, and anxiety that result in:

- Shallow breathing, feeling uptight and shoulders, neck, back, and leg muscle tension.
- Certain recognized situations that make the individual tense or anxious.
- Learnt beliefs or behaviours that link association to pain.

Self-management strategies encourage the individual to recognize their ability to relieve anxieties related to perceived threats to health status.

Simple relaxation and breathing strategies that can be used any time, any place, any where include deep breathing (see Box 10.2).

Box 10.2 Deep-breathing advice for patients

- Sit or stand up straight.
- Relax your shoulders.
- Place a hand on your tummy just below your ribs.
- Take a slow, gentle deep breath in through your nose, feel your hand and tummy rising and your chest to expand fully.
- Slowly breathe out through your mouth, feel your tummy and hand gently sink.
- Repeat this for 4 or 5 deep breaths, then rest and breathe in a normal relaxed way for a couple of minutes.
- If necessary repeat the exercise for 5–10min.

Managing exacerbations of pain and inflammation for patients

- Rest, do not take to your bed, but avoid or reduce activities that aggravate your pain (i.e. prolonged standing, walking) for a couple of days until the pain subsides.
- Use heat, cold, or whatever you find eases your pain, several times each day.
- Practice deep breathing and relaxation techniques if you feel anxious and tense to help relax, calm down, and reduce anxiety.
- Resume exercising gently once the pain starts to settle; if you do not move, your joints will stiffen up very quickly and your muscles will weaken and tire quickly.
- Gradually ↑ your activity levels.

Expert patient and voluntary sector education and support

There are many sources of education and support in the community for people with MSC, particularly to provide information based on a general support for problems related to LTCs or aspects of 'arthritis' (the lay term to describe all forms of joint pain). They can be helpful in providing generic information about managing the symptoms and how to cope on a day-to-day basis. The community and voluntary sector now play an increasingly important role in providing information or support for patients.

Education programmes include:

- Arthritis Care: run programmes to help people self-manage. Local courses can be found at: http://www.arthritiscare.org.uk/InyourArea— choose region and select self-management. 'Challenging Arthritis': a group 6-meeting programme focuses on a programme that would provide components such as: understanding arthritis, managing pain, fatigue, emotions, symptoms, exercise and making changes—led by trained arthritis volunteers. Other courses include the 'You can break the pain cycle' which is a 1-day course. Both have been proven effective.
- The EPP—run by a Community Interest Company and developed from 'Challenging Arthritis' with similar content. A course that includes 6 meetings for people with LTCs. Proven effective and available throughout the UK: www.expertpatients.co.uk/public/default.aspx —select 'find a course'.
- Regional Primary Care commissioned education modules.

Voluntary organizations

There are numerous opportunities for a number of community-based services or voluntary organizations to complement the healthcare services. Examples include:

- The National Rheumatoid Arthritis Society (NRAS) volunteer network. Developing volunteers from the patient group who may be able to provide a 'buddy system' or be trained to provide telephone support (for example the NRAS Volunteer Network).
- Classes to improve their health and well-being (e.g. swimming or exercise classes provided by the local leisure centre, funded by a charity but delivered in the community).
- Dietary advice and cookery classes on healthy eating options.
- Local pharmacy programmes to encourage simple screening (e.g. of blood pressure) or information access points on medication queries.
- Facilitating meetings or events that enable people to meet with others who have the same condition or similar problems.
- Community-based education programmes providing general advice for all people with a LTC (e.g. the EPPs).
- Enabling patients who have become 'experts in their condition' to work as lay teachers in a structured educational programme.
- Patient educators – where patients are trained to educate healthcare professionals on joint examination techniques.

- Regional networks where patients can become an important member of an expert panel on the needs of the local community (e.g. the national network of Arthritis and Musculoskeletal Alliance (ARMA) groups)

Support groups

- NRAS: campaigning support group with many resources on website, telephone support, local networks of support, as well as a regional volunteer/coordinators. http://www.rheumatoid.org.uk/
- Arthritis Care: a campaigning support group which has local branches, web access to educational resources, telephone support, and language translation. http://www.arthritiscare.org.uk
- Healthtalkonline: www.healthtalkonline.org Search 'arthritis'. Video and audio clips of people discussing their experiences of diagnosis, treatment and living with arthritis. Highly rated site – informative, helps people feel 'not alone'.
- ARMA: an alliance of patient and health professional organizations. http://www.arma.uk.net/member.html Membership includes musculoskeletal charities e.g. back pain, SS, lupus, or children with arthritis with links to the organizations and local groups. The website also provides accessible information for patients on the standards of care they should expect from their healthcare provider, these include:
  - IJD
  - OA
  - Back pain
  - Metabolic bone disease.
  - CTD
  - Soft tissue disorders.

Chapter 11

Care in the community

General practice: practical tips

Painful joints

Patients will often present in 1° care with problems related to joint or muscle pain and this can be daunting for the new practice nurse with little or no experience of MSC. Patients may also present for other investigations or treatment and may refer to their joint problems at the same time. Individuals with symptomatic conditions affecting the joints may be reticent about seeking advice as they believe 'nothing that can be done to help their joint pains'. Support and advice offered by the practice nurse will be invaluable to those who are symptomatic.

This chapter will focus on how the patient can be assessed and referred appropriately to the right HCP and help that can be offered during the consultation (Box 11.1).

The ranges of MSC can span mild self-limiting, acute, chronic and reoccurring chronic conditions. In older patients, the commonest problems is symptomatic OA or gout; the prevalence of inflammatory conditions ↑ in middle age; and in the young, systemic conditions are more likely.

📖 Also see Introduction, p.1; 📖 Assessing the patient, p.271.

Observe ROMs and examine the affected joint for:

- Position at rest.
- Gait.
- ROM.
- Deformity.
- Signs of active inflammation (synovitis).

📖 Also see Assessing the patient, p.271.

Nursing aspects to consider

- Listen to their story and show empathy.
- Document the patient-reported experiences and problems.
- Assess the impact the pain has on their day-to-day life:
  - Consider referral to GP; confirm diagnosis if indicated.
  - Explore current pain-relieving strategies and efficacy (pharmacological and non-pharmacological) e.g. rest position heat/ice (📖 see Symptom control, p.289).
- If appropriate consider investigations e.g. CRP, ESR, RF, HB, urate.
- Offer written information or recognized website access.[1]

📖 Also see Care in the community, p.333.

Reference

1. For example: ⏁ http://www.arc.org.uk ⏁ http://www.rheumatoid.org.uk for RA; ⏁ http://www.arthritiscare.org.uk

Red flags in history taking and assessment

- Fever.
- Pain that wakes them at night.
- If one joint is red, very hot, intensely painful, with limited ROM, septic arthritis must be excluded—GP intervention. ⚠ Septic arthritis is easy to miss with a patient with coexisting RA and may be mistaken for a flare-up of their RA
- Patients with arm pain—might be due to other causes other than arthritis, such as angina or cervical nerve root compression. It is important to ensure that these concerns are appropriately explored.
- Patients on MTX and other specific DMARDs must have regular blood tests including LFTs, FBC, and an ESR.
- Patients failing to understand that MTX is to be taken once a week. Ensure that no more than 1 month's supply is dispensed at any time.
- Rarely can develop blood dyscrasias (🕮 see Monitoring and treatment side effects, Chapters 16 and 17).
- Mouth ulcers may be a sign that folic acid is not being taken.
- Patients should be aware that while they have a flare exercise should be modified.

Box 11.1 Questions to ask all patients with joint pain

- Which joints are affected?
- Is this a new problem?
- How long have you had the pain?
- How does it affect you day to day?
- Does the pain wake you at night?
- What have you tried to relieve it?
- What exacerbates the pain?
- Have they consulted with anyone about this before and are there any plans to deal with this?
- Occupation?

Managing patients with comorbidities and joint pain

The general health of individuals in wealthy economies has greatly improved in the last century and as a result life expectancy has ↑ significantly. However, ↑ longevity can come at a cost for the individual and society as life is extended but with a growing number of incurable conditions and additional health problems. Many of these incurable conditions are categorized as a 'long-term condition'. These LTCs can affect many body systems. Examples include:

- Cardiovascular disease, e.g. peripheral vascular disease, congestive cardiac failure, and hypertension.
- Diabetes.
- Neurological conditions, e.g. Parkinson's disease, multiple sclerosis.
- Respiratory conditions, e.g. asthma and COPD.
- Musculoskeletal, e.g. OA, RA, JIA, scleroderma.
- Mental health, e.g. depression.

The 1° diagnosis of a LTC can be compounded by additional comorbidities. Individuals with 1 or more comorbidities face numerous challenges over the course of their disease, impacting on the individual's physical, social, and psychological well-being (Box 11.2).

📖 Also see Education, social and psychological issues, pp.318, 320; 📖 Assessing the patient, p.271.

For the nurse providing care for those with LTCs, planned reviews and management is essential to ensure appropriate care is provided and treatment adheres to recognized standards and guidelines in care. These management decisions experience additional complexities particularly for:

- The frail and elderly who require additional health needs assessments.
- Those with 1 or more co-morbidities will present:
  - Challenges in prescribing appropriate pain relief.
  - Concordance with exercise regimens.
  - Treatment monitoring and side effects related to different drugs.
  - The additional factors related to social and psychological impact of >1 comorbidity.

Assessments must adequately account for patient needs, particularly as:

- Pain is the predominant reason for those with joint problems to seek advice from their doctor or nurse. Simple practical information, appropriate pain relief and signposting to information or referral are an essential aspect of nursing care.
- Functional limitations (e.g. OA of knee or hip) may be the key limiting factor in achieving exercise tolerance, weight reduction, or positive health behaviours.
- Self-efficacy can be enhanced by addressing patient identified needs in relation to changes in functional ability, social activities, independence, and quality of life.
- Health awareness and a positive approach to achieving a bone health lifestyle can be enhanced by demonstrating a positive 'can do' attitude in all care settings reducing the risk of learned 'helplessness'.

📖 Also see Symptom control, p.289; 📖 When to refer to the multi-disciplinary team, p.363.

Box 11.2 Comorbidities and pain: management approach

- Full holistic nursing assessment and screening questions for MSC.
- If unsure about diagnosis seek medical opinion to confirm underlying pathology (e.g. OA not PsA or mild, self-limiting conditions). Referral if required, to specialist teams.
- Identify aggravating or relieving factors for pain (and functional problems in relation to pain).
- Assess pain using VAS for pain—review after a 2-week treatment plan.
- Provide written and verbal information on how pain works and why *regular* simple analgesia is more effective in managing pain than sporadic dosing.
- Provide information (written and verbal) on non-pharmacological self-management approaches to support pain relief (e.g. rest, pacing, joint protection or cold packs, hot baths). Use as an adjunct to pharmacological measures (📖 see Symptom control, p.289).
- In prescribing consider:
  - Contraindications and drug interactions/cautions in relation to current medications and proposed pharmacological options.
  - Frail/elderly/renal or liver impairments/cautions and contraindications in prescribing and reduce dosages or selecting most appropriate drug.
  - Analgesia (simple and compound) regular dosing and optimal doses to achieve pain relief.
- If first step approach to achieving pain relief fails to adequately control pain review other prescribing options (📖 see Symptom control, p.289).
- Consider psychological and educational needs in relation to pain and underlying pathology.
- Encourage access to voluntary organizations/additional resources.
- Review pain assessments and prescribing plan/referral where necessary.
- Identify changes/benefits to LTC/comorbidities.

Functional limitations

- Identify functional limitations in relation to lifestyle, social support, and level of need/distress/pain.
- Provide practical advice on simple aids and devices if appropriate.
- Consider referral for functional assessment with PT and/or OT (for joint protection and assessment on functional ability in the context of ADL).
- Discuss risk factors in relation to changes in functional ability—risk of falls, loss of independence.
- Management plan and review of function/pain/goal setting.

Skin integrity, continence, and caring for the carers

Some MSCs can impact on the normal ROMs, functional ability, and distribution of weight. Other factors include changes to tissues as a result of the disease process (e.g. scleroderma) or drug therapies (e.g. corticosteroids). These changes may affect skin integrity, continence, and function by:

- Causing friction or rubbing from abnormal movement or weight distribution (e.g. Trendelburg gait, use of crutches).
- Inhibition (in ability or pace) to access toilet facilities or manage clothing (functional limitation to gait or manual dexterity— e.g. scleroderma changes that cause tight and contracted skin tissues).
- Poor disease control resulting in ability to mobilize at particular times of the day (gelling after inactivity in OA or EMS in RA). Flares of the disease can result in a systemic illness with fever, pain, and systemic effects such as fatigue.
- Disease-specific changes that result in ulcerations due to auto-immune responses, e.g. vasculitis.
- Medications that affect skin integrity, e.g. corticosteroids.

Consider a formal assessment for those at risk.

Caring for the carers

The practice nurse will often have contact with carers of those diagnosed with arthritis and may find themselves in a position to counsel, advise, or perhaps just listen to the carer. Providing good support is important. Although the patient may receive enough support the carer may not and they may feel inadequate, isolated, and frustrated at not knowing how they can help.

The practice nurse may recognize psychological and emotional reactions especially at initial diagnosis of a partner or close relative.

Nursing interventions

- Encourage the carer to talk about their feelings and anxieties.
- Offer information.
- Encourage the carer to give emotional support.
- Include the carer in decision making.
- Highlight the areas the patient might be experiencing concerns with, in relation to loss of independence, altered body image, reduced self-esteem and low mood, concerns regarding medication side effects.
- Encourage the carer to act as a link and information provider to others involved in the patient's care.

Encourage the patient to acknowledge their own needs and seek appropriate guidance and support.

Musculoskeletal conditions in the frail and elderly

Care for the frail and elderly

The frail or elderly patient may be receiving support in a care home or sheltered housing or may be living independently. Pain and functional limitations are likely to alert the nurses to a potential musculoskeletal problem (MSC) (Box 11.3). The level of trained nursing support may also vary and patients may have inter-related health and social care needs. Pain is a common feature and frequently under-treated in the frail and elderly.

Nurses play an important role in enabling the individual to maximize their general health status and quality of life. The single assessment process for older people has been advocated and now used routinely to undertake a comprehensive assessment of need.

> ### Box 11.3 The most common MSCs affecting the elderly
>
> - Symptomatic and asymptomatic OA—commonly affecting hands, base of thumb, cervical spine, hip, and knees.
> - PMR.
> - Gout or pseudogout.
> - Osteoporosis and related low-impact fractures.
> - Inflammatory arthritides, e.g. such as RA.

The assessment

Apart from the key aspects required to assess all patients (clinical history and physical assessment), there may be specific issues to consider when assessing individuals who are frail or elderly that will require a more in-depth exploration to identify those vulnerable or frail individuals who have additional complex needs. This may include:

- Functional ability in the context of:
  - Achieving optimum in quality of life and activities.
  - Risk of falls.
  - Maintaining independence.
- Cognitive ability and/or any sensory impairments:
  - Visual or hearing deficits may ↑ risks and reduce quality of life.
- Social and psychological needs:
  - Social isolation.
  - Economic issues.
  - General physical and mental factors that effects psychological functioning, e.g. bereavement, isolation, depression.
- Symptom control:
  - Some individuals may be more accepting of their condition (an inevitable consequence of ageing) or not wish to be seen as a nuisance.
- Personal care needs.
  - Physical ability and cognitive aspects may reduce independence and the ability to carry out some aspects of personal care.

- Tissue viability:
  - The ageing process and skin damage may result in fragile or friable tissues vulnerable to damage.
- Dignity and choice:
  - Individuals may require support and guidance on maintaining treatment options and their independent roles.
  - Impairment (physical or mental) should not be a barrier to maintaining choice and dignity.
- Pharmacological aspects:
  - Ageing kidneys do not excrete drugs so effectively and prescribing decisions need to take into account the patient's age and ability to absorb, metabolize, and excrete drug therapies.

Assessing pain

The assessment of pain is discussed in 🕮 Assessing pain, p.292. Individuals with pain (particularly if cognitively or sensorial impaired) may present with agitation, disorientation, poor sleep patters, depression, anxiety, or anorexia. Pain will frequently affect mobility and ability to self-manage, e.g. ↑ pain may present challenges for the individual in maintaining continence. In those with dementia, assessing pain presents additional challenges. Ideally, patient self-reported pain tools should be used. Evidence suggests that even those with a Mini Mental State Examination score as low as 6 are able to verbally report pain using self-report tools.

Management

🕮 Refer to Chapter 6, Chronic non-inflammatory pain; 🕮 Chapter 9 Symptom control: using pharmacological and non-pharmacological methods; 🕮 Chapter 15 Pharmacological management: pain relief; and 🕮 Chapter 16, Pharmacological management: disease-modifying drugs.

Key pharmacological issues in prescribing for the elderly

Generally, the majority of drug therapies result in greater and prolonged effects in those of ↑ age due to physiological changes in the older person. These changes can be seen in:
- Changes in the fat to muscle ratio.
- Muscle volume and power are ↓.
- Ageing heart, kidney, or liver leads to less efficient/poor function.
- ↓ in collagen, e.g. in the elasticity of the skin.
- Less acidity in the gut—acidity falls with ↑ age and motility reduces.
- Chronic kidney disease can be identified by measuring the GFR. Some drugs may be contraindicated with chronic kidney disease and other may require a reduction in dosing regimen to avoid the risk of drug toxicity.

Further reading

Arthiritis research Campaign website:⏎ www.arc.org.uk

Department of Health (2003). *National Service Framework for Older People*. DH, London.

Hutt E, Buffum MD, Fink R et al. (2007). Optimizing pain management in long term care residents. Available at: ⏎ www.medscape.com

National Osteoporosis Society website: ⏎ www.nos.org.uk

The Royal College of Nursing (2004). *Nursing assessment and older people*. RCN, London.

Telephone advice line support

Telephone advice lines (sometimes referred to as helplines) provide prompt and effective support to individuals who require healthcare advice. Helplines are valued by patients, form a significant proportion of the workload for many nurse specialists, and frequently prevent hospital admissions or requests for specialist consultations.

Helpline services vary depending upon whether it is a generic rapid access service with the aim of prompt triage for those that require urgent care or is provided by a specialist team managing specific disease areas or conditions. Some examples include:

- *NHS Direct.* A decision support systems manned by nurses who provide generic support for a wide spectrum of individual calls in relation to all health problems.
- *Voluntary or charitable organizations.* Provide non-medical guidance and support. This is often within a specific disease area or set of conditions (e.g. Continence Services or RA).
- *A rheumatology or musculoskeletal advice line service.* Provided for those with a musculoskeletal diagnosis who require LTC guidance in relation to exacerbations or side effects.
- *1° care services.* Some provide telephone triage prior to referral to a GP or rapid access support that allows targeted triage system that enables the individual to see the most appropriate clinicians, effectively manage resources, and provide patient choice.

Individuals with a LTC value support provided by telephone advice line services because:

- Advice and support can be accessed from their own home in the context of their specific needs. This approach has the potential to enhance self-management principles if used effectively as a training tool.
- Specialist support in specific disease areas is valued by individuals who develop a therapeutic relationship with a team or service who understand the complexity of their condition.
- Continuity of care—a thorough audit trail and access to patient records allows specific advice for some patients.
- They can report side effects and problems with monitoring promptly.
- The consequences of the telephone advice line decisions are part of the overall specialist team's management plans for the specific condition.

Core principles of advice line support must include:

- Knowledge and competencies of those providing telephone advice.
- Clarity for all about the aims and objective of the service and times when available. This should include how long to wait for a return call if using an answerphone service.
- Documentation and effective communication about decisions/advice provided.
- Risk management and recognition of dangers of non-verbal prompts. This should include risks related to potential flaws in patient self-reported information and patient recall on advice given.

Further reading

RCN (2006). *Telephone advice lines for people with long term conditions.* RCN. London.

Equipment aids and devices

Assistive technology (AT): what is available to help?

There is a huge range of AT including equipment, aids, devices, and support designed to help the elderly and people with disabilities maintain independence and function. Patients can have practical difficulties with a number of daily activities, e.g. personal care, household activities such as cooking, housework, and shopping, work (paid or voluntary), study, social and leisure activities (e.g. hobbies, gardening), mobility (e.g. driving, walking, stairs, and public transport). Presume there is something that could help. Staying independent and actively engaged in work and leisure makes for a healthier person physically and psychologically.

Where can I get help with daily activities and work?
(Table 11.1)

OTs have particular training in helping people remain independent through using rehabilitation and AT. They work in the NHS, Local Authority Social Services (LASS), Housing Associations, Independent Living equipment companies and voluntary sector. Support available includes:

- OT assessments for functional needs and practical advice enabling aids to be reviewed before purchase: 'try before they buy'. OTs may be able to arrange free provision if the person is eligible.
- Housing adaptations and large personal care equipment e.g. for bath, toilet, stair lift, or rails, can be provided free by the LASS. Some may be means tested.
- The Disabled Living Foundation (DLF) has regional centres with extensive equipment displays from small kitchen gadgets, to bath and toilet aids, chairs, mobility aids, stair lifts. Ring for an OT appointment in advance for independent advice.
- Environmental control systems (e.g operating lights, curtains, doors, electrical equipment) exist for people with more severe disabilities.
- Many small aids and devices can be purchased.
  - Increasingly, small gadgets are available in High Street stores.
  - The DLF has helpful online advice and fact sheets in selecting equipment to suit all needs.

Work related issues: what help is available?

If your patient has problems coping with work because of arthritis act quickly. OTs can provide lots of practical help—see Table 11.1.

- If the person has disclosed their condition to their employer the OT can do a work visit and on-site ergonomic assessment.
- If they go on long-term sick leave/unemployed it is much harder to get people back into work. Additional financial and psychological problems can result.

Further reading

Useful information: *I want to work—a guide for people with arthritis.* Available at:
🖰 www.rheumatoid.org.uk

Information leaflets on aids and devices can be seen at 🖰 www.arc.org.uk

Table 11.1 Sources of help for aids and devices

Small gadgets for meal preparation	High Street kitchen stores—look for light products, larger non-slip handles, lever action. 'Good Grips' range.
Finding out about gadgets and equipment available	Any NHS OT or LASS OT for detailed assessment and help.
	DLF Centres (free professional independent advice from OTs). To locate centres and 'try before you buy' go to: www.dlf.org.uk/public/findaproduct.html and also click on 'Ask SARA' for online advice and to download factsheets
	www.arc.org.uk/arthinfo/patpubs/—select 'Living with Arthritis'
	www.direct.gov.uk/en/DisabledPeople/ HomeandHousingOptions/index.htm—advice on where to get information; benefits; practical help with housing adaptations etc.
Free provision of aids and equipment	LASS departments—eligibility criteria may apply.
Specialist shops and equipment providers	www.keepable.co.uk—stores and online
	www.independentliving.co.uk—provides links to various suppliers
Driving and mobility (cars, scooters, and powered chairs)	www.mobility-centres.org.uk—independent OT advice on car adaptations/driving with a disability.
	www.motability.co.uk—for financial assistance if eligible for mobility benefits.
Work	Coping at work: refer to OT for work advice, ergonomic assessment and getting help with changes.
	www.jobcentreplus.gov.uk/JCP/Customers/ HelpForDisabledPeople/AccesstoWork
	'Access To Work' scheme provides financial help with work adaptations.
	Employers' occupational health department

Case scenarios for the practice nurse

Box 11.4 Case scenario 1

Mrs. C comes to see you for her blood pressure check. While she is removing her coat she seems to be in significant pain from her upper arms and finds it difficult to raise her arms. She confides to you that she has had pain in her shoulders for a few months and it is getting worse-she puts it down to old age.

Questions to ask

- How does it affect you day-to-day?
- What have you tried to relieve it?
- How does it affect your ADL?
- Occupation?
- Hobbies?
- Does it keep you awake at night?
- Any pins and needles?

Note the type of pain

- Location.
- Intensity.
- Frequency.
- Precipitating factors.
- Exclude referred pain or other underlying pathology, e.g. referred pain from the neck.
- Document the subjective information from the patient, in his or her own words.
- Note the patient's position while talking to you.

Nursing intervention

- Temperature.
- Blood pressure.
- ESR/CRP and FBC.
- Appointment with GP after blood results are received.
- Encourage patient to take simple analgesia until their GP appointment.
- Provide information on non-pharmacological pain relieving strategies, e.g. use of cold or heat packs.

Differential diagnosis

- PMR.
- OA in the shoulder.
- Simple muscular strain.

Box 11.5 Case scenario 2

Miss B has recently been diagnosed with RA and started on MTX. She is 18 years old. She is being monitored at the local hospital rheumatology department. She comes to see you for her contraceptive check. She bursts into tears and after listening to her it becomes apparent she is worried about the consequences to her life; for instance, will she ever be able to have her own children or is she going to end up in a wheel chair like her grandmother?

How can you help?

Nursing interventions

- Listen and empathize.
- Tease out all her concerns—remember she has probably been told not to drink alcohol which can be tricky if she is young and possibly wants to be out with her peers in clubs (☐ see Pharmacological management, Chapter 16).
- Explain the principle of intensive treatment at the start of the diagnosis is to prevent damage and complications in later life (☐ see Pharmacological management, Chapter 16).
- Reassure that RA is better understood today and the treatment is much more effective than when her grandmother was diagnosed.
- Advise her that with a bit of careful planning of her treatment with her specialist team she will be able to consider having a family at some point (☐ see Pregnancy and fertility, p.391).
- Encourage exercise governed by how she feels day-to-day.
- Explain pacing to ensure she can manage her job.
- Encourage her to explain her problems to her friends and reassure her that she will have good and bad days to start with when she may feel more tired, and that the medication might take a few months to reach full potential.
- Encourage concordance related to medication and blood monitoring.
- If available, advise her of the specialist telephone advice line service .
- Suggest she contacts the specialist nurse for additional advice on her RA if indicated.

For practical advice on osteoporosis and osteoarthritis see ☐ Chapter 2, Osteoarthritis; ☐ Chapter 3, Osteoporosis.

Box 11.6 Case scenario 3

Mrs H comes to see you for a blood test as she has been prescribed MTX to help modify her recently diagnosed RA.

She is in a 'bit of a state' as she couldn't hear very well when the doctor at the hospital told her about the medication. She is very worried she is not talking her medication correctly and thought the doctor said something about cancer drugs—but she can't remember what was said.

How can you help?
- Reassure her that you will be able to help and you will be able to write down the instructions for her.
- Explain that in much larger doses MTX is used in cancer care as well as for RA.
- Explain that the MTX must only be taken once a week.
- Ensure that she has also been prescribed folic acid 5mg—also to take once a week on a different day to the MTX.
- Re-enforce the message about monthly blood tests.
- Ask if she has been referred to the OT for joint protection advice—arrange referral if not so that the OT can also assess for aids and/or adaptations to the home to help maintain independence.
- Assess and ask the patient about any mobility problems they may have.
- Check that analgesia has been prescribed and that she understands how to take these to their full potential.
- Explain that the medication can take some time to modify the RA and that it is sometimes possible to have a steroid injection to settle things down while the medication is taking effect.

Ensure Mrs H has a contact number to phone for advice—either at the surgery or the specialist nurses at the hospital.

Principles of exercise for musculoskeletal conditions

The importance of muscle and physical activity

Physical activity is essential for muscle, joint, general physical, psychological and social health, function, and well-being. Muscles play a vital role in the health and function; they:

- *Contract* to move joints.
- *Allow functional stability* so that they maintain mobility.
- *Protect* from injury by preventing excessive harmful movement.
- Act as *shock absorbers* attenuating harmful forces during gait.
- Aerobic exercises (those that cause your heart and lungs to breathe faster) help to *main body weight*, *control blood sugar* and *improve mood*.

Prolonged inactivity is bad for joints; if a joint is not moved through its full range of movement regularly:

- Movement becomes restricted.
- Muscles become weaker, tire quicker, fail to prevent harmful movement.

For muscles to work efficiently a combination of factors must be applied including maintaining a joint through an adequate but full ROMs. When assessing patients consider:

- If adequate use of the joint is being maintained, including full ROMs.
- Can they demonstrate strength, endurance, and finely controlled movements?
- Are these abilities be maintained by regular exercise or physical activity?

Table 11.2 outlines functional issues to consider.

Safety issues and how to prevent injury

For the vast majority of people sensibly planned physical activity/exercise has many health benefits and few dangers. People with serious, unstable medical conditions, very deformed and unstable joints might not be best encouraged to undertake strenuous strengthening exercises, but should still be counselled to be physically active little and often, using a walking stick, etc. (Box 11.7).

Sports-related issues

Most sports injuries can be avoided:

- Through careful preparation and ensuring safe techniques.
- Warm up exercises may be helpful.
- The right equipment (including protective equipment) and appropriate shoes are imperative to safe exercising.

Sports injuries are beyond the scope of this book but consider if an acute or chronic problem. Prompt treatment to acute injuries includes topical applications of ice packs, compression, and elevation (ICE).

Table 11.2 Functional issues to consider

Joint range of movement	Move joint frequently through its full range of movement (3–4 sets of 5–10 stretches, 2–3 times a day), holding a sustained stretch (10–30sec) at the end of ROM
Strength	Perform a few contractions (5) against a high resistance (e.g. pushing against a fixed object or lifting a heavy weight), 2–3 times a day
Endurance	Perform many contractions (10 sets of 10–20 contractions), against a low resistance (light weight) 5–10 times a day.
Controlled movement	Frequent practice of specific activities so that muscle activity patterns that make up a movement become automatic.

Box 11.7 To exercise safely, effectively, and regularly people should:

- Always ensure they are stable and safe when exercising.
- Start a new exercise/activity cautiously.
- Set simple, challenging, but realistic, achievable goals—pursue them in a very focused way.
- Write an 'Action Plan' of *exactly* what, when, where, and how they will exercise.
- Progress slowly the time, frequency, and intensity of exercise.
- Work within their capabilities but 'nudge the boundaries 'of their capabilities.
- Exercise moderately—they should feel slightly warm and their heart beating a little faster but they should be able to hold a conversation while doing an activity. Blood, sweat and tears are not essential—or desirable.
- If an activity causes prolonged pain, discomfort, or swelling lasting more than a couple of days or wakes them at night, rest for a couple of days. As the pain settles resume exercising gently, gradually building up the exercises as before but leaving out activities that caused pain or adding them cautiously.
- Monitor progress. If they can't achieve a goal make it easier.
- When their goal is achieved—recognize and encourage—appreciate their achievements and benefits. Encourage them to reward themselves. Revise goals and action plans, setting more challenging goals to improve further or maintain the improvement.
- Plan for relapse—think about what might stop them exercising and how to overcome these barriers.
- Get support of family and friends.

Exercise: health benefits

As health benefits are 'dose-related', the more people do the better. In fact our usual daily physical activities—manual work, walking, gardening, shopping, housework, a day out—are 'informal' exercises that have health benefits. Almost anything that ↑ activity is good.

'Formal' exercise (exercise classes, cycling, swimming, 'aqua therapy' yoga, Tai Chi etc.) are excellent, but require effort and sometimes, equipment, facilities and supervision.

However, attaining health benefits:
- *Does not require* long bouts of exhausting, strenuous exercise.
- *Does not require* joining a gym, supervision, or expensive equipment.
- Occurs by accumulating 30min physical activity most days of the week.

> So, health improvements =
> 1 × 30min activity = 2 × 15min activity = 3 × 10min activity

It is essential to incorporate normal health benefits of exercise into the clinical using a practical approach to improve functional ability. This can be achieved by:
- Undertaking a patient-centred assessment:
  - Consider current health status and functional ability.
  - Cognitive abilities.
  - Health beliefs and behaviours.

Identify a goal setting approach with an aim of progressively improving functional ability in the context of the patient's abilities and aims.

Walking is safe, simple physical activity that can be integrated into normal routine by ↑ the amount normally taken. Provide simple practical advice for those with mild self-limiting conditions or conditions where evidence demonstrates benefits of walking. Encourage simple options such as:
- Walking rather than driving.
- Getting off a bus/train earlier and walk the last bit.
- The use of stairs rather than the lift.

Exercise is effective whether it is performed at home alone, a leisure centre or in an exercise class. The important thing is to find something that the patient finds comfortable, enjoyable, achievable, affordable and available, and they can integrate it into their lifestyle.

Exercise: nursing issues

Encouraging exercise in joint disease

An often-neglected area in management of arthritis and especially in OA and RA is exercise and the practice nurse is well placed to encourage and motivate patients. Cardiovascular risk prevention is an important factor especially for patients with RA who are 4 × more likely to suffer from cardiovascular events compared with the general population.

A gradual ↓ in functional mobility and ↑ pain and stiffness can have a negative impact on physiological, psychological, and social aspects of an individual's life. As with many MSCs the condition itself can confer risks that will result in a functional decline, e.g.:

Rheumatoid disease confers a heightened risk of
- Cardiovascular disease.
- Depression.
- Mood disturbance.
- Osteoporosis.
- Muscle wasting.
- 2° degenerative arthritis.
- Fatigue.
- Anemia of chronic disease.

These are all good indications for an exercise regimen. Patients will often ask the practice nurse 'Is it ok for me to exercise?' Most forms of exercise are safe and effective in improving function, especially if appropriately advised and gradually developed.

Exercise can be self-supervised but follow-up will encourage compliance:
- Aerobic—walking.
- Strengthening—upper and lower limb exercise, swimming, cycling.
- Gentle stretching and education about use of ice after exercise to reduce any post-exercise inflammation is important.
  Patients will need:
- Reassurance.
- Encouragement and support.
- May require involvement of therapist to support concordance for those failing to achieve goals.
- Optimized regular analgesia especially for those who are having trouble mobilizing.
- Encouraged to keep an exercise diary.

Exercise examples for patients

The following exercises should be started gently and ↑ gradually.

Knee bends

Sit on the floor, couch, or bed with your legs outstretched. Slowly bend up your right knee until you feel a comfortable stretch. Hold for 5 or 6sec. Straighten your leg out. Rest for 3sec. Repeat × 10. Repeat using the left leg.

Static quadriceps

Sitting on the floor (sofa or bed) with your legs outstretched, place a rolled-up towel under 1 knee. Push your knee down on the towel straightening your knee, pull your toes and foot towards you; feel your calf muscles stretch and your heel lift off the floor. Hold for 5sec; relax for 5sec, repeat × 10. Repeat the exercise with the other leg.

Sit-to-stands

Sitting on a chair, fold your arms. Stand up slowly without using your arms. Stand for a few seconds. Sit down slowly. Do this for 1 minute.

Step-ups

Place your right foot on the bottom step of the stairs, using the banisters for support. Step up and down with the left leg. Count and record the number of step-ups you perform in 1min. Rest for 1min, and then repeat the exercise keeping your left leg on the step.

Elastic band resistance (Fig. 11.1)

Tie an elastic inner tube of a bicycle tyre or resistive exercise bands (e.g. Thera-Band™) to an immovable object (e.g. leg a chair or bed). Loop it around your right foot. Slowly straighten your knee as far as you can, stretching the band. Hold for 5sec. Control the band so that your leg is slowly pulled back to the starting position. Repeat for 1–2min. Repeat using your left foot.

Self-resistance (Fig. 11.2)

Sitting on a chair; cross one leg behind the other. Push forward with the back leg as if to straighten it, but prevent this happening by pushing back with the front leg. Push as hard as possible for 5sec, and then relax completely for 3sec, repeat, and after 6 contractions rest for 1min. Repeat this procedure until you have done 4 sets of 6 contractions 24 contractions in total). Repeat exercise with the other leg in front.

Trunk rotations (Fig. 11.3)

Lie on the floor or bed with your knees bent. Keeping your knees together slowly let your knees fall to the right. Stop when you feel a gentle stretch in your lower back and left thigh. Hold for 5–6sec. Return to the starting position. Now let your knees fall gently to the left. Hold for 5–6 sec. Repeat × 10. Rest for 30sec. Repeat × 5.

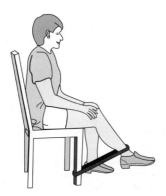

Fig. 11.1 Elastic band resistance. Reproduced with kind permission from the ARC.

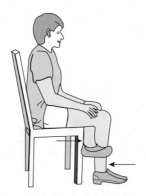

Fig. 11.2 Self resistance. Reproduced with kind permission from the ARC.

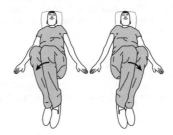

Fig. 11.3 Trunk rotations. Reproduced with kind permission from the ARC.

Hugging knees to chest (Fig. 11.4)

Lying on your back with bent knees, lift 1 leg and hold on to it with 1 hand and then lift and hold the other leg. Pull both knees gently closer to your chest, hold for a count of 5, then relax your arms but don't let go completely. Repeat the hug and relax.

Half push-ups (Fig. 11.5)

Lie on your front on a firm surface. Push up slowly straightening your elbows, lifting your head and shoulders, look up at the ceiling feeling a stretch in your lower back, breathe out, keep your hips on the floor. Hold for 5 seconds, gently lower yourself down. Repeat 5 times

Leg stretches (Fig. 11.6)

Lying on your back with your knees bent, lift one knee and hold your thigh with both hands behind the knee. Gently straighten the knee that you are holding and hold for a count of 5. Repeat with the opposite leg.

Arching and hollowing (Fig. 11.7)

Start on all fours, hands under shoulders, knees under hips. Arch your back upwards, letting your head drop, and hold for a count of 5. Then reverse this posture: lifting your head and looking up, relax your tummy and stick your behind out, holding for 5 seconds.

Hip extensions

Lie on your tummy on the floor (or bed). Without turning or twisting your back, slowly raise your right leg up behind you about 3–4 inches (~7.5–10cm). Hold for 4–5sec. Slowly lower it to the floor. Relax. Breathe out. Repeat 5 times. Repeat with left leg.

Hip abductions

Lie comfortably on your right side on the floor or bed. Keep your knee straight, slowly raise your left leg about 2 feet (~60cm). Hold for 5–6sec. Slowly lower it. Relax. Repeat × 10. Turn over and repeat exercise using the right leg.

Hip rotations

Place your right hand on the front of your right hip. Hitch your right hip so that your right foot is an inch or two off the ground (~4cm). Turn your foot inwards to the left as far as it will go (as you do this feel your hip turning inwards to the left under your hand). Hold for 5–6sec. Turn your foot outwards to the right (feel your hip turn outwards under your hand. Hold for 5 or 6sec. Repeat × 10.

Head turns

Preventing your head from tilting to the side, keeping your shoulders relaxed; slowly turn your head to look over your right shoulder. Feel a gentle stretch and tightness in your neck. Breathe gently. Hold this position for about 5–6sec. Now turn to look over your left shoulder. Hold for 5–6sec. Repeat 5 or 6 times.

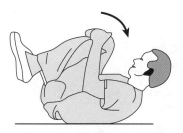

Fig. 11.4 Hugging knees to chest. Reproduced with kind permission from the ARC.

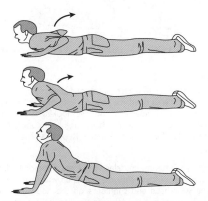

Fig. 11.5 Half push-ups. Reproduced with kind permission from the ARC.

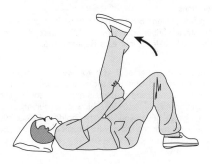

Fig. 11.6 Leg stretches. Reproduced with kind permission from the ARC.

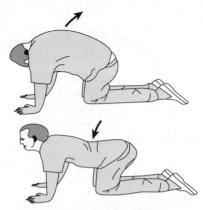

Fig. 11.7 Arching and hollowing. Reproduced with kind permission from the ARC.

Head rolls

Looking forwards, drop your chin onto your chest so you are looking at the floor. Slowly roll your head in a wide circle to the left, bringing your left ear close to your left shoulder, with your eyes looking at the direction your head is moving and coming down with your right ear coming close to your right shoulder. Relax. Repeat 3 or 4 circles. Repeat circling to the right.

Sit ups

To strengthen your tummy muscles lie on the floor or bed, place your hands on your thighs. Slowly run your hands up your thighs towards your knees, raising your head and shoulders off the floor. Hold for 5–6sec. Breathe out. Relax down slowly. Rest for 5–6sec. Repeat × 5–6.

Exercises examples for shoulders

Shoulder rotations

Clasp your hands behind your head. Gently push your elbows outwards. Feel a gentle stretch under your arms. Hold for 5sec. Breathe out. Bring your forearms back close to your ears. Repeat × 5–6.

'Drying back'

Roll up a small towel and grasp it as if you were drying your back, your right arm over the top of your right shoulder and left arm in the small of your back. With your left hand gently pull the towel down feeling a gentle pull in your right arm. Hold for 5–6sec. Now with your right hand pull the towel up, feel a gentle pull in your left arm; hold for 5–6sec. Repeat × 10. Repeat with left arm over the top of your left shoulder and your right hand in the small of your back.

Windmills

Stand relaxed with your arms by your sides. Slowly raise your arms up in front of you until you are reaching upwards. Slowly lower them to the side and behind you. Relax. Repeat 5–6 circles. Reverse the direction of the circle, going up behind and to the side and lowering them in front of you.

Figures reproduced with kind permission from the Arthritis Research Council.

Further reading

Keep Moving leaflet, available at: ⁀🖑 www.arc.org.uk

Social and voluntary sector

Historically health, social care, and voluntary sector provision all worked separately with little in the way of a strategic approach to provision of funding and numerous barriers to achieving a flexible approach to the provision of services for those in need. Excellent services were provided by a number of organizations although many were forced to work in silos (financially or organizationally). The provision of healthcare should encompass all spectrums of health and illness. In the future it is advocated that care will be improved by providing a system wide transformation built upon genuine local partnerships between:

- NHS.
- Primary Care Services.
- Local Authorities.
- Voluntary and social enterprise organizations.
- Other statutory agencies.
- User and carer communities.

The provision of a whole systems approach for a community will be achieved using local Service Level Agreements (SLAs) ensuring an agreed allocation of budgets based upon collaboration with all organizations. The strategies are developed in the context of national policies but based upon community-based health needs assessments for each region. This will enable greater interdependence between work, health, and well-being in the context of the needs of the individual. These should include recognizing:

- Their wish to live independently:
  - Encourage independent living, e.g. for older people, those with a chronic condition, disabled, or mental health problems.
- Stay healthy and recover from illness.
- Exercise and maintain control of their lives.
- Sustain family communities.
- Equal citizenship—economically and socially.
- Optimize their quality of life.
- Retain their dignity and respect.

A wide spectrum of policies and services need to identify the strategy to ensure each community has the services that are required through all stages of health and illness:

- Public health policies, e.g. infection control and falls prevention.
- Hospital care including strategies to ensure effective discharge management.
- Intermediate care.
- LTCs management.
- Packages of care that consider health and nurse care needs.
- Community equipment services.
- Informational resources—that have universal use and value for all members of the population.
- Carer support including public and patient involvement, e.g. recognizing the expertise of the carer and the role in healthcare provision.
- Systems to manage poor performance/complaints of care provided.

Social Services

A number of services are provided under the auspices of Social Services. Many of these focus specifically on those who need additional support including:

- The fail/older person.
- Physical, sensory, or learning disabilities.
- Mental health problems.

Support provided is extensive and can include support such as:

- Care homes and care services at home.
- Meals on wheels.
- Equipment and adaptations.
- Day care services.
- Social worker support and advice (children/adult needs):
  - Disability services.
  - Support for vulnerable children and their families.

Voluntary sector

There are many voluntary or social enterprise organizations that have provided essential and much valued services, often developed as a result of shortfalls in the provision of services funded by the NHS or local social services. These services are often provided by volunteers directly to patient groups or within a specific community. Examples include:

- Library services in hospitals.
- EPP—Social enterprise.
- 'Meet and Greet' volunteers in hospital and medical centres.
- Social support and information sharing for individuals with long-term conditions, e.g. RA.
- Alzheimer's Society helpline, research and support.
- Assist—impartial advice and support for the disabled.
- Carers UK helping carers recognize their needs.
- The DLF provides information and advice on disability equipment and ways of managing disability.
- The Samaritans provides a range of completely confidential services for those who are suicidal or experiencing emotional distress.
- Educational and training opportunities activities for those with medical conditions—range of voluntary sector organizations.

Many of the voluntary sector organizations provide websites, literature, telephone advice line support and local meetings/activities.

Nurses should ensure that they have a good understanding of services available within the community and proactively voice new ways of working that will encompass all social and voluntary organizations.

Further reading

Department of Health (2007). *Putting people first. A shared vision and commitment to the transformation of adult social care.* DH, London.

Volunteering England (2006). *Volunteers across the NHS.* Volunteering England. London.

Care Services Improvement Partnership (2007). *Integration for Social Enterprise.* Care Services Improvement Partnership, London.

Ward-based care and referral to the multidisciplinary team

Ward-based care: overview

As 20% of the UK population have to cope with a MSC at any one time it will be inevitable that nurses in all care settings will come across individuals with a MSC. The costs of MSC are felt by the individual and society as they have the potential to affect work-related incapacity and the use of health-care resources. It is ∴ highly likely that you will encounter such patients during your work on the ward. The benefits of understanding MSC and providing nursing expertise will be in aiding the patient's physical and mental rehabilitation whilst working as part of a MTD.

The common MSCs include:
- OA.
- Osteoporosis.
- Trauma and soft tissue injury, e.g. rotator cuff rupture in the shoulder, meniscal tear in the knee, and RTA causing fracture.
- Inflammatory joint conditions such as RA, PsA, AS, and CTDs. These conditions have systemic and long-term effects.

📖 Also see Classifying joint disease, p.4; 📖 Orthopaedic management, p.239.

New models of care such as triage, rapid assessment, and proactive reviews of patients with MSC, coupled with the advent of new targeted drug therapies, has accelerated changes in the work of rheumatology services. Rheumatology is predominantly an outpatient and day case-based specialty and is delivered by a MDT. Yet despite all these developments MSCs have a major impact on the individual, affecting not only function and quality of life but with some long-term inflammatory conditions the disease can result in systemic effects on major bodily systems such as the heart, lungs, skin, and kidney and cause deformity and damage to joints. Dedicated rheumatology inpatient beds are in short supply and in many circumstances patients are admitted according to the organ involvement (e.g. respiratory or cardiology wards). Hospital admissions may be required for:
- Management of an exacerbation of the disease (flare) and rehabilitation.
- Underlying comorbidities as a result of the systemic effects of the disease, e.g. cardiovascular disease.
- Toxicity/adverse events of treatment, e.g. MTX pneumonitis.
- Blood and imaging investigations.
- Assessment by other medical specialists and members of the MDT.
- Planned surgical procedures.
- Day case treatments.
- Respite care.

Key points for nurses to consider in ward-based care
- Symptom control needs:
  - Patients with IJD experience EMS.
  - Pain and analgesia needs.
- Functional needs of the patient in relation to the environment, e.g. chair raisers, tap turners, or other assistive devices.
  - Patients may have problems with independent activities, particularly postoperatively, as they may be unable to lift themselves up, get on and off a bedpan, or reach for a drink, unlike the more mobile patients.

- Knowledge of drug therapies commonly prescribed, monitoring, and potential side effects.
- Referral points and when and how to access specialist or MDT support.

Also see Orthopaedic care, p.239; Pharmacological management, p.419; Symptom control, p.289; Multi-disciplinary referrals, p.372.

Ward-based care and day case issues

Nurses must consider the needs of the patient in the context of a holistic and patient-centred assessment regardless of the care setting, although needs may vary significantly depending upon the diagnosis and treatments. Depending upon the knowledge and skills of the nurse managing patients with MSC, the level of additional specialist expertise required will vary, as will the environment where the care is being delivered.

Many new drug therapies are administered by IV infusion and this has resulted in the expansion of day case services and the development of protocols for the specific drugs.

Patients attend for treatments usually as a day case for:

- Administration of biologic drugs such as infliximab or rituximab.
- Bisphosphonates such as pamidronate and zoledronic acid.
- Epoprostenol infusion (a prostaglandin used to treat high blood pressure in the vessels associated with the lungs)—for shorter infusions over 5 days but some units admit patients fully for longer infusions over 3 days.
- Steroid infusions.
- Cyclophosphamide infusions.
- Joint injections—when a number of joints are being injected.

📖 Also see Pharmacological management, p.419.

Care as a day case: general issues

Patients attending for a day case infusion, particularly for the first time, require reassurance and clarity about what they should expect during the day. Treatment should ensure that:

- Pre-admission information should have been provided about the planned treatment and specific blood tests and investigations undertaken prior to day case admission. Where these have not been undertaken treatment should be reviewed and discussed with prescribing physician.
- Test results should be double checked and any abnormalities discussed with the prescribing physician.
- Any patient-held treatment records should be completed and returned to the patient.
- Specialist teams may wish to review the patient whilst a day patient.
- A day case unit visit is an opportunity to provide additional information and advice. Some units have volunteers or lay helpers who can facilitate communication and information on voluntary and social sector advice.

Treatments

IA and soft tissue injections

- Patients will require information about the procedure and clarification that there are no contraindications to receiving treatment.
- Often patients attending either as an inpatient or a day case will require joint and soft tissue injections. The procedure can be uncomfortable for the patient but the results are rapid reduction in pain, swelling, and disability.

- The nurse can support the patient through the procedure.
- Afterwards the patient will be advised to minimize mobility in the specific joint for up to 48 hours.
- Steroids may make the blood sugar rise and so diabetics are advised to be aware of this in their post-injection monitoring.
- Patients should be provided with information on how to manage post-injections, e.g. what to do if they experience problems and what activities are advised post injection.

📖 Also see Joint injections, p.494.

Addition of new disease-modifying drug therapy

Patients attending the ward and receiving interventions may also be reviewed and decisions made to change or add in a new treatment. If this is the case, nursing support should provide:

- Drug information leaflets for any proposed change of drug treatment; allow them to read the information and discuss and clarify the information with them.
- Outline the drug treatments, the drug preparation, how to take the drug, how to get a further supply, the benefits and side effects and what to do if side effects occur, monitoring requirements, alcohol allowance, contraceptive and breastfeeding precautions, vaccinations, and arrangements for follow-up. Alternative options should be discussed if the patient wishes.
- A patient-held record (shared care card) with baseline haematological and biochemical results should be provided.
- Access to and advice on use of a rheumatology telephone advice line.

📖 Also see Blood tests and investigations, p.461.

General care issues

When a patient is admitted to hospital it is an ideal opportunity to look holistically at all aspects of their care, using a problem-solving approach to achieve optimum disease control and rehabilitation to facilitate discharge and support ongoing care management plans.

Assessment of ADL

- The nurse makes a full assessment to include past medical history, current drug therapies and previous drug history, reason for admission and level of disease activity, social history encompassing living conditions, social support, work, and leisure pursuits.
- Physical assessment of joints and skin.
- Mobility status and use of walking aids and, if required, availability of toilet and chair raisers, tap turners, etc. on the ward.
- Pain status to identify the patient's methods of coping with pain.
- Psychological status to identify the patient's coping methods and current concerns.

Investigations

- A range of tests will be required from blood tests, imaging, urine, faeces, sputum, synovial fluid, and skin biopsy.
- The nurse can ensure, if personally responsible for collection of samples, that these are obtained and sent with appropriate documentation as soon as possible.
- The nurse can obtain the results so they are available for review and explain the meaning of the results to the patient.

Pain management

- The patient's pain should be reviewed regularly using an objective pain measurement tool such as a 10cm VAS or pain diary to collect information on the nature, severity, and frequency of pain. This facilitates modification of analgesia and evaluation to achieve optimum pain control.
- Where patient self-administration of medication is possible and appropriate patients should be supported in self-administration of their medications. Timing of medications is important to patients who have self-managed their conditions for many years.
- Care should be taken to establish how the patient wants to be lifted as manhandling can cause significant pain.
- Assess the frequency of bowel movements as analgesia cause constipation.
- Periods of quiet time should be incorporated into the patient's care plan to facilitate a balance of rest and relaxation.
- Observe the patient's sleep pattern to ensure that pain is not disturbing sleep.

Psychological support

Patients cope better psychologically when their pain is recognized and support provided in controlling the symptoms. The nurse needs to talk and listen to the patient over all aspects of care, especially when decisions about changes to treatment and management have taken place. This can help to clarify salient points, alleviate anxiety, and allow the patient's views to be taken into account.

Rehabilitation and discharge planning

- Immediately following the patient's initial assessment, a plan for discharge should be prepared. This will allow for all social issues that might prevent a timely discharge from hospital to be addressed.
- Early referral to relevant MDT members for assessment, programme of rehabilitation, and guidance on discharge needs.

Hygiene and toileting

- Care must be taken to provide privacy and dignity wherever possible whilst respecting the person's wish for independence, particularly for toileting and hygiene needs. This can be a specific problem for those with damaged joints or experiencing a flare.
- It is good practice to ask the patient what they can do for themselves and what they require help with. Patients experience EMS so it is preferable to allow this to ease off, and immersion in a bath or shower later in the morning can help significantly ↑ independence.

Tissue viability

- Patients often have paper-thin fragile skin (often steroid-related) and this, coupled with ↓ mobility, leads to higher objective measurement of pressure score risk. Be aware of vulnerable areas such as elbows and heels.
- Tissue viability can be improved by regularly inspecting the skin to detect potential breakdown and by keeping the skin moisturized. Good diet and fluid intake should be encouraged. Injury from sharp objects such as rings and watches should be avoided. Pressure should be regularly relieved by moving and mobilizing the patient and by using pressure relieving devices.
- Many drug therapies can give rise to rashes. These should be reported promptly and managed to avoid tissue damage.
- Report signs of abnormal bruising, bleeding, or discoloration of digits.

📖 Also see Primary systemic vasculitis, p.150.

Diet

- Assess normal dietary intake and preferences.
- Refer to the dietician if the patient has become emaciated prior to their admission, for advice regarding a build-up diet and also seek advice for patients who would benefit from losing weight.
- Ask and support the patient if assistance is required with feeding, e.g. cutting up meat, getting the tops off containers. Equally, referral to an OT may be able to facilitate greater independence using aids and devices (such as special cutlery).
- Don't overfill water jugs and ensure that it is accessible.

Risks related to inpatient care

Patients with long-term musculoskeletal/functional limitations are prone to falling

- Recurrent inflammation leads to loss of muscle bulk and stretching of tendons, ligaments, and the capsule that support joints.
- Osteoporosis is induced by the inflammatory process, immobility, and long-term use of steroids. Falls often result in fracture of the humerus, wrist, thoracic spine, pelvis, or femur.
- Steroid use thins the skin and falls often result in soft tissue injury, such as full tissue skin tears and chronic ulceration.
- Patients may be on a combination of several drugs thereby ↑ the likelihood of drug interactions and confusion so ↑ the risk of falling.
- Falls and significant injury greatly ↑ the risk of premature death, loss of confidence, and mobility leading to greater disability.
- Careful assessment and support to mobilize patients must be considered, e.g. the use of a walking aid might be appropriate in order to reduce the risk of falling and injury.
- Provide a safe, clutter-free environment and ensure the nurse call button is accessible.

Infection

- Immunosuppressant drugs such as MTX, biological agents, and steroids are commonly prescribed. In some circumstances bone marrow suppression may make the patient more susceptible to infections, sometimes fatally.
- Unusual infections such as TB, osteomyelitis, and septic arthritis can occur.
- Infection can accelerate very quickly. Concomitant steroid therapy can mask the onset of infection and the patient can become rapidly overwhelmed.
- Regular monitoring of patients general well-being, temperature, and vital signs are paramount in early detection and treatment of infection.
- If infection occurs, they may need a combination of aggressive antibiotic therapy.
- Ideally immunosuppressed patients should be isolated from other patients with infection.
- Effective hand washing and disinfecting procedures are crucial to avoid cross infection from 1 patient to another.

Points to consider in drug therapies

Disease-modifying drugs need to be taken on a regular basis. If a patient fails to continue their DMARD for several weeks it is highly likely that they will relapse.

- On occasions drug treatment can be accidentally discontinued, e.g. patients routinely stop their DMARD for surgical procedures such as hip replacement and there is a failure to inform the patient that the drug should be recommenced. An ideal way to counteract this difficulty is to ensure that the DMARD is prescribed in their medication to take home on discharge.
- Discharge from hospital can be a risk to the patient as they are often lost to follow-up or receive no monitoring.

- Following hospital admission, patients may relapse very quickly and therefore it is good practice to ensure that the patient receives a review in the clinic within 6 weeks.
- Monitoring arrangements should be confirmed before discharge. GPs may be unable to provide monitoring and it will be necessary to arrange for a follow-up appointment with the rheumatology nurse specialist.
- It is helpful to ensure that monitoring blood tests are taken and checked prior to the patient discharge—optimizing the interval before they have to return to the hospital or their GP.
- Rarely patients will be on subcutaneous MTX. If the patient or carer is unable to inject then a nurse competent in administration of cytotoxic drugs should be identified to administer this medication.
- Patients who hold shared care monitoring booklets should have information updated and returned to the patient prior to discharge.

Points to consider for patients attending as a day case

Day case patients attend usually for a short period ∴ all relevant information needs to be conveyed about the treatment to be given and actions to be taken at home, especially when an invasive procedure has been administered such as carpal tunnel release, injection, or infusion treatment.

Multidisciplinary team referrals

Referrals to the MDT will be required at times when patients are admitted with a MSC. The rheumatology nurse specialist is often in a key position to coordinate MTD referrals and can therefore advise ward-based nurses on the most appropriate referral for the patient.

Rheumatology nurse specialist

- Acts as an expert resource for ward and teams managing patients with complex, long-term MSC.
- Can, in many cases, undertake an assessment of disease activity in relation to the MSC.
- Educates patients about the disease, treatment, and facilitates development of coping skills.
- Provides nurse-led clinics for review and tight control of patient's disease activity.
- Offers telephone support for patients, carers, and HCPs.
- Coordinates referrals to the MDT.

PT

- Teaches patients exercise regimens to build muscle strength and maintain a full range of movements in joints.
- Provides targeted treatment to joints or muscle groups, e.g. for frozen shoulder, and some give joint injections.
- Offers other treatments such as acupuncture and TENS.
- Manages hydrotherapy, OA, and back pain classes and falls clinics.
- Provide musculoskeletal triage services working as extended scope PTs.

OT

- Educates patients on joint protection, e.g. using assistive devices such as a helping hand or kettle tipper and energy conservation by planning and pacing daily activities.
- Supplies and fits custom-make hand and finger splints.
- Assesses patients in the home or workplace, advising on the organization of the environment to enable tasks to be performed more easily.
- Provides wheelchair assessments.

 Also see Equipment aids and devices, p.344.

Podiatrist

- Assesses the function of the lower limb in order to make orthotic appliances such as a metatarsal support to redistribute loading, reduce pain, and facilitate mobility.
- Educates on foot care.
- Provides joint injections to the lower limb and performs minor surgery under local anaesthetic, such as tenotomy and excision of metatarsal heads.

Orthotist

Measures and provides a wide range of orthotic appliances such as insoles, bespoke footwear, knee braces, hand splints, and cervical collars. Works in conjunction with the podiatrist on provision of lower limb appliances.

Dietician

- Provides expert advice on specific dietary needs in the context of a condition, e.g. calcium and vitamin D intake for those at risk of osteoporosis.
- Provides education on healthy diet and important food groups to be included in reducing and weight-gain diets.
- Advises and supports patients on the use of dietary supplements and exclusion diets.

Clinical psychologist

- Assesses the impact of the condition to help resolve personal and emotional issues and aid in the development of effective coping. One such strategy is CBT which enables patients to alter their thinking and gain control.
- Advises on use of anti-depressant drugs.

Pharmacist

- Educates patients on drug treatments, checks the safety of drugs prescribed, supports patients entering drug trials, and provides drug information and support to prescribers.
- Reviews poly-pharmacy and identifes potential drug interactions/side effects.
- Medicines management for discharge from hospital.

Social worker

Advises on social issues of self-care, respite care, housing, aids, adaptations, and benefits.

Medical referrals

A specialist opinion is often required about the systemic effects of arthritis. In complex cases, the patient might be referred to the following specialties: renal, hepatology, respiratory, cardiology, neurology, dermatology, haematology, urology, ophthalmology, rehabilitation, and pain team.

Surgical referrals

Surgical opinions are often required and these range from vascular, plastics, hand, foot, arthroplasty, and spinal surgeons.

Self-management, monitoring, and patient-held records

It is recognized that the patient must be central to care in order that they can adjust to and live with their long-term MSC. This is to enable the patient to navigate their way through the healthcare system, make decisions about how their condition is managed, improve their concordance with treatment, utilize health resources appropriately, and enjoy improved health outcome and quality of life. Patients are increasingly being recognized as consumers and are being consulted on redesign and delivery of services.

Self-management

The patient can only develop self-management skills if they are:
- Informed about the importance of their involvement and the role they are to play.
- Given access to full, transparent, and unbiased information about their condition, prognosis, treatment interventions, and the service that they can expect to receive.
- Given consistent and unconflicting advice from all health professional groups.
- Able to build a rapport with their HCPs.
- Offered a range of treatment options over which they feel they have a choice.
- Aware of the next steps in their treatment plan and so it is good practice to provide a copy of clinic letters to patients in order that they can ensure plans are acted up with their carers, community health professionals, other hospital specialists, and employer.
- Given helpline support and can gain rapid access for reassessment.
- Given early support from diagnosis and this support continues throughout their care pathway.
- Provided with access to support groups in the voluntary sector.
- Provided access to nurse-led clinics for review and tight control of disease activity.
- Offered telephone support for patients, carers and HCPs.
- Provided by access to members of the MDT.

📖 Also see Self-management, p.324; 📖 Patient education, p.318.

Patient education

- Is a set of spontaneous or planned activities aimed at facilitating the acquisition of knowledge, self-management skills, coping, improvement in mood, pain control, and health behaviour.
- Can take place on a one-to-one basis by the bedside, in clinic, over the telephone, or by email.
- Can take place alongside the patient's carer.
- Can be delivered in small groups in a classroom, covering topics such as aetiology of the disease, management of pain and coping with a flare, diet, joint protection strategies, exercise, and drugs.
- Can be in the form of a leaflet or booklet, especially to back up a verbal discussion.

Patient pathway

- Increasingly patients are entering pathways of care that coordinate care across acute and 1° care settings and time interventions to improve health outcomes.
- Regardless of the aim of care pathways, patients with arthritis face constant uncertainty and unplanned exacerbations are a constant factor in their lives. The nature of the disease is of remission and relapse and it is important for patients to know what the next steps in their pathway will be. This helps to alleviate anxiety, enabling them to plan, mentally prepare, and recognize that options have not run out

Monitoring of drug therapy

DMARDs can result in a range of minor to extremely severe side effects so monitoring is vital. The side effects and the frequency of monitoring vary for each drug and these have been set out in national guidelines.[1] The term 'monitoring' is not just about identifying side effects but also about monitoring the patient's well-being, disease activity, and response to treatment.

- Patients need to be taught how to self- monitor and about the action they must take should a side effect occur.
- Monitoring usually takes place in the rheumatology clinic and GP surgery, but it might also need to be done on the ward initially, if the patient has commenced a new DMARD as an inpatient.
- Rule of thumb is to monitor FBC, liver and renal function tests initially and based upon national DMARD guidelines (2–4-weekly may be required) for most drugs. This helps to identify trends in blood results, indicating development of immunosuppression, anaemia, liver and renal abnormalities.
- Blood tests to measure levels of inflammation such as ESR and CRP help to gauge level of disease activity alongside a physical examination of the patient.
- Urine tests and blood pressure monitoring is required for some drugs as they can cause proteinuria and hypertension.
- Assess the patient and ask about symptoms of mucositis, stomatitis, herpes simplex, rashes, infection, dyspnoea, nausea, vomiting, diarrhoea, hair loss, bruising and bleeding, and anything new or unusual about their health.
- Seek advice over any monitoring concerns from an expert rheumatology practitioner.

Also see Pharmacological management, p.419.

Reference

1. Chakravarety K, *et al.* (2008). BSR and BHPR Guidelines for Disease-modifying anti-rheumatic drug therapy (DMARD) in consultation with the British Association of Dermatologists. *Rheumatology.* Available at: www.rheumatology.org.uk

Patient-held record (shared care card)

It is good practice to issue a patient-held record/patient-held monitoring booklet if patients are receiving regular treatment that requires monitoring of blood results. The most important group is those patients who are treated with a DMARD. Examples of DMARDs include MTX or leflunomide.

If patients attend as a day case or inpatient and bring along their patient-held monitoring record it is a record that belongs to the patient (Figure 12.1). It needs to be returned to them. It is an important aspect of their care and they will appreciate relevant blood tests or treatments being recorded in this document, e.g. an injection of Depo-Medrone®.

This information will be helpful to the specialist team reviewing the patient at the next clinic appointment but, most importantly, continue the principles of:

• Self-management and patient knowledge about blood monitoring and trends in blood results.
• Reducing potential risk related to treatments and changes in blood results.
• Providing an important aide memoir for the patient of treatments received, e.g. treatment, dose, and date administered.
• Reinforces to the patient the value of close monitoring of their treatment

The patient-held blood monitoring booklet:

• Details the baseline and sequential monitoring blood results, drugs, and dose titration, important instructions for patients, and rheumatology department contact numbers.
• Enables identification of worrying trends and action to be taken.
• Facilitates information exchange and communication between care settings.
• Gives the patient information to provide to any healthcare worker and shows evidence of improvement and deterioration.
• Patients need to be educated about the details that are recorded.

Further reading

Department of Health (2006). *Musculoskeletal services framework*. Department of Health, London.

Hill J (2006). *Rheumatology a creative approach*. John Wiley & Sons Ltd: Chichester.

CURRENT BIOLOGIC: _____

DMARD: _____

PREVIOUS DMARDs	DATE STOPPED	IN COMBINATION WITH
PREVIOUS BIOLOGIC:		

DATE							
HB							
WCC							
NEUTROPHILS							
PLATELETS							
McV							
ALT							
ALK PHOS							
ESR/CRP							
VIS							
B/P							
URINE HAQ SCORE							
DOSE CHANGES							
DAS							
COMMENTS							

Fig. 12.1 Example of a shared care monitoring booklet.

Chapter 13

Rapid access and emergency issues

Infections in musculoskeletal conditions

Introduction

Patients may have infections unrelated to their arthritis. However, there are various inflammatory mechanisms and infections that are linked to MSC, e.g. septic arthritis, ReA, rheumatic fever. Patients with MSC may be more susceptible to infection—either bacterial or viral—and these may be systemic or local. Susceptibility may be related to drug therapies or confounding diseases.

Corticosteroids, DMARDs, and biologics all have the potential to ↑ infection risk and potentially mask the signs of infection. Immunosuppressive therapy may mask the normal signs and symptoms of fever.

▶ Infections must be diagnosed early in order to prevent the onset of systemic infection.

▶▶In the event that infection is suspected DMARDs should be stopped and prompt advice sought.

Some conditions such as inflammatory and connective tissue disease have a strong association with pulmonary infections. There should be a strong index of suspicion if patients present with symptoms suggestive of TB, particularly for those being treated with anti-TNFα therapies as there is the potential for re-emergence of latent TB (📖 see New disease-modifying drugs: biologic therapies, p.456).

If patients present with viral herpes zoster/varicella and are taking immunosuppressive therapy, this should be stopped and referral made for specialist advice. Shingles may present following a high-dose steroid infusion in those previously exposed to the varicella virus. Treatment is urgently required with anti-zoster therapies such as acyclovir.

In ideal circumstances patients should be screened for their immune status and immunization should be planned prior to them starting DMARDs, but particularly newer biologic therapies; however, this has to be balanced against the need to start prompt treatment.

For specific guidance on children and young people see 📖 New disease-modifying drugs: biologic therapies, p.456).

Nursing care issues in management

The nurse in 1° care or rapid access clinics should be vigilant to the signs of infection.

▶ Be aware that patients with inflammatory conditions taking DMARDS and biologics are at higher risk of infection.

For systemic infection (see Box 13.1) check for:
- Fever, aches and pains, rigor, nausea/vomiting.
- URTI—cough, short of breath, chest pain, sputum.
- UTI—burning/stinging, frequency/urgency, lower abdominal pain.

For local infection check for localized pain, swelling, redness, pus, and sometimes fever.

Review

Monitor resolving signs and symptoms of fever, ESR, CRP, and WBC. Assess the patient thoroughly to ensure resolution of symptoms. Careful monitoring and review of treatment benefits and investigations will be essential.

Social and psychological impact of infections

Patients can feel anxious and concerned about the infection but also fearful about the consequences to their condition generally. If their underlying condition is usually treated with immunosuppressive therapy they will also be concerned that their treatment is stopped and their disease will flare. To allay fears and ensure patients are adequately informed, they should be provided with information about investigations and treatment plans, together with general advice and support to improve outcomes and concordance.

Box 13.1 Systemic infection

Presentation
- Fever

Diagnostic considerations
Differential diagnoses e.g. ReA, osteomyelitis, PAN.
- Septic arthritis (🕮 see Septic arthritis, p.384).
- Viral infection.
- Rheumatic fever.

Investigations
- WBC, CRP, ESR, U&Es, and LFTs.
- Sputum/urine specimen for culture and sensitivity.
- Chest auscultation.
- If septic joint suspected, joint aspiration for Gram stain and culture prior to starting antibiotics (if an arthoplasty in situ this will require urgent referral to orthopaedic surgeon).
- Blood cultures.
- If non-articular sepsis, appropriate swabs should be taken, i.e. skin or oral/urethral swabs.

Treatment
- If patient is taking an immunosuppressive therapy (e.g. DMARDS/biologics) stop treatment and contact 2° care rheumatology team.
- Patients with inflammatory conditions have a lower threshold for treatment for chest infection or UTI and usually need >3-day course of antibiotics.
- If patient is systemically unwell consider urgent admission.

⚠ Surgeons require biologic therapies to be stopped before surgery (according to the half-life of the drug) and will be restarted once there are no risks related to infection.

☛ In some cases MTX is also withheld prior to surgery.

Accessing key management information in caring for those with musculoskeletal infections

- Communicate with rheumatology team. Use rheumatology nurse specialist helpline as point of contact.
- Liaise with rheumatology team to access monitoring protocols and advice regarding trends/abnormal values and when to stop treatment.

Points to note

- Concerns exist regarding the ↑ risk of TB with biological therapies. Biologics are used in the treatment of RA, PsA, AS, and some forms of vasculitis, mixed CTD. Patients should carry a biologics alert card is receiving anti-TNFα (Fig. 13.1).
- DMARDs and biologics can be continued during surgery unless a specific risk of infection is identified.
- Signs and symptoms of pneumonitis (which can be related to MTX), such as SOB, cough, and fever must not be confused with infection. Patients require prompt investigation (HRCT lungs and PFTs) and stop MTX immediately.

📖 Also see Septic arthritis, p.384.

Further reading

British Society for Rheumatology (2006). *Guidelines for the management of rheumatoid arthritis (first 2 years)*. British Society for Rheumatology, London.

British Society for Rheumatology (2006). *Guidelines in the management of hot swollen joints*. British Society for Rheumatology, London.

Hakim A, Clunie G, Haq I (eds) (2006). *Oxford Handbook of Rheumatology*, 2nd edn. Oxford University Press, Oxford.

Arthritis Research Campaign
BIOLOGICAL THERAPY ALERT CARD

To health professionals:

I am a patient on BIOLOGICAL treatment.

**This therapy can increase the risk of infection
and may mask commonly recognized signs
and symptoms such as fever and pain.**

arc 0870 850 5000
www.arc.org.uk
Committed to curing arthritis

Patient's name:

Current biological therapy:

Consultant's name:

Hospital:

Hospital phone no:

Arthritis Research Campaign, Copeman House, St. Mary's Gate, Chesterfield, Derbyshire S41 7TD

Fig. 13.1 Example of a Biologic Alert Card. Reproduced with kind permission from the Arthritis Research Council.

Septic arthritis

Introduction (Box 13.2)

⚠ If a patient presents with a hot swollen joint, which is not trauma related, the most serious differential diagnosis is septic arthritis which is considered a medical emergency. Other potential diagnoses are ReA, monoarthritis, or crystal arthritis (gout).

In the patient who presents with a hot swollen joint <2 weeks with a restriction of movement, treat as for septic arthritis until proven otherwise.

Social and psychological impact

Patients can feel extremely anxious, unwell, and fearful of diagnosis. Early treatment and pain relief can help to overcome anxiety. Reassurance and clear explanation can help ease fears.

Nursing care issues in management

Nurse review should include clinical examination and history to ensure prompt diagnosis, immediate commencement of appropriate antibiotics, and joint aspiration. Advice includes resting the affected joint and ensuring non-weight-bearing until the inflammation and pain settle. Mobilization should then be encouraged as soon as possible. Refer for inpatient physiotherapy to support mobilization and passive and active exercise.

Treatment with antibiotics is normally dictated by local treatment policies on the use of antibiotic therapies—refer to local guidelines/seek advice from the microbiologist and bacteriologist.

Follow-up post infection until fully resolved.

Response to treatment

Swelling should subside and blood cultures become negative. If no improvement seek advice regarding antibiotic therapy, causative organism, or alternative foci of infection. Also consider further investigation, e.g. MRI for osteomyelitis.

Review

Monitor signs and symptoms, ESR, and CRP. Improving results can support the decision to stop antibiotics

Skin and soft tissue

Superficial infection, i.e. cellulitis covering the swollen joint, is also treated with antibiotics.

⚠ Under no circumstances should IA steroids be used. Bursal infections commonly of the olecranon and pre-patellar are managed with serial aspirations and oral antibiotics. However, if no response IV antibiotics should be used.

Box 13.2 Septic arthritis: overview

Presentation
- Hot swollen joint.
- Fever.

Diagnostic considerations
- Differential diagnoses, e.g. ReA, monoarthritis or crystal arthritis (gout).
- In the absence of fever but with a high evidence of clinical suspicion treat as septic arthritis.
- If a prosthetic joint refer to orthopaedic surgeon.

Investigations
- Joint aspiration for Gram stain and culture prior to starting antibiotics.
- Blood cultures.
- WBC, CRP, ESR, U&Es, and LFTs.
- If non-articular sepsis, appropriate swabs should be taken i.e. skin or oral/urethral swabs.

Treatment
- Antibiotics are given intravenously for 2 weeks, or until improvement and then oral antibiotics for 4 weeks (consider local antibiotic policy).
- IV penicillin is 'best fit' antibiotics whilst awaiting culture results.
- No risk factors—use IV flucloxacillin 2g qds.
- High risk—elderly, frail, UTI, add IV cephalosporin, e.g. cefuroxime 1.5g tds
- MRSA risk—IV cephalosporin and IV vancomycin.

Further reading

British Society for Rheumatology (2006). *Guidelines in the management of hot swollen joints*. British Society for Rheumatology, London.

Coakley G, Mathews C, Field M et al. (2006). BSR and BHPR, BOA, RGCP and BSAC Guidelines for management of the hot swollen joint in adults. *Rheumatology* **45**, 1039–41.

Hakim A, Clunie G, Haq I (eds) (2006). *Oxford Handbook of Rheumatology*, 2nd edn. Oxford University Press, Oxford.

Rapid access and emergency complications

This section advises the practitioner on clinical issues that require prompt early specialist medical opinion.

Drug toxicity

MTX pneumonitis

MTX pneumonitis, generally thought to be the result of a sensitivity reaction, occurs within the first 6 months of commencing the drug. If suspected, MTX should be stopped immediately and urgent specialist referral made. This complication can progress rapidly and may be fatal if not detected and treated early.

Presentation
- Sudden dry cough.
- Shortness of breath.

On examination
- Sometimes fever.
- May have fine crackles on auscultation.

Investigation
- FBC—eosinophilia.
- PFTs.
- HRCT lungs.

Treatment
- Prednisolone at high dose, 60mg/day.

▶ Drug-induced pneumonitis can present with other medications.

Overdose of MTX

In the case of accidental overdose potentially causing acute toxicity, treat with folinic acid 15mg every 6 hours for 24 hours and monitor LFTs, U&Es, and FBC. The pharmacist can provide guidance on management.

Leflunomide toxicity

In the case of severe toxicity affecting LFTs and skin, stop leflunomide and administer washout procedure, colestyramine 8g administered 3 × a day usually for 11 days. Alternatively, 50g of activated, powdered charcoal may be administered 4 × a day. Monitor LFTs.

Respiratory complications

Lung disease and respiratory complications are a common complication of RA. This may be part of the disease process or due to the toxicity of the medication prescribed.

Rheumatoid lung disease

Rheumatoid lung disease is manifested as interstitial lung disease or restrictive lung disease. The single most important advice to patients is to give up and stop smoking.

Differentials

- Lung disease related to drug toxicity.
- Infection.
- Other coexisting medical conditions.

For investigations, chest examination and treatment—see 📖 MTX pneumonitis, pp.380, 476, 480. However, a lung biopsy may also be considered.

Pneumonitis

This basically translates to inflammation of the lung tissue and chronic inflammation can lead to irreversible scarring known as pulmonary fibrosis. Presentation, chest examination, and management—see 📖 MTX pneumonitis, pp.380, 476, 480.

Respiratory infections

Chest infections may be acute or chronic (e.g. those seen with COPD) and are usually bacterial. Pleurisy however is different as this is infection of the lining of the lung rather than the airways.

Causes of chest infection in patients with RA

- Immune system response reduced due to immunosuppressive therapy.

Presentation

- Chesty cough.
- Discoloured sputum (yellow/green).
- SOB.
- Chest pain.

On examination

- Fever.
- Coarse crackles on auscultation.

Investigations

- ESR and CRP.
- Sputum specimen for C&S.
- Chest x-ray.
- HRCT lungs may be required.

Treatment

- Antibiotics.
- Analgesia.
- Fluids.
- Oxygen.
- Advise patients to stop smoking and review of therapy may be required.

Further reading

Dawson JK, Graham DR, Lynch MP (2002). Lung disease in patients with rheumatoid arthritis. *CPD Rheumatology*, **3**, 38–42.

Joint Formulary Committee (2008). *British National Formulary*, 56th edn, British Medical Association and Royal Pharmaceutical Society of Great Britain, London.

Breathlessness

Breathlessness is a relatively common problem seen in patients with rheumatological disease. It is worth having a framework to enable you to undertake a good clinical history and make a management plan.

Framework

Breathlessness could be due to:
- A cardiac or respiratory complication of their condition.
- Lung disease related to drug toxicity.
- Pulmonary infection as a result of immunosuppression, e.g. penumonia.
- A comorbidity, e.g. asthma, COPD, heart failure.

▶▶ The most important thing to rule out immediately is infection.

Initial assessment: history

- Pattern of symptoms.
- Symptoms to suggest infections—fever, chills, night sweats, productive purulent sputum.
- Duration of breathlessness—worsening rapidly?

Initial assessment severity

- Vital signs—TPR and breathing pattern.
- Oxygen saturation.
- ↓ in exercise tolerance from their usual.
- Evidence of other system involvement, e.g. hypertension, ankle oedema, poor urine output.

Initial assessment: drug history

- ▶ Many drugs can cause pulmonary complications, e.g. SAS and MTX pneumonitis.
- On immunosuppressant?
- On drugs that cause lung toxicity.

Initial assessment: coexisting disease

- Smoking history.
- Cardiovascular disease, e.g. hypotension/hypertension, ischaemic heart disease.
- Respiratory disease, e.g. asthma, COPD.
- Ask the patient 'does the problem present in a similar way to previous exacerbations?'.
- Recent immobility or major surgery, e.g. lower limb linked to pulmonary embolism.

📖 For underlying condition, e.g. hypertension or asthma, refer to appropriate treatment guidelines.

Observations and investigations for those with infection

- TPR.
- Oxygen saturation and, if asthmatic, peak flow.
- Bloods—FBC, CRP.
- Chest x-ray.

- If patient reports purulent sputum—specimen for culture (to identify organism).
- Consider blood culture if acutely ill.

At the end of this process you will have an idea of whether this is:

- Infection—urgent assessment and treatment required.
- Worsening of coexisting disease—manage according to treatment for underlying condition.
- Is this a new problem requiring a medical assessment?
- Severity and pace of change of breathlessness.

⚠ If following assessment the patient appears severely ill or there is rapid deterioration—seek urgent medical advice.

⚠ If a patient is on a biologic DMARD they may not present with classical signs of infection

📖 Also see Pharmacological management, p.419; 📖 Assessing the patient, p.271; 📖 Rapid access and emergency issues, p.379.

Frequently asked questions

What if an infection does not settle?

The diagnosis should be reviewed and the patient reassessed. Medical advice should be sought for those with polypharmacy or complex disease presentations. If patients are being treated with biologic therapies it is essential that they get an urgent medical opinion.

When should a GP/community nurse refer to 2° care?

Refer any patient with suspected septic arthritis, or systemic infection urgently to 2° care or emergency services. If patients appear systemically unwell and the disease activity increases specialist advice should be sought to guide management.

Do DMARDs, steroids, biologics mask infection?

Yes, these drugs may mask infection showing a normal WBC count and lack of fever. Patients who are on these therapies are immunosuppressed and have an ↑ risk of infections so a high index of suspicion should be maintained.

How can I tell the difference between a chesty cold and drug-induced pneumonitis?

If a patient is prescribed a drug recognized to cause pneumonitis (e.g. MTX or gold) you need to seek medical advice if there is any doubt. The cough can come on suddenly or gradually, will be unproductive, and may or may not be accompanied by breathlessness. Additional questions to exclude a cold may be helpful (e.g. have they had a runny nose and sore throat?). However, if there is any doubt whatsoever medical advice should be sought and the patient should be advised to withhold treatment.

Chapter 14

Fertility, pregnancy, and relationships

Fertility and conception

Fertility and issues related to conception and child-bearing are important for those of child-bearing age. For the clinician the challenges are those of wishing to control the disease with the patient's wishes to become a parent. For patients parenting a child, decisions are even more complex, particularly when drug regimens are needed for life and may impact upon fertility, conception, and pregnancy decisions. Treatment may be potentially harmful to the unborn child. Patients need careful counselling and support especially for those who are of child-bearing age and may not have a family of their own. Specialist guidance should be provided on:

- Contraceptive advice.
- Long-term strategy on family planning, e.g. treatments may ↓ fertility (e.g. storage of eggs or sperm prior to starting treatment).
- Pre-conceptual counselling for those with Anti-Ro and Anti-La antibodies (↑ risk of delivering babies with neonatal skin rash, and in subsequent pregnancies, congenital heart block).
- Clinical decisions on maintaining disease control and well-being (without medication) whilst attempting to conceive and during pregnancy.

As a number of rheumatic diseases (particularly LTCs) predominately affect ♀ of child-bearing age, discussions often focus on ♀ and particularly issues related to pregnancy but ♂ with a LTC who may be fathering a child must also be counselled and advised. The welfare of the mother and unborn child must be considered as many treatments may pass through the placental barrier. All patients on drug therapies with the potential to affect the unborn child must have:

- Appropriate information and advice about the treatment prescribed.
- Contraceptive advice and long treatment term strategies.

The most significant conditions that face these challenges include:

- RA, APS, PSV (☐ see relevant sections).
- SLE, especially those with APAs (☐ see relevant sections).
- Scleroderma also called systemic sclerosis, especially those diagnosed with pulmonary hypertension or ♂ with erectile dysfunction
- SS in those with antibodies to Anti-Ro and Anti-La (☐ see Sjögren's syndrome, p.130).
- Marfan syndrome—pregnancy carries an ↑ risk of aortic and cardiac problems.
- Rarely, hyper mobility can ↑ the risk of maternal and fetal mortality related to post-partum bleeding.

Fertility and contraceptive advice

- RA, SLE, PSV, SS—not known to directly affect fertility.
  - Evidence suggests ↓ fertility when disease is poorly controlled or when additional disease complications (e.g. lupus nephritis may associated with amenorrhea).
  - APS may be associated with infertility.
- Specialist support may be required to select contraceptive (e.g. hand function difficulties fitting Dutch cap/use of intra-uterine coil).

- Some conditions are sensitive to hormone levels (e.g. lupus may flare - during menstrual cycle)—for lupus patients with APAs or associated with APS—contraceptive should be progesterone (there is an ↑ risk of blood clots with combined oestrogen-containing types of contraceptive pill).
- Ovulation induction and in vitro fertilization (IVF) have identified ↑ risks (fetal and maternal) including:
  - Lupus flares.
  - Ovarian hyper stimulation.
  - Thrombosis similar to the risks in later pregnancy (APS only).
- Medication reviews prior to conception and when breastfeeding.
- Research on drugs affecting infertility have been poorly researched but current guidance suggests that drugs such as MTX may reduce ♂ ♀ fertility (may be reversible on stopping treatment).
  - SAS—♂ reduced sperm count (reversible on cessation).
- MTX and SAS deplete folate—provide folate therapy.
- ♂ with erectile dysfunction may require specialist advice.

Drug therapies: fertility and safety issues

- Pre-conception treatment plans (3–6 months prior to plans to conceive/father a child) should be carefully considered in consultation with the patient and clinician. A general principle is that all drug therapies should be avoided whilst attempting to conceive/father a child the potential risk to the patient (of stopping treatment) has to be balanced against potential risk to the unborn child.
- Many conditions are treated with cytotoxic therapies that must be avoided during pregnancy (e.g. MTX, leflunomide). Evidence reveals ↑ risks related to 1st trimester exposure, e.g. congenital abnormalities.
- Some drug therapies that may be continued during pregnancy (based on risk/benefit discussions) include:
  - Hydroxychloroquine sulphate.
  - Sulfasalazine.
  - AZA and ciclosporin A (although limited data available).
- High-dose corticosteroids may cause menstrual irregularities/anovulatory cycles.
  - Avoid prolonged systemic treatment unless risks to the patient are higher than those to the unborn child.
  - Pulsed therapies may be considered for some patients.
- Cyclophosphamide continued with acute multi-system episodes. Associated with ovarian failure but dependant on:
  - Age of ♀ at start of treatment (younger the patient the ↓ risk).
  - Cumulative dose and route of administration—IV probably safer than oral.
- Avoid NSAIDs at 3rd trimester—after 28 weeks of gestation (risks of premature closure of ductus arteriosus and some evidence on impairment of fetal renal function).
- ⚠ All new drugs (black triangle) are contraindicated in pregnancy.
- Preliminary observational data on accidental pregnancies while treated with new biologic DMARDs ('black triangle' drugs—adalimumab, etanercept, and infliximab) are reassuring.

Key point: improved outcomes for mother and unborn child if conception and pre-natal phase achieved whilst disease activity is quiescent

Pregnancy and long-term conditions

There are a number of MSCs that are systemic, and in some cases potentially life-threatening, that may require long-term medications to control the disease. The most significant of these include:

- RA.
- Spondyloarthropathies, e.g. AS.
- SLE.
- PSV.
- Scleroderma/systemic sclerosis.
- APS.

There are therefore important issues for patients (♂ and ♀) to consider before planning for a family (📖 see Fertility and conception, p.392).

Pregnancy

2–3% of *all* pregnancies in the normal population result in serious fetal malformations and a further 6% have minor malformation. Early fetal development is the most vulnerable time of gestation in relation to malformations and drug toxicity issues; ∴ essential pre-requisites for all patients should be:

- Initial guidance and information when starting treatment with cytotoxic or DMARDs in relation to risks and benefits of treatment and consequences of conception whilst on treatment.
- Preconception counselling for all patients receiving treatments for LTCs of child-bearing potential.

The aim of all clinicians will be to achieve remission or at least maintain optimum disease control during the pregnancy but with the minimal drug toxicity/risk of teratogenicity. Specialist support required to manage complex pregnancies includes: rheumatology, obstetric, and paediatric teams, and, depending upon the condition and potential complications, respiratory and renal teams. In RA the disease usually improves during pregnancy whilst in others careful monitoring of the patient and unborn child is required. For some conditions there are additional risks to the mother during pregnancy (e.g. SLE) and in others evidence of management and outcomes is limited (e.g. PSV). High disease activity in SLE, APS, and systemic sclerosis at conception and pre-natal phases appear to be linked with worst outcomes for the mother and unborn child.

AS and RA

- AS—no remission during pregnancy. Mechanical problems at delivery due to sacroiliitis.
- RA—remission during pregnancy (~75%).
- RA—↑ risk of premature birth, low birth weight, and pre-eclampsia.
- RA—frequently relapse of disease post-partum requiring specialist support to establish disease control.

Scleroderma: limited evidence but some reports suggest:

- Live births in ~75% of cases.
- Contraindications to pregnancy include pulmonary hypertension, uncontrolled hypertension. Diffuse scleroderma—wait until disease stable.

- Cardiology and pulmonary reviews required.
- Reflux oesophagitis and cardiopulmonary decompensation may develop.

SLE and systemic sclerosis

- Pregnancy in SLE associated with renal disease leads to ↑ risk of poor outcomes. Close monitoring necessary.
- Low C3, C4 levels, and/or high anti-double stranded DNA levels in SLE are associated with fewer live births and greater preterm births.
- Anti-Ro and anti-La antibodies in pregnant SLE and systemic sclerosis patients lead to ~2–5% risk of congenital heart block. If first child delivered with congenital heart block subsequent pregnancies are at ↑ risk of congenital heart block.
- SLE patients with APAs or patients with APS or previous history of miscarriage (>30% in 1st pregnancy) will need:
  - Anticoagulant therapy—aspirin and low molecular weight heparin should replace warfarin throughout pregnancy and post-partum.
  - Obstetric monitoring and obstetric-led birth.

PSV

- ↑ risk of thromboembolic events during pregnancy—treatment as for SLE.
- Pregnancy in Takayasu arteritis—limited evidence appears outlines:
  - 86% resulted in live births.
  - If Takayasu arteritis with abdominal aorta involvement—↑ risk to mother and unborn child.
  - Hypertension (41%) and pre-eclampsia (35%).
- Pregnancies rare in WG (older age group, rare disease). Limited evidence suggests pregnancy can be life threatening to the mother with spontaneous and therapeutic abortions and maternal death.
- Pregnancy in Churg–Strauss syndrome—despite affecting ♀ of child-bearing potential, data on pregnancy is extremely limited.
  - May require corticosteroids and AZA (with risk–benefit assessment) to main disease control during pregnancy. Rare but successful cases of immunoglobulin treatment during pregnancy.
- Pregnancy in PAN rare (older age group). Very limited evidence. Those diagnosed late in pregnancy appear to have high rates of maternal death.
- Pregnancy in MPA—extremely rare case reports. Use same management principles as for WG.

Key point

Disease control is essential for good maternal and fetal outcomes. Establish disease control ante and post-partum care and provide support to mother and family in caring for infant.

Further reading

Association of Rheumatology Health Professionals. (2006). *Clinical care in the rheumatic diseases*, 3rd edn. Association of Rheumatology Health Professionals, Atlanta, GA.

Foster R, D'Cruz DP (2007). Vasculitis in pregnancy. ◌ www.medscape.com

Joint Formulary Committee (2008). Drug toxicities and lactations. In *British National Formulary*, 56th edn. British Medical Association and Royal Pharmaceutical Society of Great Britain, London.

Breastfeeding and medications

Breast milk is an emulsion containing water, lipids, carbohydrates, minerals, and proteins. A small amount of drug taken by the mother will be excreted in breast milk; although breastfed infants may consume generally very low doses of their mother's medications it is important to consider the risks to the child.

Concentrations of drug in breast milk may be affected by:
• The amount of fat (or lipid) present in the breast milk.
• The pharmacokinetics of the mother.
• The pH of milk may also fluctuate, potentially altering the pharmacodynamics of medications excreted in breast milk.
• The molecular weight and dose and dosage intervals of the medication.
• The drug's half-life will affect how long the drug is found in the breast milk.

The changes seen during pregnancy (e.g. ↑ in body weight, body fat, GI absorption, and enhanced hepatic metabolism) will also affect drug absorption and metabolism. In practical terms this has little relevance in affecting the drug therapies prescribed for rheumatic diseases or for the mother but may be important when having to consider drug dosages passed on via breast milk to an infant.

The amount of drug excreted in breast milk can be reduced by considering the timing of breastfeeds and medications (e.g. ensuring that oral drugs are taken just before breastfeeding where there will be insufficient time for drugs to concentrate in breast milk). Key issues in relation to some commonly used drugs in rheumatology include:
• There is limited information on the risks to the breastfed child whilst the mother is taking medication and ∴ the general rule is that all drug therapies should be avoided whilst breastfeeding.
• Patients should be advised to avoid breastfeeding whilst on anti-rheumatic drugs such as MTX. MTX levels excreted in breast milk are said to be <10% of those in plasma; however, as little is known of the harmful and cumulative effects on the developing child, MTX should be avoided if breastfeeding.

For detailed information regarding the risks of medications whilst pregnant or breastfeeding refer to the SPC of medication or the drug data sheet/*BNF*.

Sexuality

Sexual problems are very common for patients, but offering emotional support and practical solutions can radically improve the patient's quality of life.

Spot possible causes

Physical causes consider:
- Joint pain.
- Joint stiffness.
- Fatigue.
- ↓ or altered sensation or poor blood circulation causing erectile or orgasmic dysfunction; dry vagina causing dyspareunia.
- Medications triggering loss of libido, erectile dysfunction, anorgasmia.

Psychological factors

Psychological factors play an important role in perceived:
- Feelings of unattractiveness or poor body image.
- Low esteem affecting libido.
- Helplessness lowering desire and affecting performance.

Relationship

Illness and ensuing dependency may cause guilt, resentment, withdrawal by partner, couple conflict.

Offer emotional support

Be aware... that sex may be an important part of an individual's life independent of illness, age, or marital status.

Subtly mention the problem... in the right environment try to take the initiative so the patient doesn't have to. You can make this less of a big issue by normalizing 'Is arthritis affecting your sexuality in any way?'.

Normalize... explain that the problem is common and acceptable. Consider using examples such as this, 'Many patients with your condition find it's difficult to make love'.

Create emotional space... support by allowing patients to express anxiety, guilt, and anger. Consider open questions such as 'Do you want to talk about how you feel?'

Empower... so patient feels more hopeful and in control. Offer statements such as 'There's lots you can do to improve things'.

Offer general solutions

- Examine list of medications and treatment plans; identify any medications that may be the source of sexual problems.
- Discuss with the patient possible support such as painkillers or erectile dysfunction medication.
- Encourage the patient to be physically affectionate with their partner, to offset lack of sexual contact.
- Suggest options such as relationship-building strategies, such as better communication. If necessary suggest seeking additional support.

Get patient using sex-specific solutions

- Identifying times of day when pain level is lower.
- Suggest resting before and after sex to lower fatigue.
- Encourage them to ensure the room is heated well to avoid getting cold during sex.
- Before sex, easing pain with hot bath, massage, painkillers.
- Raising libido through erotic magazines or DVDs.
- Applying lubricant to offset vaginal dryness.
- Shortening foreplay if pain or stiffness builds.
- Using sex toys such as vibrators.
- Choosing more pain-free techniques—oral or hand sex may be easier than intercourse.
- Experimenting to find more comfortable sexual positions; 'Further reading' includes suggestions for publications.

Further reading

Regard is an organization for gay men and lesbians: ⌖ www.regard.org.uk

Arthritis Care: *Relationships, Intimacy and Arthritis*. Available at: ⌖ www.arthritiscare.org.uk.

Arthritis Foundation: *Guide to Intimacy with Arthritis*. Available at: ⌖ www.arthritis.org.

Arthritis Research Campaign: advice on sexuality and arthritis. ⌖ www.arc.org.uk

For problems that require specific support/advice on relationships suggest seeking additional support from Relate: ⌖ www.relate.org.uk Phone: 01788 573241 or see directory for local service.

Arthritis Research Campaign: patient information leaflets on sexuality and arthritis. Available at: ⌖ www.arc.org.uk

Furst E (2006). Sexuality and scleroderma, *Scleroderma Voice* 2006, Issue 2. Contact: ⌖ www.scleroderma.org

National Institute of Arthritis: *Musculoskeletal and Skin Diseases: Sex and Lupus Patient Information Sheet*. Available at: ⌖ www.niams.nih.gov.

National Rheumatoid Arthritis Society has some interesting and useful pieces about sexuality and RA. Available at: ⌖ www.rheumatoid.org.uk

Self-esteem and effect on relationships

Self-esteem is a person's own appraisal of their worth and combines personal beliefs ('I can manage to undertake normal work activities') and emotions ('my disease makes me feel like a second-class citizen'). Individuals with a LTC can face numerous challenges to their self-esteem and these effects can impact upon their personal relationships.

- The disease itself may be perceived by some members of the lay public in negative ways (e.g. AIDS) or be perceived as principally an old age condition, despite the person being relatively young (e.g. arthritis or Parkinson's disease).
  - Society perceives sexuality as belonging to the young, fit, and healthy—adding to the burden the patient may perceive about their disease.
  - The patient may feel a sense of shame about their condition, e.g. perceiving themselves as inferior in society or feeling guilty because of the adjustments that have to be made as a result of their condition and effect on their significant others.
- The consequences of the conditions may disrupt perceptions of self by:
  - The variable nature of the condition—leading to a poor sense of 'control' over life and ability to plan and manage daily activities.
  - Disrupt life with frequent reminders of the chronic disease status—e.g. numerous outpatient appointments, frequent blood tests, drug regimens, or a disease that excludes activities or social participation e.g. consumption of alcohol, sporting activities, or dietary restrictions.
  - Changes that occur to body image, e.g. joint changes seen in the hands of those with RA or obvious skin rashes in PsA.
  - Facial changes that may occur as a result of WG or butterfly rash seen in SLE.
- The condition may significantly ↑ reliance on others, e.g.:
  - Inability to complete tasks such as dressing, personal hygiene, or preparing a meal.
  - Changes that result in role reversals in relationships, e.g. traditional roles undertaken by a wife may have to be undertaken by her partner (e.g. hanging the washing on the line). For a male loss of key roles may affect their long-standing, established perceived roles as breadwinner or protector.
  - Loss of work participation may affect financial standing and security, ↑ the sense of loss that comes with changes to their perceived role in society or ability to manage/control family income.
- Changes may affect the individual's perception of attractiveness and belief in their appeal sexually. This will affect sexual relationships with their partner for example.
  - Partners who also provide a role as carer may find it hard to revert then to sexual partner
  - Changes in body image may make the person nervous of making the first sexual approaches—fearing they are no longer attractive.
  - Individuals may find it difficult to communicate their anxieties and challenges with their partner.

- Patients may worry about being seen unclothed.
- Pain and fatigue from the disease may also have a negative impact on the wish to be touched.

Social participation

Evidence suggests that those with a LTC who have a good level of social support (in the form of satisfactory relationships and financial infrastructures) have a high level of perceived self-efficacy and have improved outcomes. Individuals should be supported in coming to terms with their condition and negotiating their healthcare needs. When self-esteem is low it can be difficult for patients to effectively negotiate without an advocate.

The role of the nurse in enhancing self-esteem

- Patients will, over time, need differing levels of support and may take time to feel able to discuss issues related to relationships. Enhancing the therapeutic relationships and encouraging a holistic and patient-centred approach to care should encourage practitioner/patient communication.
- The partner or close family/friends supporting someone with a LTC may often go unrecognized or unsupported and needs to be considered in the context of the patient's self-esteem and ability to participate actively in society.

Nurses should:
- Provide an opportunity for the patient (and, if the patient consents, the partner) to be able to discuss issues of concern.
- Provide an environment conducive to discussing such personal issues.
- Be comfortable and receptive to discussing relationship issues.
- Normalize the problem. Provide reassurance and appropriate information to enable the patient to recognize their problems are not unique and support is available to them.
- Enable the patient to achieve personal goals in improving self-esteem:
  - Set goals, e.g. taking up a small part-time voluntary post.
  - Refer to OT for aids and devices for independent living, e.g. kitchen equipment or aids to enable ease of dressing.
- Advise on ways that they can participate and network where appropriate to organizations or support groups that will allow the patient access to other patients with similar experiences.
  - EPPs or voluntary network groups such as the NRAS.
- Where appropriate, provide contact details for organization such as marriage guidance for those with specific relationships problems

📖 Also see Sexuality, p.398.

Further reading

Arthritis Research Campaign. leaflet on 'Intimacy and arthritis'. Available at: 🖰 www.arc.org.uk

Hill J (2006). *Rheumatology a creative approach*. John Wiley & Sons Ltd: Chichester.

Pharmacological management: pain relief

Pre-treatment and review: prescribing issues

Pre-treatment assessment

Pain is a complex phenomenon that involves physical and mental sensations, unique to the individual experiencing pain. The presenting complaint of pain may also be linked to other factors that may heighten or precipitate the sensations of pain. These include:

- Prior experience of pain and ability to control symptoms.
- The underlying conditions—is the disease adequately controlled?
- Knowledge of underlying cause for the symptoms, e.g. knowledge of a disease contributing to inflammatory joint pain.
- Psychological aspects that may moderate perceptions of pain, e.g. heightened anxiety or denial of underlying pathology.
- Beliefs, behaviours, and cultural factors that may affect pain or perceptions of pain and controlling pain.
- Social factors that may alter the perception of symptoms.

Pre-treatment assessment of risk and benefit of prescribing analgesia

An assessment should include:

- General health status and evaluation of comorbidities or prior illness, surgical treatments.
- Current prescribed medications and potential drug interactions.
- Drug history in relation to adverse events or treatment side effects.
- The presenting history, duration of presenting complaint and causal factors to pain, e.g. chronic non-malignant pain or recent onset IJD.

Following this assessment the nurse should have sufficient information to know:

- Prior treatments and potential drug interactions/adverse events.
- The patient's previous experience of different analgesia or pain relieving strategies and benefits gained.
- Cautions and contraindications to consider, e.g. prior history of GI blood or steroid psychosis.
- The nature of symptoms, e.g. duration/intensity of pain, with an assessment of the level of pain experienced by the patient, e.g. use of a VAS.

A purely pharmacological approach to pain management may fail to adequately control pain and prescribers should explore with the patient:

- The individual's knowledge of pain and how pain relief works, e.g. to achieve effective pain control, regular dosing may be required rather than waiting for the pain to become unbearable before taking medications.
- Other non-pharmacological approaches that may be an adjunct to prescribed medications.
- An assessment of current pain scores and patient needs, expectations of symptom control.
- A planned review process to examine changes in pain scores and benefits of prescribed pain relief.

Also see Assessing pain, p.292.

The review process

If the patient is to have confidence in achieving effective pain relief they should be offered a review appointment with a specified time frame for their current drug regimen. A prescribing plan must include a review process. This will build a safety framework to ensure a thorough assessment of the treatment prescribed and subsequent prescribing plans—e.g. can an effective treatment such as paracetamol be added to their repeat prescriptions?

A number of analgesics may be considered safe and effective over a short period of time but may not be appropriate to consider as part of a long-term strategy.

Patient information

- Patients should receive information on the treatments they are prescribed, including potential risks and benefits of treatment in the context of their health condition.
- Monitoring or clinical attendance responsibilities as part of the prescribing plan.
- Access to support and advice including:
  - Written information on the underlying condition and treatment.
  - Additional information resources such as web-based, self-help groups, health and well-being activities in the community.
  - Patient self-help/support groups.

Ensure patients who have a LTC requiring access to regular pain relief are aware of:

- If prescribed pain relief to have for such episodes they should know how they should 'step up' or re-start analgesia (and non-pharmacological options) to manage symptoms.
- Guidance on when to 'step down' treatment and how to document changes in their self-medication if required.
- Advise on what to do if initial symptom control fails and they need to seek additional support. If it is likely they will require specialist support/advice—who they contact and contact details.

For those with self-limiting conditions who would not be expected to require follow-up (e.g. referral for joint injection for OA of the knee) guidance should be provided on what to do if the condition fails to resolve as planned, and what to do if they experience side effects from their treatment.

📖 Also see Chronic non-inflammatory pain, p.171; 📖 Symptom control: pain relief, pp.289, 292; 📖 Assessment of pain: red and yellow flags, p.294; 📖 Depression and fatigue, p.298; 📖 Intra-articular injections, p.494.

Further reading

For the management of neuropathic pain: Clinical Resources Efficiency Support Team (2008). *Guidelines on the management of neuropathic pain.* CREST, Belfast.

The analgesic ladder: step one

Introduction

Pain is defined as an unpleasant feeling which may be associated with actual or potential tissue damage and which may have physical and emotional components. Before prescribing analgesia it is useful to identify whether the patient's pain has 1 or more of 4 components:

- Mechanical nociceptive.
- Inflammatory nociceptive.
- Neuropathic—pain related to lesions/dysfunction of the peripheral nervous system.
- Psychological.

▶ Nociception is a neurophysiological term and refers to specific activity in nerve pathways.

📖 Also see Assessing pain, p.292; 📖 Symptom control: assessing pain, p.289; 📖 Assessment tools, p.539; 📖 Chronic non-inflammatory pain, p.640.

Chronic pain syndromes: assessing pain

The analgesic ladder as defined by the WHO for nociceptive pain outlines a step-up approach starting with non-opioid, moving to weak opioid, and then strong opioid (Box 15.1).

Discuss taking analgesia with the patient and include information on potential side effects and benefits. A common problem is that patients frequently fail to take regular analgesia and then wait until the pain has become unbearable. This can result in the patient gaining minimal benefit from analgesia as heightened pain perceptions render the analgesia ineffective or they have to wait for a further 20–30min for the drugs therapeutic benefits to be achieved. Regular analgesia may be effective but in some cases patients analgesia may be ineffective (or side effects may warrant a change) and they will need to move up the analgesic ladder. Responses to analgesia vary and some patients may experience ↑ side effects of a medication e.g. drowsiness/constipation.

Example: step one

Paracetamol (acetaminophen)

- Tablets (500mg); soluble tablets (500mg); oral suspension (120mg/5mL; 250mg/5mL); suppositories (250mg, 500mg) in a dosage of 0.5–1.0g every 4–6 hours, with a max dose of 4g (8 × 500mg tablets)/day.
- This is 1st-line treatment for acute and chronic musculoskeletal pain. The mechanism of action is thought to be inhibition of prostaglandins in the brain resulting in ↑ pain threshold.

Side effects: medication overuse headache.

Relative cautions: liver disease and severe renal impairment.

Contraindications: known hypersensitivity to paracetamol.

Box 15.1 Analgesic ladder

Step 1
Non opioid: paracetamol.

Step 2
Weak opioid: codeine, tramadol.

Step 3
Strong opioid: morphine, oxycodone, fentanyl, buprenorphine.

The analgesic ladder: step two

Example 1: step two
Codeine tablets (15mg, 30mg, 60mg), syrup (25mg/5mL)
- Codeine is metabolized in the body by an enzyme process called demethylation to morphine, with 10% of the compound converted to morphine. This process stimulates the opioid (mu and k) receptors in the CNS and causes inhibition of the spinal and central processing pain sensation.
- The amount of codeine in combined preparations varies. It is important to be aware of the different dosages and combinations available and try and match them according to the control of pain and side effects the patients is experiencing.
- Codeine may be combined with paracetamol in the form of co-codamol.
- Dosages vary between both codeine and paracetamol as outlined:
  - 8/500 = 8mg codeine/500mg paracetamol.
  - 15/500 = 15mg codeine/500mg paracetamol.
  - 30/500 = 30mg codeine/500mg paracetamol, in a dosage of 30–60mg every 4–6 hours and a maximum of 240mg/day.

Side effects
Nausea, vomiting, constipation, dizziness, sweating, dependence, medication overuse headache.

Cautions
Use as low as possible dose in elderly, and patients with hypothyroidism, hypoadrenalism, chronic hepatic disease and renal insufficiency, asthma. Pregnancy and breastfeeding.

Contraindications
Known hypersensitivity to any of the tablet constituents; respiratory depression; obstructive airways disease; paralytic ileus; head injury; raised intracranial pressure; acute alcoholism.

Example 2: step two
Tramadol
- Useful when codeine is ineffective or causes constipation. Tramadol may have less respiratory depression and is possibly less addictive than codeine.
- Tramadol works from the binding of sigma, kappa, mu opioid receptors, and inhibition of noradrenaline reuptake, and serotonin release.
- Capsules (50mg), orodispersible tablets (50mg), or soluble tablets (50mg), and modified release tablets (twice daily regimen): 100mg, 150mg, and 200mg tablets. Dosage is 50–100mg 4-hourly. Modified release twice daily preparations initially 50–100mg twice daily. Maximum dose of 400mg/day.

Side effects

As with codeine, nausea and vomiting are more common. Abdominal discomfort, hypotension, psychiatric disturbance (hallucinations), convulsions may occur.

Contraindications

Uncontrolled epilepsy, pregnancy and breast feeding.

For those patients taking regular 4–6-hourly doses of tramadol, consider a modified release preparation. If unable to tolerate tramadol, an alternative is tramacet. This may have equal potency to tramadol by combining tramadol and paracetamol, with an improved side effect profile.

Pain relief: tricyclics and other anti-depressants

Pain is a unique personal experience for the patient and for some people pain is not relieved using non-opioid analgesia and non-pharmacological approaches. Patients who have chronic pain may also experience symptoms of depression or insomnia. The use of an opioid is usually recommended for moderate-to-severe pain and may not be appropriate for patients with chronic pain. However, another option for chronic unrelieved pain can be the addition of an anti-depressant (e.g. tricyclic) which are widely used to treat non-affective symptoms of chronic musculoskeletal pain although currently this is an unlicensed indication (🕮 see Chronic non-inflammatory pain, p.171). Refer to *BNF* for full details and SPC for each drug.

The most effective older tricyclic anti-depressants (TCAs) often no longer used to treat depression are used to support pain relief and are thought to work by ↑ the chemicals (noradrenalin).

TCAs

TCAs appear to have a synergistic benefit (when prescribed with a central acting analgesic) for the patient with chronic pain or neuropathic pain unrelieved by traditional pain-relieving approaches. TCAs fall into 2 broad categories—those with less sedatives effects and those that have a sedative effect:

- Sedative effects—amitriptyline, clomipramine, dosulepin.
- Less sedative effects—imipramine, nortriptyline, and lofepramine

Evidence suggests they are most effective in conditions such as fibromyalgia to improve sleep quality, pain, and well being. TCAs used for neuropathic or chronic pain include:

- Amitriptyline (helpful in sleep deprivation) usual dose range from 10–50mg, 2 hours prior to going to bed. Evidence of benefit suggests doses of <50mg daily.

TCA dose should be started low and gradually ↑ to achieve effect and limit side effects. Pain relief benefits may take a few months whilst sleep deprivation may improve within 2 weeks.

Common side effects: dry mouth, blurred vision, low blood pressure, dizziness, drowsiness.

Cautions
- Arrhythmias and heart block can occur (sudden death has been reported).
- Convulsions—caution in epilepsy.

SSRIs

SSRIs block the uptake of serotonin involved in endogenous pain control but are generally used less for non-affective symptoms. It is important that there is a clear rationale for prescribing a TCA or SSRI, e.g. is it to treat mild depression or for non-affective symptoms? The prescription of anti-depressants appears to be ↑ in some conditions:

- Fibromyalgia.

- RA.
- Spondyloarthropathies.
- Low back pain.
- OA.

In SSRIs the onset of analgesic effect is usually faster than those expected when used for anti-depressant effects and dose required are usually lower than when treating depression.

SSRIs tend to have fewer side effects than TCAs but appear to be less effective, requiring high dosages. SSRIs used for pain relief include:

- Citalopram 20mg daily.
- Fluoxetine 20mg daily.

New generation serotonin and noradrenaline re-uptake inhibitors (SNRIs), e.g. venlafaxine, are currently unlicensed for chronic musculoskeletal pain use but may be beneficial although expensive. Evidence suggests a low side effect profile. Refer to guidelines on 1° care depression for additional information.

Common side effects include:
- Nausea, anxiety, headache.
- Sexual dysfunction.
- Constipation.
- Dry mouth.
- Urinary hesitancy.

Caution
- The elderly—regular review and careful monitoring required.
- Glaucoma.
- Cardiac disease.
- Diabetes mellitus.

Anti-epileptics—for neuropathic pain
- Gabapentin 300mg day 1. 300mg bd day 2. 300mg tds day 3; ↑ by 300mg per day to a maximum dose of 3.6g daily. Trial for a period of 3–8 weeks.
- Pregabalin 150mg daily in 2–3 divided doses increase (after 3–7 days) to a max of 600mg if necessary.

Common side effects: dry mouth, dizziness, cognitive impairment, diarrhoea, nausea.

Caution: avoid abrupt withdrawal.

Pain relief: non-steroidal anti-inflammatory drugs

Introduction

This section will discuss traditional NSAID therapies including COX-2 NSAIDs. The broad term NSAID will be used to describe both NSAIDs and COX-2 unless otherwise stated. NSAIDs can be beneficial for MSC where there is pain and inflammation (e.g. RA, OA, AS, acute articular and peri-articular disorders, cervical spondylitis, acute back pain, and acute gout) or following orthopaedic surgery. When NSAIDS are prescribed they should be at the lowest effective dose for the shortest duration and considered in the context of an overall pain-relieving approach for those conditions that have an inflammatory component. In some circumstances, NSAIDS may form part of a comprehensive approach to relieve pain which should include other forms of analgesia as well as non-pharmacological approaches

The mechanism of action is that of inhibiting the release of cyclo-oxygenase (type I and type II) suppressing the activation of prostaglandins along the pain pathway in the peripheral nervous system. NSAIDs can be broadly classified into 2 main categories

- Traditional NSAIDS may vary in their therapeutic spectrum of inhibiting cyclo-oxygenase (type I and type II).
- COX-2 inhibitors, preferentially block cyclo-oxygenase-2, the principal enzyme identified in the production of inflammatory mediators. COX-1 is an essential enzyme for constitutional functions e.g. gastro protection remain relatively uninhibited by COX-2 therapies.

Traditional or non-selective NSAIDs

- Ibuprofen, 1.2–1.8g/day in 3–4 divided doses, with a maximum dose 2.4g/day.
- Naproxen 500mg is given initially for acute pain and 750mg for acute gout followed by 250mg every 6–8 hours. In addition naproxen 250mg-500mg twice a day can be given for chronic rheumatic disease.
- Diclofenac is given to a maximum of 150mg/day in 2–3 divided doses.

COX-2 selective NSAIDs

- Celecoxib—200mg/day in 1–2 divided doses may be given for OA and elderly patients; 200–400mg/day in 2 divided doses may be given for RA.
- Etoricoxib—120mg may be given for acute gout; 60mg/day may be given for OA; and 90mg/day for RA.

Side effects

- GI bleed (traditional NSAIDs have a high risk) or dyspepsia.
- Cardiovascular events (stroke or myocardial infarction).
- Side effects related to renal impairment (poor excretion/metabolism).
- Liver impairment (hepatitis and jaundice).
- Exacerbation of asthma.

Other documented side effects include:

Nausea, vomiting, abdominal pain, flatulence, diarrhoea, peptic ulcers, perforation, fluid retention, hypertension, aggravating asthma (bronchospasm), rashes including photosensitivity. Nephrotoxicity—including interstitial nephritis, nephrotic syndrome and renal failure.

Cautions with NSAIDs

Proceed cautiously using NSAIDs in the elderly and when patients have cardiovascular, renal, and hepatic problems; patients with history of heart failure, hypertension, asthma; and patients with history of GI problems such as ulcerative colitis, Crohn's disease. Currently evidence suggests that all NSAIDs (non-selective or selective COX-2 inhibitors) can ↑ blood pressure by 3–5mmHg, ↑ risk of stroke, angina, and heart failure. Avoid NSAIDs in patients who have ischaemic heart and/or cerebrovascular disease.

Contraindications with NSAIDs

NSAIDS are not suitable for patients with a known sensitivity, active peptic ulcer disease, GI bleeding or perforation due to NSAIDs, patients with severe liver, renal, cardiac failure, and patients with ischaemic heart, cardiovascular, or peripheral vascular disease. Patients in last trimester of pregnancy.

For latest guidance refer to:
- The *BNF* and the latest CSM.
- NICE
- The European Medicines Agency (EMEA) on prescribing NSAIDs.
- Product SPC for each drug.

Topical NSAIDs

Topical NSAIDs demonstrate benefits in relieving pain particularly in treating discreet areas or for small-to-moderate size joints (e.g. OA base of thumb or knee pain) or for acute musculoskeletal injuries, such as epicondylitis, tendonitis, and tenosynovitis. Creams or gels should have the prescribed amount applied to affected area; 2–4 × daily. As long as the patient takes the prescribed dose and dosing regimen, only small amounts of the drug are systemically absorbed. Patches are usually prescribed over a period of time, e.g. 1 patch applied for 72 hours.

Possible side effects include:

Mild-to-moderate local irritation, erythema, pruritus and dermatitis, and photosensitive skin reaction. Rarely, minor GI side effects such as nausea, dyspepsia, abdominal pain, and dyspnoea.

Further reading

Madhok R, Wu O, McKellar G, *et al.* (2006). Non-steroidal anti-inflammatory drugs—changes in prescribing may be warranted, *Rheumatology*, **45**, 1458–60.

Gastric cytoprotection

Introduction

GI disorders are a common complaint for many individuals—heartburn, epigastric pain, gastro-oesophageal reflux disease, and GI bleeds. GI symptoms can present as a result of:

- Drug interactions, e.g.:
  - Aspirin and corticosteroids.
  - Nausea and GI symptoms from DMARD therapies.
- Individual patient risk factors including:
  - Previous GI disorders including dyspepsia, or peptic ulceration.
  - Lifestyle factors including high alcohol intake, smoking history, obesity, and poor dietary habits.
- Predisposing factors such as *Helicobacter pylori* status.

Treatment of GI disorders

Treatment of GI disorders must be considered in the context of the underlying pathology but the treatment options include:

- Antacids, compound alginates, or indigestion preparations.
- Antispasmodics and drugs affecting gut motility (used for non-ulcer dyspepsia).
- Ulcer healing drugs (H2-receptor antagonists and PPIs).
- Treatment of *H. pylori* infections.

GI bleeding

A GI bleed is defined as bleeding in the oesophagus, stomach, or duodenum characterized by fresh bleeding or 'coffee ground' bleeding.

NSAIDs inhibit prostaglandins and ↓ mucous production. Protecting patients from risks related to GI bleeding or ulceration must be considered in the context of prescribing for MSC. PPIs are routinely prescribed to prevent the risk of GI bleeds related to treatment with NSAIDs. GI bleeds can be related to:

- Varicose bleeding or tear of the stomach due to excess vomiting—Mallory–Weiss tear.
- Drug-induced.
- Polyps, inflammatory diseases.
- Cancer.
- NSAIDs.

Prevention of NSAID-induced GI bleeding

Traditional NSAIDs should be prescribed at the lowest effective dose for the shortest possible duration. Patients who require pain relief should be assessed to find the most appropriate treatment. Cardiovascular and GI risks should also be assessed to ensure eligibility for either a traditional NSAID or COX-2 inhibitors:

- PPIs are the most effective treatment to be co-prescribed with a traditional NSAID.
- A combination of a prostaglandin analogue (misoprostol) is combined with some NSAIDs for gastro-protection.

- Patients who have no cardiovascular risk factors but identified risks related to GI bleeds should be considered for a COX-2 inhibitor.

PPIs

PPIs act by inhibiting gastric acid secretion by blocking the enzyme secreting system (proton pump) of the gastric parietal cells. The ↓ gastric acidity means that the gut is less effective at preventing bacterial infections such as *Campylobacter* or *Clostridium difficile*.

PPIs are prescribed for:

- Short-term benefit for treatment of gastric and duodenal ulcers and are used as part of the eradication therapy for *H. pylori* in combination with antibacterial therapy.
- Prevention and treatment of ulcers associated with NSAIDs.
- Control excessive gastric acid secretions.

Cautions

- Liver disease.
- Breastfeeding.
- May mask symptoms of gastric cancer.

Side effects

- Nausea, vomiting and abdominal pain including flatulence and diarrhoea.
- Headaches and dizziness.

H2-receptor antagonists

Histamine H2-receptor is blocked and as a result gastric acid secretion is reduced.

H2-receptor antagonists are prescribed to:

- Heal gastric and duodenal ulcers.
- Relieve symptoms of gastro-oesophageal reflux disease.
- Treat NSAID-associated ulcers.

Cautions

- Renal impairment.
- Pregnancy and breastfeeding.
- May mask symptoms of gastric cancer.

Side effects

- Diarrhoea, abdominal discomfort.
- Headaches and dizziness.
- Changes in LFTs (rarely liver damage).

Further reading

NICE (2004). *Management of dyspepsia in adults in primary care*. NICE, London.

NICE (2008). *Management of osteoarthritis*. NICE, London.

Joint Formulary Committee (2008). Gastro-intestinal system, section 1.1; Musculoskeletal and joint diseases section 10.1. In *British National Formulary*, 56th edn. British Medical Association and Royal Pharmaceutical Society of Great Britain, London.

Topical therapies

Topical therapies are sometimes used as an adjunct to other pain-relieving strategies for acute or chronic pain although the evidence supporting their use currently remains limited. They may also be used for those who are intolerant to oral analgesics. The rationale for topical therapies is that by applying topically the systemic effects will be reduced. Rubefacient is a term that may be applied to such topical agents, however terminology does differ and clarification may be needed to ensure whether NSAIDs are considered part of this category or not.

A systematic review to explore quality, validity, and effect size of topical non-steroidal anti-inflammatory therapies has shown a modest short term benefit (2 weeks) in pain relief for conditions such as acute sprains and OA. Topical therapies used as analgesics for MSC include:

- Rubefacients containing salicylates or capsaicin.
- NSAIDs, e.g. diclofenac, ibuprofen, piroxicam.
- Local anesthetics (e.g. lidocaine)—chiefly used for post-herpetic neuralgia or where allodynia is prominent.

Rubefacients

Rubefacients include a wide range of different chemicals. The broad term of rubefacients frequently includes salicylates (that are pharmacologically similar to non-steroidal anti-inflammatory agents) and compounds such as capsaicin which is said to work by acting as a counter-irritant, reducing musculoskeletal pain by acting as distraction to the pain by producing an irritation to the skin. Counter-irritation is said to result in a pleasant sensation that relieves discomfort experienced in muscles and tendons as a result of altering or offsetting the pain in the sensory nerve endings.

Salicylates

Topical salicylates have shown mixed results in acute and chronic pain. Limited evidence suggests that efficacy is demonstrated in acute pain at 7 days although poor to moderate efficacy seen in chronic pain at 14 days.

Capsaicin

Capsaicin is extracted from chilli peppers and is a naturally occurring alkaloid. It appears to affect the sensory nerve endings. Available in strengths of 0.075% (post-herpetic neuralgia) or 0.025% (for OA) and are usually applied 3–4 × a day.

NSAIDs

The use of topical NSAIDs remains controversial particularly in the UK where the Prescription Pricing Authority data suggests they make up 10% of the total cost of analgesics and NSAID prescribing. NSAIDs need to be able to penetrate the skin and be actively absorbed in high concentrations so that they can actively inhibit COX enzymes before producing pain relief. Evidence suggests that topical therapies have a much lower systemic dose accounting for the reduction in side effects but also potentially the sustained therapeutic benefit (plasma concentration at 1–2 hours declines rapidly).

Issues to consider in the use of topical therapies

- Acute conditions (e.g. joint strains, sprains) are likely to gain the most benefit from topical NSAIDs.
- Chronic MSC may benefit from topical therapies in the short term (NNT 5 although evidence is weak).
- Differing terminology used to describe different topical therapies.
- Variations in concentrations of the topical agent being prescribed.
- Topical therapies may be more a more expensive option than oral analgesia.
- A number of preparations can be purchased by the patient over-the-counter, some contains NSAIDs and/or counter irritants.
- Although evidence is limited and further research is needed, topical therapies as an adjunct to other treatment modalities may enhance the patient's perception of empowerment/self-efficacy in managing the condition.
- Therapeutic effect of topical NSAIDS relies upon skin integrity and vasculature.

Advice to give the patient

- General information on the use of pain-relieving strategies and how to step-up or step-down management based upon pain assessment.
- Provide detailed information on the risks and benefits of treatment based upon individual treatment choices, based upon a patient-centred assessment.
- Topical therapies must not be applied to broken or infected skin.
- They may experience a transient burning sensation.
- Ensure they wash their hands immediately after applying the treatment.
- Patients with a known allergy to aspirin or NSAIDs should avoid topical therapies (e.g. asthmatics).
- Adverse events include:
  - Number Needed to Harm of 2.5.
  - >50% of patients experienced local adverse event (burning sensation).
  - Photosensitivity is rare (1–2 cases per 10,000 patients) with topical NSAIDs

Also see Symptom control, p.289.

Further reading

Bandolier Extra (March, 2005). Topical analgesics. Available at: www.ebandolier.com

Joint Formulary Committee (2008). Rubefacients and other topical anti-rheumatics, section 10.3.2. In *British National Formulary*, 56th edn. British Medical Association and Royal Pharmaceutical Society of Great Britain, London.

Frequently asked questions

Is analgesia addictive?

In some cases the use of opiates has led to their abuse and dependence but only when used on a regular basis in an inappropriate way. Used appropriately in the context of severe pain this is not a concern.

What is meant by medication overuse headache?

Headaches can occur when analgesic levels trough e.g. the patient wakes with a morning headache. It is thought that sustained analgesia use can cause pain signalling mechanisms to become more sensitive.

Who are the most at risk group of patients for GI complications?

The highest risk group are those who are: >65 years, also using medications likely to ↑ GI side effects, e.g. anticoagulants, corticosteroids; or with serious comorbidity; or those with prior history of peptic ulcer ± complication, who may require prolonged use of or the maximum recommended doses of NSAIDs.

What is the best advice?

Use the lowest effective dose for the shortest duration. Review the pain-relieving benefits and other supporting strategies regularly. Encourage the patient to report any gastric symptoms and to take their medication with food. A traditional NSAID prescribed with gastro protection (usually a PPI) if there are no contraindications (e.g. prior GI risks) may be considered. If prior previous peptic ulceration (and there are no cardiovascular contra-indications) a COX-2 can be prescribed together with a PPI. Encourage a pharmacological and non-pharmacological approach to pain management and encourage the patient to use self-management strategies such as the use of cold packs, rest and relaxation, and joint protection.

Which NSAID would be the most effective?

NSAIDs have a highly variable effect between patients so it is vital to find one that suits the individual, allow up to 4 weeks of taking the NSAID on a regular basis for full anti-inflammatory effect. It is important to allow an adequate trial and evaluate the benefits to the patient in level of pain relief achieved. It may be necessary to have a short trial of a few NSAIDs before finding the one that provides the maximum benefit to the patient.

Chapter 16

Pharmacological management: disease-modifying drugs

Pharmacological management: pre-treatment assessment

Nurses play an important role in preparing patients before starting a new treatment. A thorough screening process should encourage concordance and reduce risks related to poor knowledge of drug therapies or anxieties about what to do if side effects are experienced.

The level of screening may vary according to the therapy being prescribed (e.g. being prescribed a short course of paracetamol for knee pain in an otherwise healthy patient will differ from a patient who has diabetes and PSV who is being prescribed cyclophosphamide). All screening should consider:

• A patient-centred approach.
• A thorough medical assessment and baseline clinical examination.

A patient-centred approach

Patients may be anxious about the treatment prescribed, or adjusting psychologically to a diagnosis or change in disease state. The patient should be actively encouraged to participate and ask question and discuss any of their personal anxieties/goals. Screening often incorporates education about the disease and the drug therapies prescribed (📖 see Blood tests and investigation, p.461; 📖 Patient consent and informed decision making, p.316).

An assessment of medical history and baseline clinical history

The nurse should ensure they undertake a review of the medical record and specific risk factors related to the proposed drug therapy and combine this with a consultation that reviews:

• General health status, previous medical and surgical history, comorbidities. Assess rate, strength, and rhythm of pulse, blood pressure, weight.
• Age, smoking status, alcohol consumption.
• Family history—including any linked to genetic predispositions.
• Previous drug history, previous allergic reactions, side effects.
• Current prescribed medication and over-the-counter treatments (including complementary therapies). Consider poly-pharmacy risks.
• Lifestyle or social issues that may affect risks to treatment , monitoring, or concordance:
  • ⚠ Discuss fertility and contraceptive use.

The body systems should be reviewed. These include:

• **Immune status**—consider general information but also:
  • Corticosteroids, biologic therapies, or disease-modifying therapies—review immunization status of TB history, hepatitis risks, and chicken pox.
  • Immunizations may be required prior to starting treatment, e.g. administration of live vaccines.
• ⚠ **Screen for infections** or risk related to re-emergence of latent infections, e.g. TB or prior septic arthroplasty where joint remains in situ.

- ⚠ *Cardiovascular:*
  - Cardiac risk factor, e.g. high density lipoprotein/↑ blood pressure.[1]
  - Underlying cardiovascular disease. Some therapies (e.g. biologic DMARDs) refer to the New York Heart Classification Criteria to exclude those at risk of developing side effects.
  - Hypertension and lipid levels may need an assessment and specific treatment before commencing a therapy, e.g. ciclosporin.
- *GI:*
  - Prior history of GI bleed, dyspepsia, or factors that predispose to risks, e.g. aspirin/steroid use in a patient requiring pain relief.
  - Gastric symptoms prior to starting a bisphosphonate for osteoporosis.
  - Risk factors may determine choice of drug e.g. COX-2 or NSAID + PPI.
- ⚠ *Haematological:*
  - FBC, U&Es including creatinine, LFTs, CRP, ESR, PV—prior results and baseline assessments.
  - Pre-screening results must be scrutinized to ensure safety of commencing treatment—refer to protocols/guidelines or seek advice for abnormal results.
  - Inflammatory markers at baseline and to inform composite scores used such as the DAS 28 (uses ESR or CRP).
- *Hepatic:*
  - LFTs will be considered with all blood tests and should be considered in the context of predisposing risk factors, underlying disease, or lifestyle factors, e.g. alcohol consumption.
  - Dermatologists sometimes request a pre-screening test to assess hepatic status—pro collagen III.
- *Musculoskeletal:* baseline assessments of composite scores, functional ability, or bone health, e.g. risk of osteoporosis. Assessments may be essential for adherence to NICE guidance.
- *Neurological:* identification of any neurological conditions or family history (e.g. demyelinating disease) should be documented. Biologic therapies may precipitate exacerbation of demyelinating disease.
- *Renal:*
  - Good renal function is essential for excretion of many therapies. Poor function may ↑ risk of toxicities. Drugs may exclude treatment if renal impairment.
  - Urinalysis, e.g. screen for infections or urinary proteins.
- *Respiratory:*
  - Interstitial lung disease, prior pulmonary TB, or poor respiratory function need to be reviewed with prescribing physician.
  - Chest x-ray or PFTs may be necessary prior to starting MTX or biologic therapy
- *Skin:* examine for signs of bacterial or fungal infections. Presence of rashes, lesions, or vasculitis changes.

Reference

1. BNF 56 (2008). BNF Cardiovascular risk prediction chart.

Screening before treatment: documentation and decisions

The screening process combined with good documented evidence of pre-treatment health status and exclusion of risk factors is an essential component to nursing support in drug therapies.

In addition to the actual screening process documentation should include:

- Evidence that the patient has been provided with written and verbal information about the treatment and has had an opportunity to explore all questions/anxieties about the treatment.
- Information including outcomes from a patient-centred consultation, documented in the notes (□ Nursing issues and the patient-centred approach, pp.312, 314).
- The patient has reviewed the information and understands their responsibilities in undertaking regular blood monitoring and concordance to treatment. That they consent to treatment.
- The patient has been provided with a patient-held monitoring booklet/ record or passport that informs them of:
  - The treatment they are prescribed, dose, timing and duration of treatment.
  - Their recent test results.
  - When they will be seen again.
  - Side effects of treatment and what to do should they develop, e.g. treatment and telephone advice line at the hospital.
  - Individual issues or risk factors identified in the assessment or as a result of the consultation.
  - What they should expect in the next few weeks of treatment and what to do if something untoward happens.

Decisions to be made when screening patients

Nurses should have the knowledge and skills to be able to screen patients, interpret the results, and recognize when to seek guidance from the prescribing physician following the screening process. The screening process may reveal:

- Previously missed cautions or contraindications to the proposed treatment:
  - Co-prescribing factors that may enhance or reduce the proposed drug dosage or route of administration.
  - Comorbidities that may be affected by the proposed treatment, e.g. exacerbation of demyelinating disease.
- Pre-screening tests may reveal factors that require further investigation, e.g. previous history of untreated TB or impaired renal function.
- Patient may decline treatment and alternative treatment may need to be offered.
- General health status may have declined or changed since referral and require intervention or review, e.g. recent infection.

Tools to support screening clinics

- Specific nurse-led drug screening/monitoring protocols and guidelines.
- Regional or national screening guidelines.
- Treatment protocols for specific drug therapies.
- Regional or national treatment monitoring guidelines.
- NICE guidelines to screen for adherence to guidance.
- Drug SPC, see: ⊕ www.medicines.org.uk
- The *BNF*: ⊕ www.bnf.org

Additional resources

- Clinical Knowledge Summaries: ⊕ www.cks.library.nhs.uk
- Medical Health Products Regulatory Agency: ⊕ www.mhra.gov.uk
- National Patient Safety Agency: ⊕ www.npsa.nhs.uk
- The National Osteoporosis Society: ⊕ www.nos.org.uk
- The British Pain Society: ⊕ www.britishpainsociety.org

Further reading

British Society for Rheumatology (2008). *BSR guidelines on disease modifying drug therapies*. BSR, London.

Hakim A, Clunie G, Haq I (eds) (2006). *Oxford Handbook of Rheumatology*, 2nd edn. Oxford University Press, Oxford.

Ryan S (2007). *Drug therapy in rheumatology nursing*. John Wiley and Sons Ltd., Chichester.

Disease-modifying anti-rheumatic drugs

A number of MSCs have an underlying inflammatory component and many of these are as a result of an auto-immune process. There has been significant progress in the last 15 years in understanding the key cell-to-cell interactions in the auto-immune pathway. This has meant that many new therapies have been developed, targeting the body's specific cell-to-cell interactions responsible for driving inflammatory auto-immune conditions, and their mechanism of action is better understood, unlike the older traditional DMARDs. Ultimately the aim is to suppress the disease and stop the resulting damage that occurs, e.g. tissue or organ damage, synovial proliferation, joint erosions, long-term disability.

Treatment options for inflammatory auto-immune driven conditions include a range of therapies but the main focus should be on achieving rapid and proactive management to ensure disease control/suppression.

- Symptom relief—analgesia and NSAIDs
- Symptom relief and modification of inflammatory component—corticosteroid therapies
- Disease modification—traditional (or conventional) disease-modifying drug therapies, e.g.:
  - AZA.
  - Ciclosporin.
  - Hydroxychloroquine.
  - Leflunomide.
  - MTX.
  - Mycophenolate.
  - Penicillamine.
  - SAS.
  - Tacrolimus.
- Disease modification—biological disease-modifying drug therapies, e.g.:
  - Adalimumab—Humira®.
  - Etanercept—Enbrel®.
  - Infliximab—Remicade®
  - Rituximab—MabThera®.
  - Abatacept—Orencia®.
  - Certolizumab—pending licence.

📖 Also see Biological disease-modifying drug therapies, p.456.

Licensed and unlicensed use of **DMARDs**

Traditional DMARDs are used in the treatment of a number of conditions **not all** of which are prescribed under their licensed indications. These include:

- AS.
- CTDs:
  - Behçet disease.
  - Vasculitidies.
- Felty syndrome.
- Inflammatory myopathies such as dermatomyositis, polymyositis.
- Pemphigus vulgaris.
- PMR
- Polyarteritis.
- PsA.
- RA
- Scleroderma
- Systemic and discoid lupus erythematosus.

DMARDs are immunological modifiers and require regular monitoring for adverse events and efficacy. They usually take a number of weeks before benefits are achieved and can cause unpleasant side effects particularly in the early phases of treatment. They vary in efficacy for the range of treatments outlined and toxicity profiles.

Traditional disease-modifying anti-rheumatic drugs

Introduction

Traditional DMARDs have been used in the treatment of inflammatory forms of joint disease for >50 years. These traditional DMARD therapies have evolved in an ad hoc way without a real understanding of the mechanisms of action.

Traditional DMARDs do not reflect the development of newer biologic DMARDs. The mechanism of action for biologic therapies is more clearly understood (e.g. the pathway of TNFα).

However, both traditional and biologic DMARDs inhibit the immunological response to an inflammatory process. Traditional and biological DMARDs require care before prescribing. The process should include:

- An assessment of the disease activity using recognized diagnostic and treatment criteria.
- Screening of the patient for underlying infections prior to treatment.
- General health screen to ensure normal function:
  - Haematology, biochemistry (liver and renal).
  - Renal function—normal renal function (or may require dose reductions).
  - Respiratory—in some cases detailed respiratory function tests.
  - Cardiac status.
  - Other comorbidities—demyelinating disease, diabetes.
- Some DMARDs may require additional screening tests:
  - AZA—thiopurine methyl transferase (TPMT) status.
  - Ciclosporin—lipid profiles.
  - Biological DMARDs—screening for TB status as well as the others listed.

Combination therapy with traditional DMARDs

It is common practice for combination therapy to be used to achieve proactive and targeted management of the condition. There is strong evidence particularly in the inflammatory arthritides (e.g. RA) to support aggressive treatment regimens. Combination therapies use 2 or 3 DMARD therapies together—e.g. MTX, SAS, and hydroxychloroquine. The combination therapies appear to have no additional risks in relation to toxicity when prescribed together (see Fig. 16.1).

Detailed information on specific DMARDs can be found in this chapter under specific drug therapies.

Further reading

BSR (2008). *British Society for Rheumatology Shared Care Monitoring Guidelines*. BSR, London. Available at: ⁀ www.rheumatology.org.uk

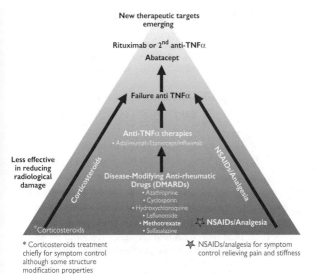

Fig. 16.1 Therapeutic pyramid of licensed indications in the treatment of RA. This pyramid highlights all therapies licensed to treat RA. To review detailed evidence of those recommended by the regulatory authorities such as NICE or Scottish Intercollegiate Guidelines (SIGN) refer to individual websites such as ⟨ www.nice.org.uk or ⟨ www.sign.ac.uk

Azathioprine and ciclosporin

AZA and ciclosporin were originally developed to prevent rejection of organ transplants but are now also used as traditional DMARDs to control the underlying immunological inflammatory response. They suppress the inflammatory processes and as a result inhibit progression of damaging joint and tissue destruction.

AZA and ciclosporin general management

- Pre-screening required for both therapies, haematological, pregnancy, and immunological status (📖 see Screening prior to DMARD treatment, p.422).
- Regular blood monitoring required (+ BP for ciclosporin):
  - FBC including WCC.
  - LFTs.
  - U&Es (including K^+), creatinine for ciclosporin.
- Vigilance for evidence of skin rashes, bruising or muco-cutaneous ulcers.

⚠ Note: a trend in blood results is as important as absolute values.
📖 Also see Blood tests and investigations, p.461.

Patients treated with AZA and ciclosporin should be advised:

- It will take up to 3 months before they feel the benefit of treatment although they may feel a benefit earlier.
- They may experience side effects during this time and these should abate. Side effects include:
  - Nausea, loss of appetite (occur in ~23% of patients on AZA).
  - Itching, rashes, or mouth ulcers.
  - Muscle aches.
- Monitoring for any side effects include tests to check bloods, liver, and renal function.
- Do not alter the dose they are prescribed.
- Report promptly any infections they experience (occur in ~9% of patients on AZA).
- They must not get pregnant while on treatment (use effective method of contraceptive).
- Blood monitoring regimens are important and will help identify problems.
- They should not have any live vaccines whilst on treatment.
- Herbal or complementary therapies—advice the doctor or nurse of any being taken as there may be interactions.
- If side effects become a problem or if they are uncertain about their treatment seek advice as there is always something that can be done to help with side effects.

Key factors in nursing management of patients taking AZA

AZA is an immune modulating drug that inhibits DNA synthesis inhibiting cell replication. It is a pro-drug metabolized by the liver, 30% protein bound, 45% excreted in urine with the remainder metabolized by 6-methylmercaptopurine (6MMP).

An inability to metabolize AZA due to an enzyme deficiency means some patients are vulnerable to serious adverse events. The deficiency of TPMT is classified as:

- Homozygous state—AZA should be avoided and can be fatal (within 6 weeks)
- Heterozygous state—may be subject to delayed bone marrow toxicity (symptoms may not be evident until 6 months after starting treatment).

Dose of oral azathioprine

A typical dose is usually 1mg/kg/day, ↑ after 4–6 weeks to 2–3mg/kg/day.

⚠ Drug interactions may ↑ the risk of toxicity (e.g. co-prescription of allopurinol dose of AZA should be *cut to 25% of original* dose.

Key factors in nursing management of patients taking ciclosporin

Ciclosporin has an immunosuppressive action on pro-inflammatory cytokines by inhibiting responses by T cells. Observe for potential side effects which can include:

- Impairment of renal function.
- ↑ in lipids (reversible).
- Observe serum: ↑ creatinine may necessitate dose reductions.
- Limited evidence in the elderly.
- ⚠ Significant drug interactions, e.g.: pharmacodynamics with co-prescriptions:
  - NSAIDs may adversely affect renal function.
  - Hepatotoxicity potential with NSAIDs.
  - Nifedipine use with caution.
  - Avoid colchicine and potassium-sparing diuretics.
- ⚠ Patient self-administered:
  - Interactions with St. John's Wort (↓ ciclosporin effectiveness).
  - Grapefruit (flesh and juice) must be avoided for 1 hour prior to taking ciclosporin ↑ bioavailability.
- ▶ Note blood trends or unexplained bruising (with or without sore throat)—withhold treatment and seek medical advice.

Dose of oral ciclosporin

Treatment is normally started as 2 divided doses of 2.5mg/kg/day and gradually ↑ after 2–4 weeks interval by 25mg each ↑ until clinically effective (maximum dose of 4mg/kg/day.) Maintenance dose usually effective at 2.5–3.2mg/kg/day (titrate according to tolerance, efficacy). Refer to SPC for licensed indications and *BNF* for prescribing information

Further reading

BSR (2008). *British Society of Rheumatology DMARD Guidelines.* Available at: ⌂ www.rheumatology. org.uk

Patient Information Leaflets on all drug therapies available from Arthritis Research Campaign: ⌂ www.arc.org.uk

D-penicillamine and sodium aurothiomalate (intramuscular gold)

General management

D-penicillamine and sodium aurothiomalate (Myocrisin®) are the older generation of DMARD therapies and have been ↓ in use as evidence to demonstrate benefit of treatment is sub-optimal compared to MTX. The occasional life threatening rash or anaphylactic reaction from sodium aurothiomalate is also an additional consideration in prescribing. However, if other DMARDS have failed to control the disease they are other therapeutic options.

- Pre-screening required for both therapies: haematological, pregnancy, and immunological status.
- Regular blood monitoring required:
  - ~50% of RA patients experience an AE in the 1st 6 months of treatment.
  - 25% will discontinue treatment.
- Urinalysis is necessary as both drugs have the potential to cause renal impairment and are excreted in the urine.
- For prescribing information and rare adverse events refer to SPC and *BNF* for prescribing information.

⚠ A trend in blood results is as important as absolute values.

📖 Also see Blood tests and investigations, p.461; 📖 Screening prior to DMARD treatment, p.422.

Patients treated with D-penicillamine and sodium aurothiomalate (IM gold) should be advised:

- It may take 3–6 months before they feel the benefit of treatment although they may feel a benefit earlier.
- They may experience side effects during this time and these should abate. However some must be reported promptly. Side effects include:
  - Nausea, loss of appetite (taking medication before bed may reduce nausea).
  - Itching, rashes or mouth ulcers (do not ignore even rashes—even those that appear late in treatment—they can be serious).
  - Abnormal taste sensations in D-penicillamine (should resolve spontaneously).
  - Abnormal bruising or severe sore throat.
- Do not alter the dose prescribed.
- Report promptly any infections they experience.
- They must not get pregnant while on treatment (use effective method of contraceptive).
- That we monitor for side effects related to bloods, liver, and kidneys and blood monitoring regimens are important and will help identify problems.
- They should not have any live vaccines whilst on treatment.
- Advise doctor or nurse if taking herbal or complementary therapies—as they may interaction with the medication.
- If side effects become a problem or if they are uncertain about their treatment seek advice as there is always something that can be done to help with side effects.

Key factors in the management of penicillamine and IM gold

▶ Note blood trends or unexplained bruising (with or without sore throat)—withhold treatment and seek medical advice.

Dose of oral D-penicillamine

A typical dose in 2 divided doses: 125–250mg/day, ↑ by 125mg every 4 weeks to 500mg/day. The dose may be ↑ to 750mg/day if response is not achieved in 3 months. Patients should be advised:

- Milk, antacids, zinc supplements or iron tablets can be taken but must be administered at least 2 hours after taking D-penicillamine as they interfere with drug absorption.
- Haematological side effects include neutropenia, thrombocytopenia, and aplastic anaemias—rapid or gradual changes in the blood picture may be seen.
- Contraindicated in moderate-to-severe renal impairment.

⚠ Drug interactions include digoxin, antipsychotic. Also consider drugs with concomitant nephrotoxicity (including sodium aurothiomalate).

Cautions

⚠ Caution if co-prescribed:

- Aspirin—may exacerbate hepatic dysfunction.
- Phenylbutazone or oxyphenbutazone—hepatic dysfunction.
- Angiotensin-converting enzyme inhibitors due to an ↑ risk of severe anaphylactoid reaction in these patients.

Contraindications include: severe renal or hepatic impairment, history of blood disorders/marrow aplasia, SLE, significant pulmonary fibrosis, porphyria. Pregnancy or lactation.

⚠ IM gold

In the elderly, renal or hepatic impairment (moderate) history of urticaria, eczema, or inflammatory bowel disease. Rare anaphylactic reactions may occur a few minutes after injection. Early signs include dizziness, nausea, sweating, and facial flushing. Treat according to policy on anaphylaxis and discontinue treatment.

Dose of sodium aurothiomalate (IM gold)

A test dose of 10mg sodium aurothiomalate should be given in the clinic/ward and patients should be observed for 30min for any signs of allergic reaction. Continue with further injections of 50mg sodium aurothiomalate once a week until a significant treatment response is seen.

Review of treatment response

Benefits should be seen at cumulative dose of at 500mg although efficacy should be assessed after a cumulative dose of 1g has been administered. Responders to treatment—↑ the interval between injections to 1 every 4 weeks (50mg dose). If no response is seen after cumulative doses of 1g consider an alternative DMARD.

Further reading

Arthritis Research Campaign: patient information leaflets, available at: ⁀🖰 www.arc.org.uk

BSR (2008). *British Society of Rheumatology DMARD Guidelines.* Available at: ⁀🖰 www.rheumatology.org.uk

Hydroxychloroquine sulfate

Hydroxychloroquine is principally used as a prophylaxis against malaria although benefits in treating RA and SLE have been demonstrated for many years. Hydroxychloroquine has a lower toxicity profile compared to other DMARDs but also a lower therapeutic benefit and is therefore chiefly confined to treating milder disease or in combination therapy.[1]

General management

Ophthalmic pre-screening is required for hydroxychloroquine. This should include visual acuity of each eye and annual review with optometrist whilst on treatment for any signs of blurred vision.

Caution
- ↑ risk of retinal toxicity if dose exceeds 6m/kg. Check visual acuity.
- Renal or hepatic impairment. Therapeutic doses may need to be adjusted for those with renal impairment (40% renal excretion).
- Patients with epilepsy—may reduce threshold for convulsions.

Contraindications
- Breastfeeding.
- Pre-existing maculopathy.

Drug interactions
These include ↑ plasma concentrations of digoxin, MTX, ciclosporin. Avoid use with amiodarone, moxifloxacin, mefloquine and quinine.

▶ Relatively safe in pregnancy—risk benefit analysis should consider relative potential harm to unborn child against the relative risks of stopping treatment.

Patient treated with hydroxychloroquine should be advised:
- To take hydroxychloroquine with food to avoid GI symptoms.
- To avoid anti-acids within 4 hours of dose.
- Side effects usually resolve with continuation of treatment but these include:
  - Nausea, diarrhoea, abdominal discomfort.
  - Blurred vision, irreversible retinal damage, headaches, and dizziness.
  - Skin reactions (rashes, itching). May exacerbate psoriasis.
  - Hair loss.

Dose of hydroxychloroquine sulfate (oral)

A typical regimen would be 200–400mg daily. Dosage may be reduced to 200mg daily depending upon clinical response.

📖 Also see Screening prior to DMARD treatment, p.422.

Reference

1. Royal College of Ophthalmologists. *Screening grid for ocular toxicity.* Available at: ⌐ www.rcophth.ac.uk

Further reading

Arthritis Research Campaign: patient information leaflets, available at: ⚲ www.arc.org.uk

BSR (2008). *British Society of Rheumatology DMARD Guidelines*. Available at: ⚲ www.rheumatology. org.uk

For licensed indications, prescribing. and rare adverse events see Summary of Product Characteristics and *BNF*.

Leflunomide

Leflunomide is one of the most recently developed traditional DMARDs. It has an active metabolite that inhibits the human enzyme dihydroorotate dehydrogenase and as a result has anti-proliferative activity and arrests lymphocyte activation. It has a long half-life (~2 weeks) and is strongly protein-bound. There is no dose adjustment recommended in patients with mild renal insufficiency.

General management

- Pre-screening required for haematological, pregnancy and immunological status (📖 see Screening prior to DMARD treatment, p.422).
- Allergic responses, toxicities, pregnancy, or severe side effects will require an urgent therapeutic washout.
- Pre-existing anaemia, leucopenia, and/or thrombocytopenia, or patients with impaired function of the bone marrow function are at risk of ↑ haematological disorders.
- Early signs of skin or mucosal reactions occur raise the suspicion of allergic reaction.
- ▶ Interstitial lung disease has developed whilst being treated—observe for cough and dyspnoea and report urgently.

Patients treated with leflunomide should be advised:

- They may experience side effects; this should abate over time. Side effects include:
  - Nausea, loss of appetite, diarrhoea.
  - Hair loss.
  - Liver impairment—alcohol should be avoided/or limited to within national limits (e.g. 4–8 units per week)
- Side effects can occur which is why we monitor to make sure the bloods, liver, and kidneys are functioning normally. Blood monitoring regimens are important and will help identify problems.
- The benefits of treatment are usually seen between 4–6 weeks after starting treatment and may further improve up to 4–6 months.
- Not to alter the dose they are prescribed.
- Report promptly any infections they experience as they may require treatment.
- They must not get pregnant while on treatment (use effective method of contraceptive). They should contact their doctor/nurse immediately if they believe they might be pregnant—a therapeutic drug washout may be required.
- They should not have any live vaccines whilst on treatment.
- Herbal or complementary therapies—advice the doctor or nurse of any being taken as there may be interactions (📖 see Ciclosporin, p.428).
- If side effects become a problem or if they are uncertain about their treatment, seek advice as there is always something that can be done to help with side effects.

Cautions

- Localized or systemic infections including hepatitis B or C.
- History of TB.

- Potential hepatotoxicity/haematotoxic issues related to co-prescription of other drug therapies (e.g. phenytoin, warfarin, and tolbutamide). MTX is listed as a caution although it is often prescribed in combination therapy with leflunomide.

Contraindications
- Severe immunodeficiency.
- Serious infections.
- Liver impairment or moderate-to-severe renal impairment.
- Hypoproteinaemia.
- Bone marrow impairment, e.g. anaemia or cytopenias.

$\triangle$ Note: a trend in blood results is as important as absolute values.

Key issues for nurse management.

▶ Note blood trends or unexplained bruising (with or without sore throat)—withhold treatment and seek urgent medical advice. Note toxicity may require washout (📖 see Blood tests and investigations, p.461).

Dose of leflunomide (oral only)

The licensed indications suggest a loading dose of 100mg once daily for 3 days (in practice often not prescribed due ↑ incidence of side effects with loading dose). Frequently patients are commenced on a maintenance dose of leflunomide 10–20 mg once daily for RA; for PsA dose is 20 mg once daily.

Further reading

Arthritis Research Campaign: patient information leaflets, available at: ◌ www.arc.org.uk

BSR (2008). *British Society of Rheumatology DMARD Guidelines.* Available at: ◌ www.rheumatology. org.uk

For licensed indications, prescribing. and rare adverse events see Summary of Product Characteristics and *BNF.*

Joint Formulary Committee (2008). DMARDs: Leflunomide. In *British National Formulary,* 56th edn. British Medical Association and Royal Pharmaceutical Society of Great Britain, London.

Methotrexate

MTX is the 'gold' standard of traditional disease-modifying drug thera-pies suppressing disease activity for IJDs. GI and bone marrow toxicities with MTX are significantly ↓ if prescribed folic acid. MTX is prescribed in oncology and gynaecology and is prescribed to prevent cell replication. MTX inhibits the activity of an enzyme (dihydrofolate reductase) responsible for the synthesis of purines implicated in cell replication (DNA) resulting in a fall of malignant and, it appears, inflammatory cells. MTX is frequently prescribed in combination with other traditional DMARDs (e.g. MTX and SAS) and co-prescribed when patients are treated with a biologic DMARD. MTX can be administered subcutaneously (better bio-availability).

General management

- Pre-screening required includes haematological, respiratory function, pregnancy, and immunological status.
- Chest x-ray (unless taken within last 6 months). If chest x-ray or risk factors indicate consider PFTs to identify pre-existing or occult lung disease. In some circumstances consider HRCT, e.g. for interstitial lung disease.
- Dermatologists may require an additional pre-screening test to monitor liver status (pro-collagen III levels).
- Regular blood monitoring required—FBC,U&E, LFTs.
- ▶ Vigilance for signs of toxicity—these can occur at any time during treatment, e.g. pulmonary pneumonitis (cough, dyspnoea)—if any suspicion, seek urgent medical advice.
- Frail and elderly require lower doses. Observe for signs of renal impairment ↑ risk of toxicity.
- ⚠ Note: a Trend in blood results is as important as absolute values

📖 Also see Screening prior to DMARD treatment, p.422.

Patient treated with MTX should be advised:

- They may experience side effects; this should abate over time. Side effects may be reduced if MTX is taken at night with full glass of water. Side effects include:
  - Nausea, loss of appetite, diarrhoea, and headaches.
  - Hair loss or skin rashes.
  - Mouth ulcers.
  - Liver impairment—seek medical advice regarding alcohol consumption whilst on treatment (should be at least <nationally recommended levels).
  - Rare but important risk of developing respiratory problems—seek medical advice for unexplained cough or dyspnoea.
  - They will also be co-prescribed folic acid 5mg—dosing regimens vary.
- If side effects become a problem or if they are uncertain about their treatment, seek advice as there is always something that can be done to help with side effects.
- MTX is prescribed *as a once a week dose*. They must not alter the dose they are prescribed. If they forget to take a dose
  - Delay 1–2 days, take dose and return to normal dosing day the following week.
  - >3 days, make a note they have missed the dose and then take their normal dose on their normal dosing day the following week.

- Side effects can occur which is why we monitor to make sure the bloods, liver, and kidneys are functioning normally. Blood monitoring regimens are important and will help identify problems.
- Report unexplained bleeding or bruising.
- Treatment can take up to 3 months for benefits to be achieved.
- Report promptly any infections as they may require treatment.
- Conception whilst receiving treatment must be avoided (use effective method of contraceptive). Seek medical advice promptly if pregnancy occurs.
- They should not have any live vaccines whilst on treatment.
- Herbal or complementary therapies—advice the doctor or nurse of any being taken as there may be interactions.

Cautions
- Localized or systemic infections including hepatitis B or C.
- History of TB
- Potential hepatotoxicity/haematotoxic issues related to co-prescription of other drug therapies (e.g. phenytoin, probencid, penicillin, tolbutamide, co-trimoxazole, trimethoprim.)

Contraindications
- Pregnancy or breastfeeding.
- Liver impairment or moderate-to-severe renal impairment.
- Suspicion of local or systemic infection.
- Hypoproteinaemia.
- Bone marrow impairment, e.g. anaemia or cytopenias.

Key factors for nursing management for patients taking MTX

- MTX *once a week dose only*. ⚠ Patients must check tablets (dosages of 2.5mg or 10mg tablets).[1]
- Folic acid is usually not administered on the day that MTX is taken.
- Side effects and toxicities can occur at any time during treatment
- ▶ Note blood trends or unexplained bruising (with or without sore throat)—withhold treatment and seek medical advice.
- If over-dosage occurs seek prompt medical/pharmacist advice to enable chemical washout.

Drug dose (oral, SC, or IM routes prescribed for MSC conditions)
These will vary according to age, renal function and route of administration but dose range from 5–25mg once a week.

📖 Also see Blood tests and investigations, p.461.

Reference

National Patient Safety Agency (NPSA): ⁀ www.npsa.nhs.uk

Further reading

Arthritis Research Campaign: patient information leaflets, available at: ⁀ www.arc.org.uk

BSR (2008). *British Society of Rheumatology DMARD Guidelines*. Available at: ⁀ www.rheumatology. org.uk

For licensed indications, prescribing, and rare adverse events see Summary of Product Characteristics and *BNF*.

Mycophenolate mofetil

MMF inhibits the pathway of active metabolites required for the synthesis of DNA. This inhibition results in a reduction in T- and B-lymphocytes as they are critically dependent for their proliferation on *de novo* synthesis of purines necessary for DNA.

General management

- Pre-screening required.
- MMF does not normally cause major organ toxicity.
- △ Note: a trend in blood results is as important as absolute values.

📖 Also see Screening prior to DMARD treatment, p.422.

Cautions

- Suspected lymphoproliferative disorders or unexplained anaemias/leucopenia and thrombocytopenia.
- Localized or systemic infection.
- Active serious digestive system disease.
- Frail and elderly.

Contraindications

- Pregnancy and breastfeeding.
- Localised or systemic infections.
- Should not be co-prescribed with AZA.

Patient treated with mycophenolate should be advised:

- They may experience side effects which are usually related to the dose. Side effects if severe will abate on cessation of treatment but include:
  - Sickness, nausea, loss of appetite, diarrhoea, vomiting, or abdominal pain.
  - Hair loss, skin rashes, bruising.
  - Mouth ulcers.
  - Urinary—urgent sensation to pass urine.
- It is important to use sun block or sunscreen and avoid exposure to strong sunlight as there is a slight ↑ in skin cancers.
- Symptoms of allergy including wheezing, SOB, swelling of face, lips, or tongue—stop treatment and seek medical advice.
- If side effects become a problem or if they are uncertain about their treatment, seek advice as there is always something that can be done to help with side effects.
- MMF is prescribed as a capsule and should be taken on an empty stomach.
- Side effects can occur which is why we monitor to make sure the bloods, liver, and kidneys are functioning normally. Blood monitoring regimens are important and will help identify problems.
- Report unexplained bleeding or bruising.
- Treatment can take up to 3 months before the benefits are achieved.
- Report promptly any infections they experience as they may require treatment.
- ♂ and ♀ patients need to be aware that conception whilst receiving treatment must be avoided (use effective method of contraceptive). Seek medical advice promptly if a pregnancy occurs.

- They should not have any live vaccines whilst on treatment.
- Herbal or complementary therapies—advise the doctor or nurse of any being taken as there may be interactions.

Key factors in nursing management

- ▶ Note blood trends or unexplained bruising (with or without sore throat)—withhold treatment and seek medical advice.
  - Severe neutropenias occur in ~0.5% for those receiving full dose.
- Drug interactions include:
  - Cholestyramine ↓ absorption of MMF by ~40%.
  - Antacids containing aluminum and magnesium hydroxide ↓ absorption of MMF by 33%.
  - Probencid ↑ plasma concentration of MMF.
  - Note: if patients have renal impairment and are co-prescribed aciclovir with mycophenolate they will have raised concentrations of both aciclovir and mycophenolate.

📖 Also see Blood tests and investigations, p.461.

Drug dosage (note oral or IV routes available)

The typical dose is 500mg twice a day, gradually ↑ over weeks until the optimum dose is achieved, e.g. if well tolerated this may be ↑ to 1g twice a day thereafter. Maximum is usually 3g/day.

Further reading

Arthritis Research Campaign: patient information leaflets, available at: ⁑ www.arc.org.uk

BSR (2008). *British Society of Rheumatology DMARD Guidelines*. Available at: ⁑ www.rheumatology. org.uk

For licensed indications, prescribing. and rare adverse events see Summary of Product Characteristics and *BNF*.

Sulfasalazine

It appears that SAS may work by inhibiting specific metabolites that have a disease-modifying effect on conditions such as inflammatory bowel or IJD. The enteric coated form should be prescribed.

General management

- Pre-screening required for haematological, pregnancy and immunological status.
- ⚠ Note: a trend in blood results is as important as absolute values

📖 Also see Screening prior to DMARD treatment, p.422.

Cautions

- Haemolysis may occur for those with glucose 6 phosphate dehydrogenase deficiency.
- Moderate renal impairment—encourage high fluid intake, may cause crystaluria.

Contraindications

- Severe renal impairment.
- Hypersensitivity to sulphonamides/co-trimoxazole.
- Acute intermittent porphyria.
- Pregnancy (a relative contraindication—depending upon risk benefit analysis of benefit and harms to the patient versus the unborn child).
- Breastfeeding.

Patient treated with SAS should be advised:

- They may experience side effects during this time and these should settle with continuation of treatment. Side effects include:
  - Nausea, loss of appetite, dyspepsia.
  - Dizziness, headaches.
  - Abnormal LFTs.
  - Itching, skin rashes, or mouth ulcers.
- It may take up to 3 months before they feel the benefit of treatment although they may feel a benefit earlier.
- Side effects that can occur include changes in the bloods, liver, and kidneys—which we will monitor especially for the 1st year of treatment.
- Do not alter the dose they are prescribed.
- Report promptly any infections they experience.
- General advice highlights the importance of not getting pregnant whilst on treatment and to use effective method of contraceptive; however, SAS has been shown to be relatively safe during pregnancy. The doctor will discuss this to ensure a risk benefit analysis is undertaken to support treatment with SAS during pregnancy
- Herbal or complementary therapies—advise the doctor or nurse so they can document these and review should there be any interactions.
- SAS may make urine a yellow orange colour. It may also affect contact lens staining them a yellow orange colour.

- If side effects become a problem or if they are uncertain about their treatment, seek advice as there is always something that can be done to help with side effects.

Key nursing issues in SAS

- Rarely eosinophilic pneumonitis can occur—dyspnoea, fever, weight loss, ↓ pulmonary function and changes suggesting infiltration on chest x-ray.
- If iron or antacids are prescribed avoid/withhold SAS administration until 2 hours has elapsed.
- Usually well tolerated.
- Slow acetylator (a genetic predisposition to be a slow or fast acetylator/metabolizer) of drug may result in drug-induced lupus-like syndrome.
- May impair folate absorption.
- ♂ should be aware of transient and reversible oligospermia.
- In some circumstances a risk–benefit analysis may mean that some patients remain on treatment whilst wishing to conceive. It may be appropriate in these patients to have a folic acid supplementation.
- Drug interactions include:
  - AZA may contribute to bone marrow toxicity.
  - Cardiac glycosides may reduce absorption of digoxin.
- ▶ Note blood trends or unexplained bruising (with or without sore throat)—withhold treatment and seek urgent medical advice.
- ▶ Rash—withhold treatment and seek urgent medical advice.

 Also see Blood tests and investigations, p.461.

Drug dosage

SAS is usually commenced at a dose of 500mg once a day for a week, ↑ weekly to gradually ↑ over weeks to a maximum dose of 2–3g per day.

Further reading

Arthritis Research Campaign: patient information leaflets, available at: ⌂ www.arc.org.uk

BSR (2008). *British Society of Rheumatology DMARD Guidelines*. Available at: ⌂ www.rheumatology. org.uk

For licensed indications, prescribing, and rare adverse events see Summary of Product Characteristics and *BNF*.

Tacrolimus

Tacrolimus inhibits calcineurin, a key component that enables message transduction in activated T cells and appears in cell cultures to inhibit IL-5 production (a cytokine). It is licensed for immunosuppression in organ transplant surgery but has been used for MSC.

General management

- Pre-screening required for both therapies, pregnancy, immunological status.
- Should not be co-prescribed with ciclosporin.
- St. John's Wort or herbal preparation should not be taken with tacrolimus ↓ blood concentrations of Tacrolimus.
- Grapefruit ↑ levels of tacrolimus.
- Should not breastfeed whilst on treatment.

Dose reduction may be required if raised blood pressure or deterioration in renal function:
- Monitor for signs of hypertension (treat hypertension).
- Monitor kidney function for signs of ↑ creatinine.
- Evidence suggests potential risk of diabetes.
- If contraception required, non-hormonal methods should be used.

📖 Also see Screening prior to DMARD treatment, p.422.

Cautions: galactose intolerance.

Contraindications: sensitivity of tacrolimus.

Patient treated with tacrolimus should be advised:

- They may experience side effects which are usually related to the dose. Side effects if severe will abate on cessation of treatment but include:
  - Flu-like symptoms.
  - Diarrhoea, nausea, abdominal pain, dyspepsia and headaches (occur in >5%).
  - Tremor.
  - Sickness, nausea, loss of appetite, diarrhoea (>5%), vomiting, or abdominal pain.
  - Skin rashes, bruising.
  - Mouth ulcers.
- It is important to use sun block or sunscreen and avoid exposure to strong sunlight as there is a slight ↑ in skin cancers.
- They must not take herbal or complementary therapies whilst on treatment as there are drug interactions.
- If side effects become a problem or if they are uncertain about their treatment, seek advice as there is always something that can be done to help with side effects.
- Side effects can occur which is why we monitor to make sure the bloods, liver, and kidneys are functioning normally. Blood monitoring regimens are important and will help identify problems.
- Report unexplained bleeding or bruising.
- Treatment can take up to 3 months before the benefits are achieved.

- Report promptly any infections they experience as they may require treatment.
- ♂ and ♀ patients need to be aware that conception whilst receiving treatment must be avoided (use effective method of contraceptive). Seek medical advice promptly if an unplanned pregnancy occurs.
- They should not have any live vaccines whilst on treatment.

Key factors in nursing management

Tacrolimus chiefly prescribed for transplant patients. Evidence suggests risks of side effects are lower with RA than in organ transplant possibly related to lower dosing regimens.

- Monitor blood pressure and renal function/creatinine levels.
- Tacrolimus may be prescribed during pregnancy in some cases—based on a risk–benefit analysis of treatment against no treatment.
- Drug interactions:
  - The dose of tacrolimus may need to be reduced when prescribed with: antifungalsl (e.g. ketoconazole, fluconazole) macrolide antibiotic erythromycin or rifampicin, phenytoin, or HIV protease inhibitors (e.g. ritonavir).
  - Carbamazepine, metamizole, and isoniazid may reduce the action of tacrolimus.
- ⚠ Note: a trend in blood results is as important as absolute values.
- ▶ Note blood trends or unexplained bruising (with or without sore throat)—withhold treatment and seek medical advice.

📖 Also see Blood tests and investigations, p.461.

Drug dosage

Tacrolimus should be prescribed as a morning, once-daily dose on an empty stomach or 2–3 hours after a meal. A typical dose might be 3mg/day for RA. The dose should be taken promptly once released from the blister pack. It may take several days before a stable dose is achieved.

Further reading

Arthritis Research Campaign: patient information leaflets, available at: ⁓🖰 www.arc.org.uk

BSR (2008). *British Society of Rheumatology DMARD Guidelines.* Available at: ⁓🖰 www.rheumatology. org.uk

For licensed indications, prescribing. and rare adverse events see Summary of Product Characteristics and *BNF.*

Corticosteroids: overview

The precise mechanism of corticosteroids and how they suppress inflammation is presently unknown. The body's naturally occurring corticosteroid hormones are produced and sustained by a complex feedback cycle involving the hypothalamus and adrenal glands. Corticosteroids consist of androgenic, glucocorticoids, and mineralocorticoids.

Corticosteroids such as oral prednisolone may be used in the treatment of RA, PMR, GCA, vasculitis, polymyositis, and SLE for disease suppression. Different preparations of steroids and routes of administration include local injections used in MSC such as soft tissue injuries and sports injuries, IV infusions, and IM injections of preparations such as Depo-medrone® (📖 see Corticosteroids: preparations and routes of administration, p.446).

The most commonly used treatments for MSC are:

- 💬 Oral prednisolone—the relative benefits and harms of oral prednisolone use in low doses as part of routine management is contentious. However, oral prednisolone is commonly used in the management of PMR.
- IM, IV, or IA methylprednisolone, hydrocortisone, or triamcinolone acetonide.

When treating with corticosteroids it is important to:

- Use the lowest possible dose for the shortest duration to minimize the risk of side effects, particularly osteoporosis. For this reason parenteral corticosteroids are often used instead of oral corticosteroids.
- During times of physical stress (health-related crisis e.g. infection) ↑ corticosteroid may be needed. Regular corticosteroid may suppress the appropriate response.
- If patients have been treated with oral corticosteroids (>3 weeks) adrenal suppression occurs ∴ corticosteroids must not be stopped abruptly; collapse or death from adrenal insufficiency can occur.

❶ Stopping oral corticosteroids abruptly can result in adrenal insufficiency.
❶ Corticosteroids may need to be ↑ at times of additional stress to maintain the same level of steroid effect.

Side effects

- GI—dyspepsia, peptic ulceration, nausea.
- Musculoskeletal—proximal myopathy, osteoporosis, avascular necrosis.
- Endocrine—adrenal suppression, weight gain, increased appetite.
- Ophthalmic—glaucoma, corneal or scleral thinning.
- Neuropsychiatric effects—euphoria, depression, psychosis.
- Other effects—bruising, striae, impaired healing, skin atrophy.

Contraindication

Any evidence of systemic infection.

Cautions

- Hypertension, congestive heart failure, liver failure, renal insufficiency, diabetes mellitus, or osteoporosis. In addition caution should be used if any prior history of severe affective disorders (particularly if a previous history of steroid-induced psychoses), epilepsy or seizure disorders, or peptic ulceration.

- ❶ A previous history of TB or x-ray changes characteristic of TB may be at ↑ risk of re-emergence of latent TB.
- ❶ Corticosteroids suppress inflammatory responses ↑ the susceptibility to infections. Normal signs of infections may be masked in patients taking prednisolone.
- ❶ Ensure patients are aware that chickenpox, although normally a minor illness, may be fatal in immunosuppressed patients. If in contact during the infective phase they should seek medical advice promptly.

Nursing management and patient advice

- A full assessment of the patient should be made to clarify their immune status, e.g. history of prior exposure to chickenpox or herpes zoster:
  - If no prior exposure patients should be advised to seek urgent medical attention if they come in close contact with an infected person. Passive immunisation with varicella-zoster immunoglobulin can be administered within 10 days of exposure.
  - All patients who have receive corticosteroids for >3 months and have completed a course of steroid treatment <3months should be considered at risk.
  - If chickenpox is diagnosed, prednisolone dose may need to be ↑.
  - Patients should also be advised to avoid exposure to measles if possible and if necessary to seek immediate medical assistance should exposure occur.
- If it is possible that corticosteroid treatment will extend to a period of 3 months or more (irrespective of dose), then the guidance on preventing corticosteroid-induced osteoporosis should be followed.

Further reading

Royal College of Physicians Guidance (2002). *Glucocorticosteriod induced osteoporosis. Guidelines for prevention and treatment.* Royal College of Physicians. London.

Corticosteroids: preparations and routes of administration

The adrenal cortex and the secretion of steroids in the body have 2 main functions:

- They allow or manage normal resting state or actions of hormones that allow normal function.
- Steroids produced in the body are also used at times of stress/fear or need for a rapid response such as 'fear or flight' as a result of a threat or danger.

The adrenal cortex releases several steroid hormones including:

- Androgens—secrete oestrogen and androgens—peripherally converted (sex hormones).
- Mineralocorticoids—manage the water and mineral balances of the body (e.g. aldosterone).
- Glucocorticoids—they have an effect on metabolic, anti-inflammatory responses, levels of awareness, and sleep patterns (hydrocortisone and cortisone)

The use of glucocorticoids can have an effect on normal circadian rhythm (normal wakefulness and sleep patterns).

Glucocorticoids are the key 'steroid' of interest in treating inflammation by reducing signs and symptoms of an inflammatory condition. Steroids are not curative and when stopped may result in a return or exacerbation of the symptoms/condition.

Corticosteroids vary in:

- The potency.
- The preparations and routes of administration:
  - Oral.
  - Topical/eye drops/creams.
  - IA/IM/IV.
  - Inhaled.
  - Rectal.

Cautions

Long-term treatment needs to consider the adverse effects of treatment against the risks of continued use.

Oral prednisolone

- Prednisolone is chiefly a glucocorticoid in activity and is the drug of choice for oral therapy.
- Usually starting at doses of between 10–20mg daily up to 60mg daily in severe disease (such as GCA or acute polymyositis).

IA or soft tissue routes

IA methylprednisolone (Depo-Medrone®) or triamcinolone (Kenalog®) is indicated for local inflammation of joints and soft tissues. Hydrocortisone is used for superficial soft tissue injections e.g. for lateral epicondylitis, to minimize the risk of skin atrophy.

- Usual doses—40mg for medium sized joints and 10–20mg for small joints or tendons.

IM route
- IM methylprednisolone (Depo-Medrone®) is used to treat symptoms related to exacerbations of inflammatory arthritis or to provide some symptom control whilst starting, changing, or escalating disease-modifying therapy.
- Licensed indication is for 40–80mg but doses are sometimes administered up to 120mg based on individual patient assessment.

IV infusion
- Methylprednisolone (Solu-Medrone®) can be administered as an IV infusion to treat exacerbations of inflammatory conditions.
- Dose usually up to maximum of 1g.

Side effects of steroids
Excessive and/or prolonged glucocorticoids results in Cushing's syndrome:
- Moon face.
- Buffalo hump.
- Hypertension.
- Cataracts.
- Avascular necrosis of femoral head/osteoporosis.
- Thinning of skin.
- Bruising.
- Muscle wasting.
- Poor wound healing.
- Tendency to hyperglycaemia.
- ↑ appetite/ ↑ abdominal fat/obesity.
- ↑ susceptibility to infection.
- Hirsutism.

New disease-modifying drugs: biologic therapies

In the last 10 years, new drug therapies developed to treat many immune-mediated LTCs have had a significant impact on patient outcomes and healthcare resources. These drugs are referred to as 'biologics' because they were developed using biological engineering. Research identified a number of important components to auto-immune diseases and the cell-to-cell interactions involved in the inflammatory responses and sustained attacks upon the individuals' tissues with the resulting destruction of specific tissues (auto-immune disease). There is now a greater understanding of the cell-to-cell interactions along the inflammatory pathways as well as clarity about the acquired (adaptive) and active (innate) immunity which are not so clearly delineated as previously thought, with more of an overlap between acquired and active immunity than previously believed.

The biologics 'targeted' approach mimics the body's normal communication processes and introduces treatments that can block these pathways. A specific example is the development of monoclonal antibodies that can communicate and capture or block important inflammatory messengers (cytokines) before they lock in to a receptor and activate an inflammatory response. In the case of IJDs specific cytokines have been identified that play a pivotal role in the inflammatory pathway. One of the first conditions to benefit from biologic therapies was RA. Other IJDs have increasingly benefited from this research and evidence continues to grow in a wide range of auto-immune driven conditions

Traditional DMARD therapies and biologic DMARDs

The traditional DMARDs, particularly MTX, have been effective to some degree in suppressing the disease in some IJDs. However, evidence (in RA) has demonstrated that radiological damage continues despite treatment, resulting in loss of function and ↑ disability. Traditional DMARDs can be effective for a significant proportion of patients in a disease group (e.g. RA) but for a small group it is erosive and progressive and traditional drug therapies fail to suppress the disease.

Traditional DMARD therapies vary in their efficacy, toxicity, and length of time that they are effective. During the course of person's disease they can easily have exhausted all traditional therapeutic options yet still have active destructive disease with the resulting symptoms of pain, fatigue, and systemic damage. Traditional DMARDs are significantly cheaper than the cost of newer therapies (e.g. the newest of the traditional DMARDs, leflunomide, costs ~£614 (E876) per annum (without any administration or monitoring costs).

The 1st generation of biologic disease-modifying drugs uses complex and expensive procedures that involve biologically engineering monoclonal antibodies. As a result many of these therapies cost between £8000–10,000 per annum, on average per patient (E11400–14200) (📕 see Disease-modifying anti-rheumatic drugs, p.424).

Benefits of biologic DMARDs (evidence in RA)

Patients with aggressive and erosive disease have new therapeutic options that can demonstrate:

- Evidence to suggest that biologic DMARDs can halt and in some cases retard radiographic progression.
- Reduction in the sustained effect of inflammatory mechanisms on endothelial tissues and ↓ risks of cardiovascular disease.
- Large observational studies which have to date demonstrated the overall safety of anti-TNFα.
- That patients treated early with biologic DMARD have shown significant benefits with greater disease control, minimal joint damage, and reduction in symptoms (pain and fatigue).

Risks of biologic DMARDs

- Biologics require a thorough assessment and screening process to reduce risks related to treatment.
- There are clear eligibility criteria for commencing and staying on treatment.

📖 Also see Anti-TNFα, p.452; 📖 Rituximab, p.454; 📖 Abatacept, p.457; 📖 Cetrolizumab pegol, p.457;. 📖 Infections in musculoskeletal conditions, pp.380, 384, 488.

Examples of biologic DMARD therapies

The term 'biologic' therapy is a general term used to describe techno-logy that biologically manipulates antibodies to enable them to be used as treatments. The composition of each therapy varies depending upon how the antibodies were developed, and the component parts that make up the antibody design (e.g. fixed and variable chains). The biologic therapies developed for MSC include:

- Adalimumab—a human monoclonal antibody: binds to inactive (tissue bound) and biologically active (soluble) TNFα.
- Anakinra—a recombinant form of human antibody. Interleukin 1 receptor agonist (IL-1ra): blocks receptors for IL-1 by actively competing with IL-1 receptors.
- Etanercept—a fully human p75 TNF receptor (fusion protein): binds to soluble active TNFα and lympotoxinα (TNF-β).
- Infliximab—a chimeric (mouse + human) monoclonal antibody: binds with transmembrane (tissue bound) and biologically active (soluble) TNFα
- Rituximab—a chimeric (mouse + human) monoclonal antibody binds to extra cellular domain of CD 20 B cells.
- Abatacept—fully human fusion protein using extra cellular portion of specific T cell receptor (CTLA-4) bound to human immunoglobulin (IgG) enabling the binding of CD80 and CD86 (CD = cluster differentiation) antigen presenting cells.

Further reading

Ryan S, Oliver S, Brownfield A (2007). *Drug therapy in rheumatology nursing*. John Wiley and Sons Ltd., Chichester.

Treatment with biologic therapies: key points

- This topic sets out the licensed biologic therapies for MSC.
- ▶ Further in-depth information should be sought from the SPC or drug information sheets of each therapy and the *BNF*.

Adalimumab licensed indications (subcutaneous administration)

Licensed indications for AS, PsA, RA, polyarticular JIA (aged 13–17 years), Crohn's disease.

- Prescribing dose for musculoskeletal indications of 40mg once a fortnight.
- Can be administered as a monotherapy when intolerant to MTX.

Key treatment considerations include:

- Mild-to-moderate injection site reactions—common>10%.
- Risk of emergence of latent infection—including TB.
- Risk of exacerbations of demyelinating diseases—review history.
- Contraindicated in those with moderate-to-severe heart failure.
- Contraindicated in those with active infections including TB.
- Combination therapy with MTX—unless intolerant of MTX.
- Blood monitoring required if on MTX monthly.
- Avoid live vaccines.

 Also see Adalimumab, pp.452, 502.

Anakinra licensed indications (subcutaneous administration)

Licensed indication for RA following failure of MTX:

- Prescribing dose of 100mg once daily.
- Must be prescribed in combination with MTX—a once a week dose.
- Should not be co-prescribed with an anti-TNFα therapy.

Key treatment considerations include:

- Neutropenia.
- Similar issues to anti-TNFα therapies although should not be prescribed for those with impaired renal function.
- Note: not recommended by NICE.

Etanercept licensed indications (subcutaneous administration)

Licensed indications for RA, polyarticular JIA, PsA, AS, plaque psoriasis:

- Prescribing dose 25mg twice weekly or 50mg weekly.
- Combination therapy with MTX for RA—unless intolerant of MTX.

Key treatment considerations include:

- As for adalimumab but no blood monitoring recommended in SPC. If on MTX blood monitoring will be required.

 Also see Etanercept, pp.452, 502.

Infliximab (intravenous infusion)

Licensed indications for RA, AS, PsA, psoriasis, adult and paediatric Crohn's disease, ulcerative colitis:
- Prescribing dose varies according to indication from 3mg/kg–5mg/kg of body weight.
- Musculoskeletal dosing regimen: 0, 2, 6 weeks then 6–8-weekly thereafter (depending upon indication).
- For RA and PsA must be co-prescribed with MTX.

Key treatment considerations include:
- Infusion related reactions—within minutes or hours following infusion (approximately 22% in research evidence versus 9% in placebo). <1% develops severe infusion reactions—rarely necessary to discontinue treatment.
- Blood monitoring for MTX.
- As for adalimumab and etanercept.
- Access to specialist infusion clinics—with resuscitation facilities.

📖 Also see Infliximab, p.518.

Rituximab (intravenous infusion)

Licensed indications for non-Hodgkin's lymphoma (NHL), RA.
- Prescribing dose for RA is 1000mg infusion (day 1 and day 15) with MTX (once a week dose).
- Pre-treatment of paracetamol 1000mg, methylprednisolone 100mg, and chlorphenamine 10 mg IV.

Key treatment considerations include:
- Allow timings to administer pre-treatment infusions (60min before rituximab).
- Withhold anti-hypertensive therapies for 12 hours prior to infusion.
- Infusion related reactions—rituximab 36% vs. 30% placebo. Mainly mild-to-moderate. Infusion reactions in RA are significantly lower in rate and severity to those seen in NHL.
- Access to specialist infusion clinics–with resuscitation facilities.

📖 Also see Rituximab, p.524.

Abatacept (intravenous infusion)

Licensed for RA co-prescribed with MTX:
- Prescribing dose dependent on weight: <60kg, 500mg; >60kg and <100kg, 750mg; or >100kg, 1000mg). Treatment 0, 2, then 4-weekly.

Key treatment considerations include:
- Infusion reactions <1%. Other nursing care issues—at present consider as for other biologic therapies until further clinical experience develops.
- Similar issues to other infusions. Early evidence suggests similar nursing care issues to other biologics until clinical evidence available.

📖 Also see Abatcept, p.508.

Anti-tumour necrosis factor alpha: overview

TNFα is an important pro-inflammatory cytokine (chemical messenger) implicated in MSC such as RA and other IJDs. TNFα is considered to be the pivotal cytokine that starts the process of an inflammatory cascade within the immune system. TNFα is released from an activated T cell to start the process of an inflammatory response. By blocking this cytokine and preventing it 'locking into' key receptors the inflammatory pathway cannot be activated effectively.

3 therapeutic options have been developed to block the mechanism of action of TNFα. These are:

- Adalimumab (Humira®) a subcutaneously administered therapy.
- Etanercept (Enbrel®) a subcutaneously administered therapy.
- Infliximab (Remicade®) delivered as an infusion every 8 weeks (once stabilized on treatment).

📖 Also see Infliximab (IV infusion), p.518;. 📖 Adalimumab licensed indications (subcutaneous administration), pp.448, 450, 502 📖 Etanercept licensed indications (subcutaneous administration), pp.452, 502.

What is anti-TNFa? All 3 current anti-TNFa therapies are developed from biotechnology using monoclonal antibodies.

Issues in treatment with anti-TNFα therapy

A national register in the UK collects evidence to examine safety and efficacy of biologic therapies (biologic register).[1] Screening and treatment eligibility criteria for anti-TNFα therapies have been developed for AS, PsA, and RA.

📖 Also see Assessing the patient, p.271; 📖 Clinical examination and history taking, pp.274, 276.

Treatment is contraindicated if there is evidence of:

- Active infections. Screening for infections (bacterial, viral, or fungal) including prior contact with/or immunization against TB must be reviewed and discussed with prescribing physician.
- Moderate-to-severe heart failure. NYHC Criteria III/IV.
- Pregnant or breastfeeding.
- Sepsis of native joint (within last 12 months).[2]
- Sepsis of prosthetic joint (within last 12 months) or indefinitely if joint remains in situ.[2]

Caution for patients who have:

- Caution for mild heart failure (NYHC I/II).
- Demyelinating disorders—caution in those with pre-existing or recent onset CNS demyelinating disorders.
- Caution for those prone to infections, e.g. chronic leg ulcers, persistent chest infections, in-dwelling catheters.
- Patient infected with hepatitis B—evidence contradictory at present. Adhere to SPC until further evidence emerges.
- Hepatitis C—appears to show no deterioration in hepatitis or viral load following treatment.
- HIV infections—cannot be advised at present; minimal evidence available.

- Caution in patients with COPD or ↑ risk of malignancies due to heavy smoking.
- ☞ Cautions in patients who have a prior history of malignancy (<10 years). International observational data will inform the debate about malignancy. Discuss with prescribing physician.

Screening patients[1]

- Fulfills eligibility criteria, patient consent to treatment, and data collection for the BSR Biologics Register.
- No contraindications as outlined earlier. Any areas of cautions review and discuss with prescribing physician and patient.
- Screen for TB and risks related to prior TB contact or travel to areas of high risk, TB history, and prior immunization.[3]
  - Undertake screening as indicated and according to identified risks. Patients may require treatment if at high risk or suboptimal treatment in the past.
  - Chest x-ray if not undertaken in last 6 months or repeat if index of suspicion for infections or lung disease.
- Blood pressure, weight, and normal blood monitoring profile prior to commencement of therapy.
- Co-prescribed MTX:
  - Evidence suggests optimal response when co-prescribed.
  - Reduces risks of antibodies against the monoclonal antibody therapy.
- Note history of atophy or previous allergic reactions—discuss with prescribing physician if patient has a history or severe allergic reactions.
- Ensure patient is using effective method of contraceptive. ♀ of child-bearing age—check not pregnant.
- Immunization status—if appropriate update immunizations before starting treatment.
- Full patient assessment re consent and follow-up management including awareness of responsibilities to monitor and report any infections.

RA eligibility criteria for anti-TNFα therapy

- Fulfils diagnostic criteria for diagnosis of RA (ACR 1987 criteria).
- Active RA with 2 DAS28 joint count scores >5.1. Taken at 2 time points, 1 month apart. (Refer to latest guidance: www.nice.org.uk.)
- Failed standard DMARD therapies 1 of which must be MTX:
  - Treatment for at least 6 months with at least 2 months on standard target dose *or* treatment <6 months—withdrawn due to intolerance or toxicity – after at least 2 months at therapeutic dose.

Further reading

NICE (2007). *Adalimumab, etanercept and infliximab for the treatment of RA*. NICE, London.

References

1. The British Society for Rheumatology Biologics Register: ☞ www.rheumatology.org.uk

2. BRS guidelines: ☞ www.rheumatology.org.uk

3. British Thoracic Society Guidelines (2005): ☞ www.thoraxjnl.com

B-cell (CD-20) depletion therapies

B lymphocytes are a vital component of our immune system. T and B lymphocytes act in different ways to enable an appropriate immune response. B cells have a synergistic effect with T cells and are identified as playing a role in:
• T-cell activation and expansion.
• Production of antibodies such as RF.
• Production of pro-inflammatory cytokines (TNFa) IL-6 and lymphotoxin.

B cells develop in sequential steps, developing from stem cells through to plasma cells that produce antibodies (Immunoglobulins). B cells proliferate and when fully developed have the capacity to react to antigens and produce plasma membrane-bound antibodies. B cells that produce antibodies are in effect the memory of the immune system, recognizing and creating a specific antibody response to antigen attacks.

Cell surface markers are expressed on precursor B cells. One of these markers, CD-20, is the focus of B-cell depletion therapy. Rituximab depletes B cell with the CD-20 marker, disabling those cells and reducing the B cells that produce antibodies. This approach does not compromise the patient's immune system as stem cells and plasma cells are unaffected. Rituximab has shown sustained benefits for RA patients with a reduction in radiological evidence, signs and symptoms, and a good safety profile. There is currently only 1 licensed B-cell depletion therapy available, rituximab.

What is rituximab?

Rituximab is an anti-CD-20 B-cell depletion therapy developed as a monoclonal antibody. Biologically engineered from part chimeric and part human antibody. It is recommended as a combination therapy with a once-weekly dose of MTX and administered as an IV infusion (📖 see Rituximab, p.524).

Rituximab in the treatment of MSC

Ritixumab has a long history in the treatment of NHL. Early evidence has demonstrated that the level of infusion-related reactions is significantly lower in the inflammatory arthritides group of patients compared to NHL:
• RA: 30–35% 1st infusion reactions—severe infusion reactions are uncommon and rarely lead to withdrawal.
• NHL infusion-related reactions: >75% 1st infusion reactions:
  • Hypotension and bronchospasm seen in ~10% of patients.
  • Cytokine release syndrome and tumour lysis syndrome are seen in patients with a tumour load.

Treatment

Rituximab is licensed for the treatment of RA. Other MSC that are the focus of early research for efficacy and safety include:
• SLE.
• ANCA-positive vasculitis.
• Sjögren syndrome.

Eligibility criteria

Patients who have been treated with an anti-TNFα will have undertaken a rigorous screening process. If patients are being considered for rituximab without prior screening/TNFα, a review of eligibility and screening criteria using the SPC and local guidelines should be adhered to.

- Severe active RA—adults only.
- Inadequate response or intolerance of other DMARDs including 1 anti-TNFα therapy.

📖 Also see Anti-TNFα therapy, p.452.

Treatment continuation criteria

- If an adequate response is achieved following initiation of treatment (day 1 and day 15 infusion). Adequate response is defined as improvement in DAS28 of 1.2 points or more.
- Re-treatment should not be undertaken more than every 6 months.

Rituximab treatment issues that need to be considered

- Optimal treatment benefits are seen in patients who have sero-positive RA.
- Currently no DAS28 criteria for commencing treatment.
- Anti -TNFα failure patients do not require additional TB screening prior to starting rituximab.
- Clinical history and screening to exclude chronic or recurrent infections/allergies. History of atophy should be noted prior to infusion.
- Review comorbidity risk factors, e.g. cardiovascular and pulmonary disease.
- Hepatitis B and C screening—evidence to date is contradictory.
- Baseline immunoglobulin levels and CD-19 levels.
- Immunization (inactivated)—administer 1 month prior to treatment or 7 months post-infusion. Live vaccines should not be administered.
- Check concordance and prescription for MTX.

Questions and evolving issues

- Place of rituximab in those unable to receive anti-TNFα therapies.
- Benefit of rituximab in other auto-immune diseases other than RA.
- Evidence of repeated treatments in relation to long-term immune status.
- Repeat treatments (after 6 months from first infusion)—optimal time frame.
- Risks and benefits of repeat long-term courses of B-cell depletion therapy.
- Recent drug safety information has highlighted the development of PML in patients who have SLE (unlicensed indication).
- Defining treatment failures and repeat treatment time frames.

Further reading

NICE (2007). *National Institute of Health and Clinical Excellence single technology appraisal. Rituximab for the treatment of Rheumatoid Arthritis (No. 126).* NICE, London.

New biologic disease-modifying therapies

There is an intense interest in new therapies for MSC following the experiences with anti-TNFα, rituximab, and, more recently, abatacept. These therapies have transformed the lives of patients and, importantly, have provided researchers with a greater insight into the disease themselves and how they can advance treatments based upon the knowledge gained.

The challenge will be to develop therapies that can reduce the not insignificant costs related to producing monoclonal antibodies that up until now have had to be administered either by subcutaneous or IV routes, adding to the cost of the treatment. In the coming years there will be some new biologic therapies that have the potential to be introduced into the UK.

Examples of unlicensed therapies in development for:

- AS: golimumab (anti-TNFα inhibitor).
- PsA: golimumab (anti-TNFα inhibitor).
- RA:
  - Tocilizumab (IL-6 inhibitor).
  - Ocrelizumab (anti-CD20 antibody).
  - Denosumab (RANKL inhibitor).
  - golimumab (anti-TNFα inhibitor).
- SLE: belimumab (B lymphocyte stimulator (BLyS)).

New biologic disease-modifying therapies: abatacept and certolizumab pegol

Overview

Abatacept is a recently licensed therapy for the treatment of RA. Abatacept is a monoclonal antibody that has been designed to block anti-specific T-cell receptor activation. The blocking of the T-cell receptor at this early stage in the immune pathway appears to prevent downstream activation of an inflammatory cascade by pro-inflammatory cytokines (such as TNFα). This is technically referred to as blocking of co-stimulatory signals by CD80/86:CD28 .

Clinical trial data shows promising results although evidence is limited at the time of going to press on the benefits and risks related to the usual clinical caseload of patients who represent the 'real' population of RA.

Also see biologic disease-modifying anti-rheumatic drugs, p.456; Abatacept (IV infusion), p.457.

Issues related to abatacept

The general principles outlined in relation to biologic DMARDs should be considered in the context of treating patients with abatacept. However, additional areas for consideration are outlined:

- Should not be co-prescribed with TNF blocking agents—monitor carefully for patients who have failed anti-TNFα inhibitors and start Abatacept (mean half-life 13.1 days) .
- ↑ adverse events in patients with COPD, including respiratory problems.
- Potential role of abatacept in the development of malignancies unknown at present.
- Caution in treating elderly due to higher infection and malignancy rates.
- May interfere with blood glucose stick monitoring levels resulting in falsely elevated blood glucose readings on day of infusion.

Certolizumab pegol

Cetrolizumab pegol is currently **unlicensed** although subject to review for benefit and cost effectiveness in the treatment of RA. Certolizumab is a humanized monoclonal antibody that binds to both soluble and membrane-bound TNFα receptors but has been developed using Fab' fragment technology. This technology uses a small fragment of an antibody containing the antigen binding site. To date there is very little information available:

- Likely to be used in the treatment of Crohn's disease and RA.
- Administered by subcutaneous injection.
- Early studies appear to show adverse events related to mild URTIs.

Follow-up care for those on biologic disease-modifying anti-rheumatic drugs

Generally speaking, patients who start biologic DMARDs gain a therapeutic benefit significantly greater than traditional therapies. These benefits appear to lift the sense of fatigue and reduce the pain—enabling patients to participate in normal ADL. Biologics also reduce radiological progression (again, generally greater than those seen with traditional DMARDs). An observational research project designed to explore safety of anti-TNFα therapies (The British Society for Rheumatology Biologics Register)[1] and other such registries across the world regularly publish preliminary data: Evidence on RA patients treated with anti-TNFα therapies to date demonstrate:

- Cardiovascular risk—appears to be reduced in those who respond to treatment.
- Pregnancy—early evidence appears to show that these therapies are not linked to infant mortality, deformity, or premature birth. However, drug information and licensing contraindicate treatment during pregnancy.
- Infections—↑ risk of skin and soft tissue infections. Some of the infections are food borne (e.g. *Listeria*, *Salmonella*).
- Infections—re-emergence of latent TB seen. Higher proportion of extra pulmonary presentations of TB. Lower rates seen in etanercept compared to adalimumab and infliximab.
- Malignancy—incidence of malignancy remain difficult to interpret because patients with aggressive RA treated with traditional DMARDs have an ↑ malignancy rate; early data suggests there are no early signs to indicate an ↑ in malignancy in anti-TNFα treated patients.
- Mortality data—it is known that patients with RA have a reduced life expectancy. Early follow-up of RA patients treated with anti-TNFα therapies still show this reduced life expectancy (compared to the general population). ♂ standard mortality rates of 1.99 and females ♀ of 1.72. However, this reflects the reduced life expectancy seen in the pre-biologics era.
- Interstitial lung disease (ILD)—patients who have baseline ILD appear to show strong predictive trends that show ↑ all-cause mortality regardless of treatment with anti-TNFα. However, those with ILD treated with anti-TNFα have higher mortality rates. Standard mortality rate for ♂ of 3.2 and ♀ 2.0.

There are important issues to be considered from the patient's and HCP's point of view in follow-up care. However, patients can feel so well occasionally they can forget the important safety issues whilst on treatment.

Patient responsibilities include:

- Having ready access to a telephone advice line or details of a 1st point of contact person in the event of a problem with treatment.
- Ensuring that they get prompt treatment of any infections.
- Attending for review appointments and blood monitoring requirements.

- Carrying a biologic 'alert card' to advise HCPs (including dentists, chiropodists etc.) that they are receiving a treatment that significantly impairs their immunological response.
- Remembering to avoid live vaccines (and for rituximab—any vaccines whilst on treatment) and plan their immunization strategies carefully with healthcare teams.
- Avoidance of conception whilst on treatment.
- Avoidance of consumption of pates, unpasteurized milk, cheese, or raw foods (such as eggs) as an ↑ risk of opportunistic infections.
- Consideration of sunscreens and sun protection (↑risk of skin melanomas particularly for PsA patients who have already been exposed to PUVA therapy).
- If co-prescribed with MTX they should stay on treatment or discuss with their doctor or nurse before stopping their co-prescription.
- They may need to stop treatment a few weeks before surgery.
- That they remain on treatment providing they continue to fulfill the treatment criteria (benefit of treatment has to be demonstrated usually using the DAS 28).

The HCP responsibilities include:

- Enabling patients to understand their treatment options throughout the course of their disease.
- Provision of an alert card and a 1st point of contact number for those on biologics.
- Provision of expert support and advice for other non specialists practitioners in relation to patients receiving biologic DMARDs.
- Ensuring that the patient fulfills the eligibility criteria (or clinical need/ exception are documented in the notes).
- Documentation of assessments, eligibility, and treatment continuation criteria.
- Undertaking of regular reviews and reassessment of treatment benefit as outlined by NICE and national guidelines.
- Reviewing blood monitoring and assess patients' general health prior to receiving treatment. If care is delivered by supporting organizations/ 1° care teams, build effective communication strategies to support review of patients' general health status and safety issues.
- Reiteratation of safety messages and review patient knowledge on additional information needs in relation to:
  - A patient's general knowledge about their disease.
  - Specific information needs about biologics.
- If treatment fails ensure patients are provided with up-to-date evidence-based information and advice on further treatment options or the next steps in their care.

Reference

1. The British Society for Rheumatology Biologics Register: ⌂ www.medicine.manchester.ac.uk

Frequently asked questions

It seems like there are many more risks related to biologic DMARDs than a traditional DMARD is that right?

Traditional DMARDs generally have stood the test of time and we know their strengths and weaknesses. They are not without risks but generally are less efficacious in the sense of reducing radiological progression and improving symptoms related to the disease compared to the newer biologics. Those who receive prompt treatment, particularly before joint damage has occurred, gain significant benefit.

Biologics are fairly new to clinical practice they are currently categorized as black triangle therapies—that is, intensively monitored in order to confirm the risk/benefit profile of the products and require detailed reporting of any adverse events. However, it is important to know that the cell-to-cell interactions in blocking the inflammatory response are much more specifically targeted and ∴ the risks related to immunosuppression are probably greater. A high index of suspicion with patients presenting with infections/problems should be maintained. Seek medical advice if in doubt.

Will there be more of these more targeted biologics in the future?

Yes. There is increasing recognition in many auto-immune (LTCs) that these biologic and more specifically targeted therapies are here to stay. Research in the development of these therapies and what we have learnt in using the treatments have helped us understand much more about the different disease mechanism and the complex immune responses. We now understand that cytokines work like hormones and communicate with many other chemical 'messengers' that communicate with each other, sustaining inflammation.

Why is MTX co-prescribed with so many of the biologics?

Evidence in clinical trials and confirmed in clinical practice demonstrate that MTX enhances the effect of the biologics. This is because the biologics are monoclonal antibodies and the body can develop auto-immune responses to the monoclonal antibody itself. These responses to the biologic monoclonal antibody can be significantly reduced when co-prescribed with MTX. If anti-chimeric antibodies develop they reduce the therapeutic benefit of the treatment.

Chapter 17

Blood tests and investigations

Investigation of the blood

Baseline investigations usually consist of a FBC, biochemical investigations, measurement of inflammatory markers, and an immunological screen. When a MSC is suspected, analysis of the blood can help to support the diagnosis. In many cases positive results may aid (but not confirm) diagnosis. In the same light, negative results may not rule out a diagnosis. For example, the presence or absence of RF in the blood does not confirm or exclude diagnosis of RA; it simply can act as 1 of many important prognostic indicators for disease severity. ~15% of the population is RF-positive yet do not have an IJD and only 70–80% of the RA population are RF-positive (	 see Rheumatoid arthritis, p.56).

It is important to assess the FBC, renal, and liver function before commencing medication to consider issues of pharmacokinetics—how the body deals with drugs, and pharmacodynamics—the likely effects a drug has on the body, as this will influence drug choice or dose prescribed.

When a diagnosis has been established and treatment has begun, blood tests are performed to monitor disease activity, assess efficacy of treatment, and to screen for unwanted, potentially life-threatening adverse drug reactions (	 see Chapter 16, Pharmacological management: disease-modifying drugs, p.424).

This section describes the most commonly requested investigations for MSC, but it is not a comprehensive account of all the tests used in clinical practice.

Why do blood tests?

- To establish a comprehensive clinical picture or fulfil diagnostic criteria. For example, if someone is sero positive for HLA B27—present in 95% of Caucasian patients with a diagnosis of AS—this only has value if the rest of the history and clinical picture fit with the diagnosis. It should not be considered diagnostic but adds to the clinical picture.
- To aid in proactive management of early disease, e.g. to identify patients with non-specific joint problems, and before obvious clinical signs of an inflammatory disease can be confirmed, e.g. the use of a new test, anti-cyclic citrullinated peptide antibodies (anti-CCP), suggests that 50–60% of patients can be detected with early RA before specific symptoms of inflammatory disease are seen.
- To identify prognostic indicators, e.g. high positive RF titres supported by evidence of joint erosions on x-ray or US are linked to poorer long-term outcomes for patients with RA.
- Adherence to treatment criteria, e.g. hypercholesterolaemia and treatment with statins.
- To address pharmacokinetics/pharmacodynamics issues that may affect drug dose or choice of drug, e.g. mild impairment of the renal function may alter the choice of drug if excreted via the kidneys or warrant a change of therapeutic approach or more rigorous monitoring regimens (e.g. NSAIDs).
- As an early indicator of toxicity or side effects related to blood or organ functions.
- Enables an ongoing review of disease control and efficacy of treatment.

Haematological investigations

Full blood count (FBC)

The most common laboratory test is the FBC (Table 17.1) to examine different components of the blood, including red cells (erythrocytes), white cells (leucocytes), and platelets (thrombocytes).

Haemoglobin (Hb)

Measurement of Hb estimates the oxygen-bearing capacity of the red blood cells (RBCs). Anaemia (a low Hb level) is an important measure to consider in reviewing blood results.

Anaemia

- Is a common feature in inflammatory conditions such as RA.
- Is sometimes attributed to disease activity—anaemia of chronic disease.
- Anaemia can result as an unwanted effect of medication or a combination of the disease and treatments, e.g. anaemia may be caused by GI bleeding from NSAIDs taken for pain relief.

Mean corpuscular volume (MCV)

This is a measure of the average size of RBCs. In patients with anaemia the MCV classifies either microcytic anaemia, where MCV falls below the normal range, or macrocytic anaemia, where the MCV is above the normal range. The MCV may aid the clinician diagnostically, e.g.:

- A raised MCV may be related to vitamin B12 deficiency.
- A low MCV can be associated with thalassemia or iron deficiency.

White blood cell (WBC) count

Leucocytes or WBCs develop in the bone marrow and lymph nodes. They are part of the body's defense mechanism against infectious disease and foreign materials. The number of white cells in the blood is often an indicator of the status of the immune responses. WBCs may also be affected by diseases or infections. Corticosteroids also raise the WBC. The WBC count measures the total number of WBCs and estimates the numbers of each type of white cell, known as the differential count; these are:

- Neutrophils—defend against bacterial or fungal infection and inflammatory processes.
- Eosinophils—combat parasitic infections and control mechanisms associated with allergy.
- Basophiles—are responsible for allergic response by releasing histamine.
- Monocytes—have a similar function to neutrophils but they have a longer life cycle. They also present pathogens to T cells allowing the antibody response to begin.
- Lymphocytes—include:
  - B cells produce antibodies and react with pathogens to enable their destruction.
  - T cells, which help to coordinate the immune response.
  - Natural killer (NK) cells which refer to a specific function rather than a specific cell type. NK cells can respond to and kill cells displaying signals of being infected by a virus or which have become cancerous.

Raised WBC counts (leucocytosis) can be present during infection and are sometimes seen in active inflammatory conditions such as RA and gout.

A low WBC count (leucopenia) can occur in certain conditions such as SLE and Felty syndrome or as a result of drug therapy.

📖 Also see Connective tissue diseases, p.113.

Platelet count

Platelets are nuclear disc-shaped bodies circulating in the blood and are involved in the blood clotting process.

- Thrombocytosis (an ↑ platelet level). Although common in active RA, it is not associated with ↑ incidence of thrombotic events.
- Thrombocytopenia (a ↓ platelet count) is a feature of conditions such as Felty syndrome and SLE. Thrombocytopenia can also occur as the result of drug therapy.

📖 Also see Chapter 16, Pharmacological management: disease-modifying anti-rheumatic drugs, pp.419–460.

Table 17.1 Normal FBC values

	♂	♀	Unit
Hb	13.5–18.0	11.5–16.4	g/dL
Red cell count (RCC)	4.5–6.5	3.9–5.6	$\times 10^{12}/L$
Haematocrit (HCT)	0.40–0.54	0.36–0.47	ratio
MCV	78–96	78–96	fL
Platelet count	150–400	150–400	$\times 10^9/L$
WBC	4.0–11.0	4.0–11.0	$\times 10^9/L$
Differential:			
Neutrophils	2.0–7.5	2.0–7.5	$\times 10^9/L$
Lymphocytes	1.5–4.0	1.5–3.0	$\times 10^9/L$
Monocytes	0.2–0.8	0.2–0.8	$\times 10^9/L$
Eosinophils	0.04–0.4	0.04–0.4	$\times 10^9/L$
Basophils	<0.1–0.3	0–0.3	$\times 10^9/L$

Biochemical investigations

Lives function tests (LFTs)

LFTs are designed to indicate the state of hepatic function. Some laboratories may perform different groups of liver enzymes to others and ranges of values may vary. Refer to local laboratories to confirm normal ranges. Elevations of LFTs may be expressed as multiples of the upper limit of normal. (e.g. 3 × upper limit of normal).

Baseline LFT's are essential to identify any prior hepatic disease which could potentially reduce drug metabolism and ↑ the risk of drug toxicity.

- Alanine transaminase (ALT), also called serum glutamic pyruvic transaminase (SGPT), is an enzyme present in liver cells. Most sensitive indicator of liver injury (rather than biliary obstruction). When a liver cell is damaged it leaks this enzyme into the blood. (See Box 18.1.)
- Aspartate transaminase (AST), also called serum glutamic oxaloacetic transaminase (SGOT), is another enzyme that can be ↑ with liver damage. AST ↑ with MI.
- Alkaline phosphatase (ALP) is an enzyme found in the biliary ducts and can be ↑ with biliary obstructions but also ↑ with a number of inflammatory conditions. ALP is also present in bone and high levels are present in Paget's disease, fractures and others diseases affecting the bones such as metastases. (See Box 17.1.)
- Total bilirubin (TBIL). ↑ levels of bilirubin can be present in various anaemias and reflect deficiencies in bilirubin metabolism such as cirrhosis or obstruction of the bile ducts.
- Gamma glutamyl transpeptidase (GGT) may be elevated even in minor levels of hepatic dysfunction or as a result of a number of non-specific causes (mild levels of raised GGT can also be seen in inflammatory conditions such as SLE or RA). High levels of GGT can be associated with alcohol toxicity or liver disease.

⚠ Grossly haemolyzed bloods will produce spurious liver function results. ALP levels ↑ slowly with storage; preferably analyze on day of collection.

Renal function

Plasma concentrations of creatinine, urea, and the electrolytes (potassium, sodium, chloride, and bicarbonate) are useful indicators of kidney function. Creatinine is a sensitive estimator of function; raised creatinine can indicate renal damage although a GFR expressed as mL/min gives a more precise indication of the state of the kidneys.

Renal disease potentially reduces the excretion of drugs. Kidney function deteriorates with age and caution should be applied when prescribing drug therapies or monitoring treatments for the older person where ↓ renal excretion can ↑ the potential for toxicities. Some therapies have an ↑ risk of nephrotoxicity and require extra vigilance in management and when monitoring.

Box 17.1 Causes of high/low levels of some liver enzymes

Causes of high ALT

- Cirrhosis.
- Alcohol abuse.
- Congestive cardiac failure (hepatic congestion).
- Liver damage (drug induced) or hepatitis B or C.
- Medication.

Causes of low ALT

- Low ALT levels are rarely seen and usually insignificant.
- ❶ Note: strenuous exercise may cause elevation.

Causes of high ALP

- Bone disease—tumours, fractures, osteomyelitis, Paget's disease.
- Liver disease—liver tumours, biliary obstruction, cirrhosis.

Causes of low ALP

- Low ALP levels are rarely seen and usually insignificant.
- Note ALP specificity.

Inflammatory markers

The measurement of inflammatory markers in the blood; ESR, CRP, and PV can be very useful in assessing the activity of inflammatory diseases. ESR/CRP is an essential component of a disease activity score used in RA. All of these acute phase proteins ↑ in serum a few hours after initiation of an inflammatory process/injury. They are a class of proteins that derive from the liver as a response to injury/inflammation. The plasma concentrations respond to tissue injury e.g. infection, trauma, malignancy, or inflammation.

📖 Also see Inflammatory joint disease: assessing the disease, p.53.

CRP

CRP is an acute phase plasma protein produced by the liver. CRP levels can rise to very high levels (>120mg/L) after injury or during an inflammatory process. This is due to a rise in the plasma concentrations of IL-6, which is produced in macrophages, endothelial, and T cells. CRP is used as a marker of inflammation, and is useful in monitoring disease activity, but it must be remembered that CRP can be elevated in many conditions—including viral and bacterial infections. Fluctuations in CRP levels occur more quickly than in other markers of inflammation.

● Normal value 0–10mg/L.

ESR

ESR is a non-specific measure of inflammation; levels are slightly higher in:
● The elderly.
● Anaemia.
● Black populations.

The test uses anticoagulated blood placed in an upright test tube. The rate at which the red blood cells fall is measured in mm/hour. If an inflammatory process is present the ↑ fibrinogen levels cause the red cells to clump together (rouleaux formation) and settle faster.

ESR can be elevated in inflammatory arthropathies such as RA, temporal arteritis, and PMR. ESR can also be elevated in bacterial infection and malignancies.

A general rule of thumb for the upper limit of normal value of ESR is
● ♂ = age divided by 2.
● ♀ = age plus 10 divided by 2.

PV

PV is another sensitive but non-specific marker of inflammation, which provides similar information to ESR. There is no specific difference in values between ♂ and ♀. PV results are not affected by anaemia (unlike ESR). PV:
● ↑ in parallel to ESR, but is not affected by anaemia or by delay in analysis.
● Is not affected by gender but is affected by age, exercise, and pregnancy.

Some rheumatologists prefer to use PV as its sensitivity and specificity is better than ESR and CRP in discriminating between active and quiescent disease.
● Normal values 1.50–1.72mPa.

Autoimmune profiles

Antibodies are proteins produced by WBCs to defend the body against toxins such as viruses and bacteria. Autoantibodies, instead of attacking the toxins, attack the body's own cells. Autoimmune diseases, such as RA, Sjögren syndrome, systemic sclerosis, and SLE are associated with circulating auto antibodies. However, these auto antibodies can also be found in healthy individuals. Autoantibodies are sometimes detected many years before the onset of signs and symptoms of disease.

Autoimmune screening includes:

RF

This is typically an IgM/IgG immunoglobulin complex found in about 70% of patients with RA at disease onset, and a further 10–15% becomes RhF positive within the first 2 years. Such patients are said to be sero-positive. However the absence of RF in the serum does not exclude a diagnosis of RA, and those patients without RF are referred to as sero-negative.

RF is present in about 5–15% of the general healthy population, and can be found in other conditions including SLE, Sjögren syndrome, chronic liver disease, and acute viral infection, for example.

RA patients who are sero-positive are likely to have more aggressive disease, with an ↑ risk of developing extra- articular manifestations.

ANA/ANF

ANA (also known as anti-nuclear factor (ANF)), are antibodies that can attack the nucleus of cells. These antibodies are present in higher numbers than normal in autoimmune diseases, particularly in SLE.

The ANA test is requested when SLE or other autoimmune diseases such as Sjögren syndrome are suspected. A positive ANA is expressed as the titre of ANA that exceeds the level found in 95% of the normal population.

- 95% of patients with lupus have a positive ANA test.
- 20–40% of RA patients have positive ANA test.

⚠ Positive ANA in isolation does not confirm a diagnosis—see ENA.

ENA antibodies

ENA is usally requested following a positive ANA test or where clinical features strongly suggest a condition (such as Sjögren syndrome). The blood sample will then be tested for reactivity using a combined ENA test. If the results are positive further testing will identify specific antibodies to individuals ENAs—which are outlined here together with the conditions they are associated with.

- Ro—Sjögren syndrome, SLE, neonatal lupus, and RA.
- La—Sjögren syndrome, SLE, RA.
- RNP—mixed connective tissue disease, SLE.
- Scl-70—scleroderma.
- Jo-1—myositis.

ENA tests (positive or negative) do not indicate disease activity although different antibody profiles are associated with specific conditions. Repeated testing of ENA is not indicated unless there is a change in symptoms. The absence of an antibody does not exclude a clinical diagnosis, as ENAs are present only in a variable proportion of patients with the above disorders.

▶Individuals with SLE or Sjögren syndrome they should be screened for ENA antibodies before considering pregnancy.

Immunoglobulins

Immunoglobulins form a major defence system of the body against foreign organisms and are divided into 5 subclasses (IgG, IgA, IgM, IgD, and IgE). Each immunoglobulin category has distinct group of proteins but also have specific features. The value of such test are chiefly to aid identification of an auto-immune disease.

Complement

The complement system is involved in the mediation of inflammation. Measurement of the complement components C3 and C4 aids in the diagnosis of immunological disorders, such as SLE, e.g. active SLE is usually associated with low complement levels. High complement levels occur as part of the acute phase response to inflammation.

▶Rare hereditary deficiencies can be a cause for low complement levels.

Anti-CCP anitbodies

The autoantibody anti-CCP should be tested in patients suspected of having RA. Anti CCP may be detected in 50–60% of those presenting with early signs of RA patients (within 3–6 months of onset of symptoms). It appears that anti-CCP may predate arthritis symptoms by several years. Studies have shown that anti-CCP positive patients with early RA may develop more erosive disease than those without anti-CCP.

The predictive value in early disease is of particular importance- ~85% of those positive for anti-CCP and RF will develop RA. Optimal outcomes are achieved if these patients receive prompt DMARD therapy before irreversible joint damage occurs. An important test to be used in Early Arthritis Clinics.

Other tests

Serum uric acid

Serum uric acid levels are age- and gender-dependent. Concentrations of uric acid ↑ with the onset of puberty in ♂ and menopause in ♀.

Uric acid is the end-product of protein metabolism and the breakdown of purines. An overproduction of uric acid is known as hyperuricaemia and this may result in gout. Hyperuricaemia is defined as serum uric acid concentration >7.0 mg/dL in ♂ and >6.0mg/dL in ♀.

However:
- Not all people with hyperuricemia have gout.
- Not all people with gout have hyperuricaemia.
- ▶This test may not be routinely available in all units.

📖 Also see Gout, pp.102, 104.

Thiopurines-methyltransferase (TPMT)

TPMT is an important enzyme required to metabolize immunosuppressive drugs such as AZA from the body. About 1 in 300 people lack TPMT and would be at high risk of bone marrow suppression if treated with AZA. TPMT is therefore measured prior to commencing treatment with AZA and avoided in TPMT-deficient patients.

There are 2 types of TPMT deficiency that need to be considered for patients *who must be* screened prior to treatment with AZA.
- Homozygous state—AZA should be avoided and can be fatal (within 6 weeks).
- Heterozygous state—may be subject to delayed bone marrow toxicity (symptoms may not be evident until 6 months after starting treatment).

▶ Patients who are TPMT-deficient are at greater risk of catastrophic low white cell count early in treatment.

▶ Patients with normal TPMT levels on can still develop leucopenia at any stage of treatment.

📖 Pharmacological management, p.419.

Human leucocyte antigen (HLA B27)

HLAs are proteins that assist the body's immune system differentiate between its own cells and harmful substances. HLA B27 is one of the HLA antigens. Estimates vary but it is thought that about 5–8% of the normal Caucasian population is HLA B27-positive. A positive HLA B27 test is linked to a greater risk of developing a seronegative spondyloarthropathy (e.g. AS).

📖 Spondyloarthopathies, p.80.

Key points and top tips in reviewing blood results

Blood tests are a valuable diagnostic tool but:
• Blood tests constitute only a part of an holistic assessment.
• A single result cannot confirm or exclude a diagnosis.
• A trend of ↓ or ↑ of values is more valuable than a single result.
• Blood tests are affected by factors other than rheumatological disease.
• Consider comorbidities and drug interactions.
• Treatment is not given on the basis of results alone.

Where possible make use of a computerized database:
• Abnormal results may be usual for a particular patient.
• Trends in results are more easily visualized.
• Can identify key factors, e.g. relevance of starting on or ↑ DMARD dose, when drug toxicity are more likely.
• If no computer database available, a monitoring register/index cards/or patient monitoring booklet are useful.
• Results outside of the normal range must be taken in context and may be of little clinical significance.

Remember:
• Vigilance is essential.
• Appropriate monitoring and action on abnormalities reduces the risk of drug toxicity.
• Trends in results may signify drug toxicity before the blood test actually becomes abnormal.
• Drug toxicity can be fatal and happen at any stage during treatment.
• If in doubt withhold DMARD until checked with prescribing clinician.

⚠ *Remember*: a trend of ↓ or ↑ of values is more valuable than a single result and can identify the early signs of toxicity

Further reading

BSR (2008). *British Society of Rheumatology guidelines on monitoring of disease modifying anti-rheumatic drugs.* BSR, London. Available at: ⏚ www.rheumatology.org.uk

Radiological investigations

Radiological investigations play an important role in the diagnosis and ongoing management and review of many MSCs. There are 3 principles of radiation protection:

- Justification of the procedure—will it benefit the patient or lead to a change in treatment?
- Optimization—using the lowest dose necessary.
- Limitation—the dose should not exceed the agreed limits.

Many nurses have undertaken additional training to request radiological investigations; usually these are confined to plain x-rays. Before requesting an x-ray nurses must:

- Undertake relevant training and continually update their knowledge.
- Consider issues related to the use of ionizing radiations.
- Adhere to local and national guidance that outline best practice in protecting staff and patients from unnecessary exposure/harm.

Key aspects of radiological management include responsibilities for the:

- Employer:
  - Written protocols for every standard investigation.
  - Referral criteria should include clarity of referral pathways, radiation dose including limits, and quality issues.
  - Ensure adequate training for all staff including continuing professional development.
- Referrer:
  - Those entitled to refer for medical exposure.
  - Responsible for providing sufficient clinical information to justify each exposure.
- Practitioner:
  - Take responsibility for medical exposure.
  - Must comply trust procedures and ensure justification for exposure.
- Operator:
  - Responsible for all practical aspects of performing procedure.
  - Authorization of procedure.

Plain radiographic x-rays

Plain x-rays; specific positions may be requested to identify pathology—e.g. standing x-rays to explore joint space narrowing on weight-bearing. Plain x-rays are helpful in identifying:

- Erosions or fractures.
- Baseline measurement, e.g. pre-treatment chest x-ray.
- Exclude underlying pathology prior to treatment, e.g. TB.
- Calcification of ligaments, e.g. spinal.
- Joint space narrowing (JSN) or avascular necrosis or bone tumours.

Limitations include superimposed structures obscuring the view to area of interest and are reliant on the difference radiographic densities and quality of x-ray films and exposure.

Research trials use radiological evidence to evaluate changes in MSCs. In some cases specific measurement tools have been developed to identify radiological changes using a composite score based on measurements at different points on a radiological films—e.g. the total Sharp's score measures key points in x-rays of the hand or feet.

Computerized tomography (CT) scanning

CT uses a moderate-to-high dose of radiation to provide an imaging technique that shows 3-dimensional (3-D) pictures of internal tissues. This is achieved by taking frequent 2-D images whilst rotating around a single axis. Contrast enhancement enables greater clarity between tissues, demonstrating differences in their physical density. CT scans are valuable in assessment of areas such as the spine enabling an estimate of the quality and integrity of inter-vertebral discs.

Magnetic resonance imaging (MRI)

MRI uses magnetic spinning and polarization of the magnetic fields to measure interactions between absorption and emission of energy to examine the tissues of the body. MRI utilizes the different densities of tissues (proportions of water or lipid/fats), using 3-D visual 'cuts' or sliced selections to produce a visual result. It is a popular method for many musculoskeletal investigations including imaging joints, soft tissue, and early bone erosions.

Ultrasound (US)

US is increasingly gaining favor as a non-invasive technique that can be used in a clinical setting by trained clinicians to aid and inform treatment decisions. US uses a Doppler tool to beam sound waves through tissues. The early identification of erosions, synovitis, ganglion cysts, or osteopenia has particular value in treating early disease, allowing prompt treatment before long-term established damage takes place.

Isotope scanning (IS)

IS uses a small dose of radioisotope that passes systemically through the body (via an oral or IV route) to scan target organs or tissues by emitting gamma rays which identify hot spots (high level of gamma rays) or cold spots (low levels of gamma rays). Time for the radioisotope to reach the target organ may vary and patients may have to wait before being scanned with a gamma camera that detects the rays emitted from the body. IS is valuable for detecting infection, inflammation, and malignancies. Rarely, anaphylactoid reactions can occur from the injection.

DEXA scan—used to detect osteoporosis

Signs of osteoporosis may be detected on plain x-ray but do not provide an objective measures of the BMD. Dual energy x-ray absorptiometry uses low energy x-rays to measure the density of bone. The results are given as T- or Z-scores in relation to calculated averages BMD scores (see Osteoporosis, p.33).

Further reading

Department of Health (2007). The Ionising Radiation (Medical Exposure) Regulations 2000 (amendment 2006). DH, London. Available at: www.dh.gov.uk

Dougherty L, Lister S (eds) (2006). *The Royal Marsden Hospital Manual of Clinical Nursing Procedures,* 6th edn. Blackwell Publishing. Oxford.

Also see Local trust policies.

Respiratory investigations

This section outlines some of the standard tests for respiratory disease. For guidance on the different aspects of respiratory complications with MSC refer to 📖 Respiratory system, p.484.

Peak flow

Rarely useful as it is a measure of airways obstruction and has a wide normal range.

Spirometry

A simple test which can be performed in the clinic or ward. Will detect airways obstruction and also a restrictive problem due to ILD. Spirometry is often normal in early ILD.

Nursing point: test should not be performed immediately after a full meal. If the patient is on an inhaled bronchodilator they maybe asked to withhold this before the test.

Full PFTs

Generally a combination of a more complex description of lung volumes ('spirometry plus'), 'transfer factor', or 'diffusion coefficient'. A ↓ in transfer factor is usually the earliest indication of developing ILD.

Nursing point: tests are undertaken in a pulmonary function laboratory. Similar preparatory issues to spirometry

Mouth pressure

A measure of the maximum negative pressure (inspiration) or positive pressure (expiration).

Blood gases and oxygen saturation

Always record inspired oxygen. This could be the room air or percentage of oxygen or flow rate + device used.

Pulse oximetry

Measures oxygen saturation of arterial blood in the fingertip or ear lobe —the SaO_2 (oxygen saturation). Simple to perform, non-invasive and can be repeated as required. SaO_2 is variable and may fluctuate, e.g. at times of anxiety. Serial readings are ∴ helpful. Reduced in more severe ILD but often normal in mild-to-moderate disease.

Nursing point: poor circulation in the fingers (e.g. systemic sclerosis, Raynaud's) may prevent satisfactory recording from fingers—consider measuring from ear lobe. Nail varnish may also affect results.

Pulse oximetry on exercise

A fall in SaO_2 on exercise is a more sensitive test of mild ILD.

Nursing point: as for pulse oximetry. Usually a PT or nurse will undertake this investigation. Appropriate exercises need to be considered in the context of the patient. Record SaO_2 at rest, on cessation of exercise, and the lowest recorded level during observation, together with the exercise undertaken (e.g. distance travelled).

Arterial blood gases

Arterial blood samples are analyzed for O_2. Carbon dioxide acid–base status (pH, bicarbonate) rarely required in the outpatient context, unless coexistent COPD or severe respiratory muscle weakness. These might cause ventilatory failure, and therefore rising blood carbon dioxide ($PaCO_2$). Important in the assessment of the acutely ill patient as arterial blood gases can detect metabolic acidosis.

Nursing point: arterial blood gases are obtained via a needle from an artery usually radial artery at the wrist. Collected in a pre-heparinized syringe. Samples should be processed immediately or sent to the laboratory on ice. Once the sample obtained inform the pathology department immediately that sample to avoid delay in processing.

Radiology

Plain chest x-ray

An essential investigation for respiratory symptoms. May demonstrate evidence of pleural disease (effusion, thickening); parnchymal (lung tissue) abnormalities of cardiac disease. However, usually normal in pulmonary hypertension (seen in systemic sclerosis or muscle disease) often normal in milder ILD.

CT

CT pulmonary angiogram (CTPA). Now the usual method to detect or exclude pulmonary hypertension.

MR scan

Rarely helpful in lung disease.

Isotope lung scan

Used less frequently than CTPA in diagnosis of PE. Gives less information than CTPA but normal isotope lung scan does exclude PE. In the presence of other lung disease less accurate in the diagnosis of PE.

Exclude cardiac involvement

The most usual set of initial investigations to rule out cardiac causes for breathlessness are:

- Chest x-ray.
- ECG.
- Echocardiogram.

Screening for tuberculosis

Human TB is an infection caused by the bacterium *Mycobacterium tuberculosis*. In the last 2 years TB in England has risen by 15% with 350 people dying each year. In some parts of the UK there are 40 cases of TB per 100,000 population. 60% of all cases are of TB are pulmonary in the UK. Rates are higher in certain communities chiefly because of their links with areas of high TB prevalence around the world. The majority of TB is concentrated in certain areas of the UK, particularly cities.

As a result of the ↑ TB issues it is important to assess the patient's lifestyle or family history to identify potential TB risk, e.g.:
• Living in an area of high incidence or prevalence of TB.
• Frequent travel to overseas areas with high prevalence of TB (either person or family contacts).
• Have an occupational risk (e.g. laboratory or health workers, prison workers, or those accommodating refugees and asylum seekers).

Specific patients at risk

The risks of TB are related to re-emergence of latent TB or progression of newly-acquired active disease. TB is not always completely eradicated from the body but contained by the host defense mechanisms within granulomatous lesions in the body, ∴ specific factors should be considered in the context of patients who have:
• Systemic illness affecting the patient's ability to manage infections (e.g. HIV).
• Immunosuppression (e.g. MTX, AZA, mycophenolate, or high doses of steroids) or specific biologic therapies drug that can alter the body's ability to contain any traces of mycobacterium (e.g. TNFα, an important cytokine in containing granulomatosus structures within the body).

TB and anti-TNFα therapies (adalimumab, etanercept, and infliximab)

The introduction of anti-TNFα therapies revealed an ↑ incidence of TB in RA patients treated with a TNFα inhibitor. It has ∴ been essential for patients to be adequately assessed before starting treatment and to be aware that the risk of reactivation is higher in this group of patients.

Assessment and screening for TB prior to anti-TNFα therapies
• Full clinical examination and history taking:
  • Examine chest including auscultation.
  • Focus on any prior TB.
  • Any current lifestyle of work-related issues that ↑ risk related to TB.
  • Question re any signs suggestive of TB.
• If patient cannot recall prior Bacillus Calmette-Guérin (BCG) vaccine check for scar. Note: BCG vaccine introduced in 1953. BCG is no longer routinely administered to all children.
• Chest x-ray—unless chest x-ray performed within the last 3 months (review x-ray and report).
  • Any abnormal results—refer to specialist in TB.
• Review any evidence suggestive of past TB (e.g. on chest x-ray) or history of prior extra pulmonary TB. If prior treatment for TB:
  • Review with specialist to ensure previous treatment adequate.

- Monitor regularly.
- Symptoms suggestive of TB—refer to prescribing physician.

Testing for TB

Some patients once screened will be eligible for skin testing, e.g. patients who have a normal chest x-ray and no prior history of TB. The accuracy of tuberculin skin tests is significantly compromised if patients are taking immunosuppressive therapies (e.g. MTX or steroids). If patients stop treatment a skin test can be considered valid if 1 month (for steroids) or 3 months (for other immunosuppressive therapies) has elapsed.

👉 Recently blood tests have been introduced to detect latent and active TB. These include the T-Spot-TB® test and QuantiFERON® assay.

Mantoux purified protein derivative (PPD) tests should not be given to those who have a previous reaction of 15mm or greater or those who have had previous TB. Mantoux testing measures the degree of hypersensitivity to tuberculin and correlates with future risk of developing TB. The results of skin test should be read between 48–72 hours after administration. Interpretation of results must be considered with the clinical history and examination. Results of Mantoux indurations:

- <6mm negative.
- If no identified risks 6–15 mm—likely to be due to previous BCG.
- If identified high probability >6mm likely to be TB.
- >15mm unlikely to be due to previous exposure to TB or environmental factors.
- False negatives if immunosuppressed, renal failure, severe TB disease, old age, or poor handling or administration of Mantoux test.

Referral to specialist in TB treatment

Patients who have active TB cannot receive treatment with anti-TNF or rituximab (or other biologic disease-modifying drug therapies) until they have completed a full course of standard chemotherapy. Treatment is normally prescribed by a consultant specializing in TB. In some circumstances the specialist in discussion with rheumatologist (and patient) may decide on an appropriate treatment strategy based upon the individual patient risks and benefits. However, guidelines suggest that at least 2 months of full compliant treatment should be taken before considering starting treatment with a biologic.

📖 Also see Pharmacological management, p.419.

Further reading

British Thoracic Society Standards of Care Committee (2005). BTS recommendations for assessing risk and for managing *Mycobacterium tuberculosis* infection and disease in patients due to start anti-TNF-alpha treatment. *Thorax*, **60**, 800–5.

Department of Health (2007). *The Mantoux test: Administration, reading and interpretation*. DH, London. Available at: ⏚ http://www.immunisation.nhs.uk/files/mantouxtest.pdf

Royal College of Nursing (2004). *Assessment, administration and review of biologic therapies*. RCN. London.

The disease in context with treatment monitoring and side effects

The disease in context with treatment

Most nurses will have heard patients say 'I don't like taking tablets; I worry about side effects'. While it is true that many drugs for MSCs are potentially toxic, this must be considered against the risk to the patient if the arthritis is left untreated. It is necessary to explain that the aim of treatment is to relieve symptoms, but, most importantly, to control and slow progression of the disease, which if left untreated, will have 'side effects' of its own, such as irreversible joint damage, functional decline, and other related conditions such as cardiovascular disease or osteoporosis.

The role of the rheumatology nurse is to educate and empower patients about their condition and the various treatment options. Much time is spent discussing the likely benefits of treatments and also the potential risks of side effects that are sometimes experienced. Patients have a right to know about side effects, but we have to try and present a balanced picture, empowering patients to make informed choices. It is important to instigate treatment soon after diagnosis as erosive damage can occur very quickly, and it is worthwhile taking time with patients to find a treatment with which they feel comfortable and which fits in with their lifestyle.

When discussing medication, the nurse should try to reassure the patient that although there are risks associated with all drugs, by having the appropriate monitoring, potential problems would be detected early. Nevertheless some patients find having blood tests every couple of weeks very intrusive, so the importance of regular monitoring must be explained and reinforced at clinic appointments.

Some patients need a lot of support and counselling to maintain treatment, and many will try several different preparations before finding one that suits them and is effective.

Why is monitoring so important?

The principal purposes of monitoring are patient safety and efficacy of treatment.

Rheumatology conditions are, by nature, unpredictable. It is very difficult to foresee how a patient will respond to treatment, or whether they are likely to develop side effects from medication.

By monitoring patients closely it is possible to:
• Assess disease activity.
• Screen for toxicity.
• Detect trends in blood tests—e.g. a gradual fall in WBC count.
• Support the choice of medication.
• Adjust drug dosage according to disease activity.
• Ensure the patient is not over-medicated.

Many rheumatology patients are subject to polypharmacy and drug regimens may be complicated. For example, a fairly typical drug regimen for a patient with RA might include:
- MTX taken once a week.
- Folic acid taken once a week—3 days after the MTX.
- Hydroxychloroquine daily (note: the total dose of HCQ is calculated by body weight and might not be taken every day; be aware of possible variable doses).
- Prednisolone 5mg and 7.5mg on alternate days.
- A bisphosphonate taken once-weekly on an empty stomach in the middle of a fast.
- Analgesics taken when necessary.
- PPI to protect the stomach.

In terms of DMARD monitoring, most adverse reactions occur early, usually within the first few months of initiation of treatment, and ∴ monitoring is usually more frequent in the initial stages.

▶ Side effects may develop at any time and may be be precipitated by the addition of a treatment affecting the pharmacokinetics of the original prescribed DMARD. In general, once treatment is established and monitoring is stabilized, the frequency of monitoring can be reduced, but must be continued as long as the patient is taking the DMARD.

Shared-care monitoring

It is important to ascertain who takes responsibility for DMARD monitoring:
- Ideally 'shared-care' guidelines should be established, between 1° and 2° care.
- This sets out who is accountable for monitoring:
  - The type and frequency of tests required.
  - What to do when abnormalities are found.

Patients who take DMARDs are given shared-care monitoring booklets and educated about the medication they are taking and how often and why the blood tests are needed.

📖 Also see Pharmacological management: disease-modifying drugs, p.419; 📖 Nursing care issues in patient-centred care, pp.312, 314.

Blood test monitoring

When a patient comes to a monitoring consultation, the blood test results are examined for improvements, or trends that may indicate adverse reactions to drugs. This helps to decide whether a medication should be changed or the dose adjusted.

Many rheumatology patients have results that fall outside of the normal range. It is necessary to determine whether this is due to the patient's rheumatological condition, other co-morbidities, or due to the medications the patient is taking.

Haematological side effects

- *Anaemia* has a variety of causes, e.g.:
  - Anaemia of chronic disease—where the cells are normal in size and colour (normocytic, normochromic) and the degree of anaemia seems to correspond to the activity of the arthritis.
  - Anaemia due to DMARDs—e.g. due to bone marrow suppression with MTX, AZA, and sodium aurothiomalate (IM gold) or folate deficiency with MTX and AZA.
  - Iron deficiency anaemia—microcyic, hypochromic, may be a consequence of poor diet or from GI bleeding due to NSAIDs
- *Leucocytosis* ↑ white cells can be related to:
  - Active inflammation such as RA or gout.
  - Infection.
- *Leucopenia*—reduction of white cell has many causes including:
  - Conditions such as SLE and Felty syndrome.
  - Side effects of DMARDs (can be life threatening).
- *Agranulocytosis*—an acute condition due to bone marrow suppression leading to severe leucopenia, often attributed to medication.
- *Thrombocytopenia*—↓ platelets.
  - Thrombocytopenia is sometimes a feature of Felty syndrome and can less commonly be seen in RA.
  - Related to many of the DMARDs.
  - Idiopathic thrombocytopenic purpura (ITP)—thrombocytopenia of unknown cause.

Biochemical side effects

Abnormal LFTs can include:
- Mild transient ↑ in the liver enzymes are relatively common with DMARD use.
- DMARDs should be withheld in marked ↑ in liver enzymes.
- Raised ALP and GGT—may also be raised in inflammation.

Abnormalities in the U&Es associated with leflunomide and ciclosporin, penicillamine, and NSAIDs.

Key point: trends in results

It is important to observe for gradual changes in results over time. For example, there may be a slow fall in the white cells, although the white cell count remains within the normal range; the trend in results highlights the possibility of an adverse drug reaction. Vigilance and close monitoring is required as it may be necessary to withhold the drug.

Respiratory system

The baseline investigations of rheumatology patients will usually include a chest x-ray. This is because pulmonary involvement in RA is relatively common, and includes interstitial fibrosis and pulmonary nodules. Pleurisy and pleural effusions can develop due to inflammation of the pleura. The lungs can also be adversely affected by some treatments used in rheumatology and baseline evaluations are useful. Any abnormalities found on chest x-ray will need to be investigated prior to treatment and will influence the choice of DMARD.

Drugs affecting the respiratory system

- *MTX*—pneumonitis is uncommon and pulmonary fibrosis is a rare complication of MTX. Pulmonary toxicity is a rare but serious side effect of MTX and can occur at any stage during treatment although it is more likely during the 1st year. Presents as dyspnoea and unproductive cough. Full PFTs may be required. Pneumonitis should be excluded by HRCT scan.
- *Sodium aurothiomalate* (IM gold)—hypersensitivity pneumonitis, dyspnoea, cough, pleuritic chest pain.
- *SAS*—eosinophilic pneumonitis, dyspnoea, fever.
- *D-penicillamine*—rare; bronchiolitis obliterans, dyspnoea late in therapy.
- *NSAIDs*—exacerbation of asthma, pneumonitis reported with naproxen.
- The emergence of latent TB has been associated with *anti-TNFα* therapies. It is ∴ essential to ensure adequate screening before initiating treatment— this includes a chest x-ray, TB prior contacts, risks and immunological status for TB.
- ILD—evidence suggests that ILD is a possible risk factor of poor outcome when treated with *anti-TNFα*. Patients will need to be reviewed by a clinician and may require referral to a respiratory consultant before being considered for treatment.

Patients treated with DMARDs—in particular MTX or gold—complaining of dry cough, possibly accompanied by dyspnoea, should be urgently investigated to exclude drug-induced pneumonitis. Medication should be withheld until pneumonitis has been ruled out.

Patients presenting with a productive cough, accompanied by a raised white cell count is indicative of a chest infection, which will require investigating and treatment as necessary.

Nurses should be vigilant about all forms of infection (including respiratory) for those treated with anti-TNFα therapies as prompt treatment is essential.

📖 Repiratory investigations p.476.

Cardiovascular side effects

In recent years there has been ↑ interest in the correlation between IJD and cardiovascular risk. RA is associated with ↑ mortality, almost half of which is due to diseases of the heart and blood vessels, mainly heart attack and stroke. This appears to be attributed to early and more advanced blood vessel damage, due to high levels of inflammation in RA. In many rheumatology departments, annual cardiovascular risk assessments are performed.

Patients are encouraged to adopt healthy lifestyle measures such as stopping smoking, losing weight, eating a healthy diet, and taking measures to lower their blood pressure or cholesterol levels. Management of cardiovascular risk increasingly includes prescribing of anti-hypertensive and statin therapy.

In addition some medication commonly used in rheumatology practice can have an adverse affect on the cardiovascular system.

NSAIDs and COX-2 inhibitors

- COX-2 inhibitors are associated with an increased risk of thrombotic events (e.g. MI and stroke).
- NSAIDs may also be associated with a small ↑ risk of thrombotic events when used at higher doses and with long-term treatment.
- The lowest effective dose of NSAID should be given for the shortest period to control symptoms.
- Patients taking NSAIDs or COX-2 inhibitors long term should be reviewed at regular intervals.
- These drugs are contraindicated in patients with ischaemic heart disease, cerebrovasular disease, or severe heart failure.
- NSAIDs and COX-2 inhibitors should be used with caution in patients with risk factors for heart disease.
- Evidence is continually being reviewed on traditional NSAID versus COX-2 risks/benefits.

Also see Non-steroidal anti-inflammatories, p.412; COX-2 inhibitors, p.412.

Corticosteroids

- Influence electrolytes—imbalance leads to oedema and hypertension from water and sodium retention, leading to cardiac failure.
- Influence lipid and cholesterol production—imbalance leads to hyperlipidaemia and hypercholesterolaemia.

Also see Corticosteroids, p.444.

Leflunomide

- Hypertension is a recognized side effect of leflunomide.
- Blood pressure should be monitored twice before starting treatment (2 weeks apart) and blood pressure >140/90 should be treated before commencing treatment.
- Monthly monitoring of BP thereafter or at least at every visit—every 2 weeks for the first 6 months then once every 8 weeks.

Ciclosporin

- Hypertension—blood pressure should be measured prior to treatment, and continue regularly during treatment.

- Discontinue if hypertension develops during treatment that cannot be controlled by antihypertensive therapy.

📖 Also see ciclosporin, pp.487, 492.

Biologic agents

- Patient's cardiac status should be screened prior to treatment with anti-TNFα (contraindicated in NYHC III/IV).
- Anti-TNFα should be used with caution in heart failure (NYHC I/II) and should be discontinued if symptoms develop or worsen.

📖 New biologic disease-modifying therapies, p.456.

Rituximab (MabThera®)

- Hypertension and hypotension have been reported.
- Patients who normally take antihypertensives should withhold them for 12 hours prior to infusion.
- Rituximab should be used with caution in patients with known heart disease.

📖 Also see Intravenous therapies, p.507.

Further reading

British Society for Rheumatology Guidelines for Disease Modifying Antirheumatic Drug Therapy (DMARD) in consultation with the British Association of Dermatologists (2008). Available at: ⁿ www.rheumatology.org.uk

Infections

Suppression of the immune system ↑ the risk of infections. The immu-nosuppressive nature of many drugs used in rheumatology means ∴, that patients are potentially vulnerable to infection, and these risk factors must be considered when prescribing. Here are examples of immunosuppres-sive agents where extra vigilance for infection is required.

MTX

- Seek medical advice if infection suspected (particularly in the elderly) as treatment may need to be discontinued.
- Contact with herpes zoster or herpes varicella—patient may need treatment with anti-herpes immunoglobulin.
- MTX should not be given in combination with trimethoprim or co-trimoxazole.

Cyclophosphamide

Patients susceptible to broad spectrum of infections, including severe infection such as septicaemia.

Anti-TNFα

- ↑ risk of reactivation of latent TB—patients should be assessed for TB risk prior to commencing treatment. Prior treated TB infection is not a contraindication but TB prophylaxis may be required prior to treatment with anti-TNFα
- Serious infections, including fatalities, have been reported with the anti-TNFα therapies currently used in rheumatology practice. Patients should be screened for infection prior to treatment with anti-TNFα and advised to report any infections promptly.
- Patients who are treated with anti-TNFα who develop severe infections need to have biologic therapy temporarily withheld until infection is treated and resolved.
- ☛ It can be difficult to know when to seek advice re infections. However, patients treated with anti-TNFα do not always display the classic signs of infections (e.g. absence of pyrexia). If in doubt seek advice.

Corticosteroids

Can cause the patient to be more susceptible to infections including viral and fungal infections and TB

📖 Also see Infections in musculoskeletal conditions, p.380.

Further reading

National Patient Safety Agency website: ⌀ www.npsa.nhs.uk

Other side effects

The major adverse reactions to rheumatology drugs have been detailed elsewhere (📖 see Pharmacological management pp.403–460). There is, however, a wide range of other recognized side effects; briefly this includes:

GI tract
- Wide variety of GI upset with DMARDs, see Table 17.2.
- Analgesics—constipation.
- NSAIDs—indigestion and peptic ulceration. All NSAIDs are associated with GI toxicity, especially in the elderly. Selective COX-2 inhibitors have a lower risk of upper GI side effects than non-selective NSAIDs. All NSAIDs and COX-2 inhibitors are contraindicated in patients with active peptic ulceration.

▶ Note: risks and benefits of NSAIDs including cardiovascular risks are discussed in 📖 Pain relief NSAIDs p.412.

Skin (drug reactions)
- DMARDs—rashes and pruritis, see Table 17.2.
- NSAIDs—hypersensitivity– rashes can be severe.
- Corticosteroids—atrophy, bruising, acne, striae.

Headaches
- Most DMARDs—stop drug if severe.

Eyes
- Hydroxychloroquine (HCQ), see Table 17.2.
- Corticosteroids—cataracts, glaucoma.

Hypersensitivity
- Most DMARDs, see Table 17.2.
- Anti TNFα/rituximab.

Malignancy
- DMARDs, e.g. AZA, ciclosporin.
- Cyclophosphamide—↑ risk of haemorrhagic cystits and bladder cancer. The higher the cumulative dose the greater the risk.
- Anti TNFα—theoretical ↑ risk
- ☞ Lymphomas risk appears to be related to contributing factors such as uncontrolled inflammation, duration, and aggressiveness of disease rather than drug therapy.

Fertility
(📖 see Pharmacological management, p.419 for detailed information.)
- Limited evidence for most DMARDs with regard to fertility and pregnancy outcomes—must be discussed in detail with prescribing clinician.
- SAS—oligospermia.
- MTX—avoid pregnancy, contraceptive measures for ♂ and ♀—potential fetal abnormality, may induce spontaneous abortion.

- Leflunomide—effective contraception is vital during treatment and for 2 years following treatment for ♀ and 3 months for ♂. Drug washouts may be necessary
- NSAIDs—long-term use is associated with reversible but reduced ♀ fertility. Can affect closure of fetal ductus arteriosus in utero and the possibility of pulmonary hypertension of the newborn. May cause delayed onset of and ↑ the duration of labour.

📖 Also see Pharmacological management, p.419.

Metabolic disturbance

- Corticosteroids—hyperglycaemia may occur due to the effect of corticosteroids on the metabolism of glycogen. Known diabetics may require an adjustment of their diabetic therapy.
- Cushingoid features—e.g. 'moon face'.

Musculoskeletal

- Corticosteroids—osteoporosis, muscle wasting.

This is not a comprehensive list of all the known adverse reactions to rheumatology drugs. More in-depth information can be found in individual drug data sheets and the *BNF*.

Table 17.2 Examples of drug side effects

Drug	Side effects
AZA	• Hypersensitivity reaction: including malaise, dizziness, vomiting, diarrhoea, fever, rigors, rash, hypotension, interstitial nephritis • Serious effects: liver impairment, blood dyscrasias, rash, mouth ulcers
Ciclosporin	• Very common: renal dysfunction, hypertension • Common: burning sensation hands and feet, tremor, abdominal discomfort, gum hyperplasia, anorexia, ↑ hair growth • Uncommon: neohrotoxicity, hepatotoxicity
D-Penicillamine	• Uncommon: metallic taste, rash, nausea, anorexia • Serious effects: proteinuria, blood discrasias, myostis, myasthenia gravis, mouth ulcers, thyroiditis
HCQ	• Uncommon: indigestion, diarrhoea, rash, pruritis depigmentation of skin and hair • Rare: retinopathy, ECG changes, convulsions, leuopenia, hepatotoxicity
Leflunomide	• Common: diarrhoea, nausea, mild ↑ in blood pressure • Less common: mouth ulcers, weight loss, headache, dizziness, hypertension, alopecia, rash, asthenia, parasthesia • Serious effects: anaphylaxis, hepatotoxicity, toxic epidermal necrolysis • Other: potentially teratogenic
MTX	• Common: diarrhoea, nausea, stomatitis • Uncommon: headaches, drowsiness, blurred vision • Serious effects: acute hepatic, pulmonary, and bone marrow toxicity • Other: risk of fetal abnormality due to teratogenic effect
Sodium aurothiomalate (IM gold)	• Common: skin reactions, skin pigmentation on prolonged use, mouth ulcers, proteinuria • Uncommon: pneumonitis, diarrhoea, nausea • Serious effects: blood discrasias, proteinuria, nephritic syndrome, jaundice, agranulocytosis
SAS	• Common: diarrhoea, nausea, abdominal pain, headache, tinnitus, fever, photosensitization, orange urine, stain soft contact lenses • Serious effects: blood discrasias, hypersensitivity reaction • Other: oligospermia

Intra-articular, subcutaneous, and intravenous therapies

Intra-articular injections: overview

In specialist rheumatology practice experienced nurses are increasingly training to be able to inject joints. This allows for a more holistic approach to the patient with the complete episode of care delivered by one person.

When undertaking new roles nurses need to be aware of their professional code of conduct and ensure that their organization has recognized their extended role and are providing vicarious liability. The following few pages provides an outline of IA injections and are aimed at giving the nurse on a ward or a clinic area, working in the role of assisting in the administration of joint injections, more of an understanding of the principle and practicalities.

Joint aspiration is the removal of fluid from the joint space. Aspiration and injection is an essential procedure for the diagnosis and treatment of joint disease.

Indications for joint aspiration and injection

- Diagnostic to identify the cause of the problem, e.g.:
  - Sepsis.
  - Crystals—monosodium urate, calcium pyrophosphate.
  - Haemarthrosis.
- Treatment:
  - To reduce IA pressure by removing fluid this relieving pain and increasing mobility.
  - To inject steroid.
  - Recurrent aspiration for sepsis.
  - The use of IA steroid may avoid the need for systemic use.

Key issues in preparing the patient for joint or soft tissue injection

Before undertaking the procedure the person performing the aspiration and/or injection should provide a full explanation to the patient outlining the procedure and gaining the patient's consent. This should include:

- A full explanation of the procedure, to include the effects and possible side effects of IA injection.
- A clear discussion on the expected level of discomfort to be expected during the procedure:
  - This is usually minor and short lived; in experienced hands a joint injection should be no more painful than venepuncture.
  - It is helpful if the patient can be more relaxed as perceptions of pain may be reduced.
- The effects of the injection should be seen fairly quickly; if local anaesthetic is used there is an immediate effect. However, this wears off in 2–4 hours and patients should be advised to take additional analgesia before the steroid effects are felt.
- The steroids usually take effect within 24 hours and may persist for 2 months or more. In a small minority of patients it can take up to a week to see the full effect of the steroid injection

- Rest is advocated for between 24–48 hours, particularly in weight-bearing joints, so that the patient gets the maximum benefit from the steroid.
- Some patients can experience a post-injection flare. This may be as a result of a reaction to the microcrystalline suspension of the corticosteroid used. The patient should be given information to deal with this, such as rest following the injection, using analgesia as the local anaesthetic wears off. Ice or hot packs to help relieve post-injection flare pain may be helpful.
- The potential benefits of IA injection can last up to 2 months or longer.
- It is generally recommended that a joint is not injected more frequently than once every 3–4 months.
- A full explanation of potential side effects of IA injections should be given.

Side effects of IA steroid injections

- Post-injection flare is seen in 1–2% of patients.
- Facial flushing 12%.
- Joint infection is rare if aseptic technique is used (risk of 1 in 70,000).
- Rarely, subcutaneous fat atrophy can occur (more frequent with periarticular injections) and is seen as a whitening or depigmentation of the skin. This does resolve with time.
- Tendon rupture can occur if the drug is injected into a tendon.
- Some ♀ may experience disruption of their menstrual cycle, with either spotting, prolonged menstrual bleeding, or may miss a period as a result of steroid being injected.
- Patients with diabetes can experience a temporary rise in blood glucose levels and should be warned that this can happen and to adjust their diet and medication if necessary.

Drugs used in administrating intra-articular injections

Steroids are the most commonly used preparation for IA injections frequently administered with a local anaesthetic such as lidocaine.

IA steroids

- Have an anti-inflammatory effect.
- Superior to NSAIDs.
- Rapid onset, reliable, and effective for treating synovitis.
- Reduce pain and deformity, ↑ mobility and function.
- Useful in patients where systemic steroids would normally be contraindicated e.g. diabetes and osteoporosis.

Commonly used injectable steroids

There are a number of IA steroids on the market; they are relatively insoluble and as a consequence are longer-acting and not absorbed systemically to a great degree.

The commonly used preparations are listed here in order of ↑ potency and length of action:

- Hydrocortisone acetate 25mg/mL (Hydrocortistab®).
- Prednisolone acetate 25mg/mL (Deltastab®).
- Methylprednisolone acetate 40mg/mL (Depo-Medrone®).
- Triamcinolone acetonide 40mg/mL (Kenalog®).
- Local anaesthetic.

Prevents pain by causing reversible block of nerve conduction along nerve fibres.

Lidocaine

This is probably the most effective and commonly used local anaesthetic for the following reasons:

- Rapid onset of action.
- Lasting effect of between 2–4 hours.
- Incidence of side effects is low in local injection.
- Available in a range of strengths from 0.1–2%.

Most common side effects are headache, light headedness, and drowsiness. Rarely, numbness of the tongue, anxiety, restlessness, blurred vision can occur.

Other drugs used in IA injections

Yttrium-90

Yttrium-90 is a radioisotope used for the treatment of severe, chronic synovitis when IA steroids have failed to help. It is infrequently used nowadays and the value of such an approach remains controversial.

- Yttrium is used as an alternative to surgical synovectomy.
- The joint is aspirated, injected with steroid, followed by Yttrium-90.

- Strict immobilization of the joint is required to prevent extra-articular leakage of the radioisotope.
- The joint is splinted following the procedure and the patient is kept on bed rest for 48 hours following the procedure.

Hyaluronic acid (HA)

A high molecular weight polysaccharide that is a major component of synovial fluid and cartilage.

- In OA the molecular weight and concentration of HA is reduced.
- 'Viscosupplementation' with an IA injection of HA, it is claimed, helps to normalize the viscoelasticity of the synovial fluid.
- HA is licensed for symptom relief in OA of the knee when other conservative treatments have failed.
- In about 2% of patients there is an ↑ in pain and swelling following injection.
- A recent NICE guideline for OA does not recommend the use of HA.[1]

Reference

1. NICE. Guidelines for OA. NICE, London.

Preparation and management of those receiving intra-articular joint injections

Nurses and allied HCPs involved in assisting with an IA joint aspiration and injection have important roles to play in the procedure in the following ways:
- Preparation of the equipment.
- Preparation of the patient.
- Care of the patient during and after the procedure.
- Dealing with samples and disposal of fluid.

Preparation of equipment

An aseptic, no-touch technique is mandatory for any joint aspiration and injection

Assemble equipment needed:
- Alcohol swabs for cleaning the skin.
- Syringes—an assortment of various sizes depending on the joints to be injected.
- For the injection either a 2 or 5mL syringe is used for the injection.
- If the joint needs aspiration a 10–30mL syringe may be required.
- Needles—21-gauge green needles for large joints, 23 or 25-gauge (blue or orange) for smaller joints.
- Specimen bottles for the aspirate.
- Local anaesthetic—lidocaine 1 or 2% depending on the preference of the operator.
- Steroid for injection—a selection is best so that the person performing the injection can choose the most appropriate steroid for the joint to be injected (2 registered practitioners should check the prescription).
- Gloves may be worn to protect the operator, especially in high-risk situations.
- Swabs, adhesive dressings.
- Alcohol hand gel.
- Anaphylaxis kit.

Preparation of the patient

- The nurse should put the patient at ease by explaining the procedure and checking that the patient fully understands what will be happening to them and confirm the patient's identification and the prescription.
- Consent would normally be taken by the person performing the procedure and can be in the form of written or verbal consent but must be clearly documented.
- If necessary the patient should be helped to undress and expose the area to be injected, whilst maintaining their dignity.
- The patient should be positioned on a couch with the area to be injected exposed and, if necessary, supported sufficiently so that the muscles are relaxed.
- Tense muscles can make the injection impossible; for this reason it is extremely important to try and get the patient to relax. If guided imagery is used this can give the patient a pleasant image to focus on, aiding relaxation.

Care of the patient during the procedure

- The nurse should remain with the patient throughout the procedure for moral support and reassurance as required.
- The nurse can assist the injector as necessary with opening of packets, passing equipment as necessary.
- Most procedures are uneventful but occasionally the patient may feel a little faint following the procedure; if this happens lie the patient down and where possible elevate the feet.
- Following the procedure offer the patient assistance to dress if necessary.
- Written information should be provided on aftercare following the injection.
- The nurse should reinforce information regarding rest following the injection and provide a contact number for the patient to ring should there be any concern or complications.

Dealing with samples of synovial fluid

- If the joint is aspirated it is usual for the fluid to be examined for colour, clarity, and viscosity.
- If there is inflammation, such as RA, within the joint, the fluid is much more yellow and volume is high.
- In OA, the volume of fluid is often lower, the fluid more clear, and much more viscous (like egg white).
- The amount of fluid aspirated should be recorded as this can give an indication of the amount of inflammation that was present in the joint.
- Low volumes, however, do not necessarily indicate that there is no IA process; in some cases, when there is a large amount of inflammation the synovial membrane is thrown up into villous-type folds and the fluid becomes loculated or trapped in these folds. Fibrin and rice bodies and other debris may hinder aspiration
- Specimens can be sent in a universal container for Gram stain, microscopy, culture and sensitivity, as routine; these investigations are mandatory if infection is suspected. (Request a Gram stain, MC&S on the microbiology form.)
- The universal container should be labelled with patient name, date of birth, hospital number, and description of the site of fluid aspiration and other essential information requested by the laboratory.
- Polarized light microscopy is the routine examination in an acute red joint as this identifies crystals. (Requested as crystals on the microbiology form.)
- Gout crystals (monosodium urate) show up under polarized light as long needle-shaped crystals that have a strong (negative) birefringence.
- CPP crystals are seen as short, thick, rhomboid-shaped rods and show a weak (positive) birefringence.

Contraindications to intra-articular steroid injections and post-treatment advice

It is important to assess patients prior to undertaking or supporting the administration of a joint injection. Patients should not receive a joint injection if there is:

- Evidence of any active infection e.g. fever, coloured sputum, UTI, skin infection as the infection can spread to the joint.
- Joint sepsis—aspiration of the joint is mandatory, with specimens being sent for Gram stain, culture and sensitivity.
- Previous infection in the joint to be injected in the past 6 months. There is a risk of continued presence of a small pocket of sub-clinical infection which may flare as a result of the steroid injection.
- Patient currently taking antibiotics.
- Broken, damaged, or ulcerated skin near or at the injection site, as there is a route in for infection and therefore the patient is at ↑ risk of infection.
- Prosthetic joints are never injected in routine clinical practice.
- Unstable coagulopathy, patients on warfarin need a stable INR.
- Planned surgery in the next 2 weeks.
- Unstable diabetes (warn diabetic patients of the potential effect on the blood glucose).
- Fracture in or near the joint as steroids can impair the local healing process.
- Active TB.
- Ocular herpes.
- Acute psychosis or strong history of previous steroid psychosis.
- Severe local osteoporosis near the joint.
- When joint destruction is severe and there is marked instability.
- Hypersensitivity to any of the components of the injection.

▶ Pregnancy: a recent review on the use of corticosteroids state there is no convincing evidence that systemic corticosteroids ↑ the risk of congenital abnormalities. Therefore the use of short term treatments such as IA injections should **not** be considered a contraindication. Treatment as with all patients should be taken by the prescribing clinician based upon a risk benefit analysis (refer to *BNF*).

Subcutaneous therapies: overview

Medications can be delivered via a number of different routes depending upon the pharmacodynamics of the drug and the prescriber must consider:
- How the drug is absorbed and distributed.
- The processes involved in metabolizing and excreting the drug.

The subcutaneous route is used to enable a slow but sustained absorption of a drug therapy. However, the rate of absorption will depend upon the site of the injection. Diffusion through the tissues and removal/transportation of the drug by local blood supply are essential for the drug to have the planned treatment effect. Absorption from the abdomen is considered the fastest route. However, it is essential that injection sites are rotated to prevent fat atrophy, induration, or scarring. Sites that can be used for safe subcutaneous administration include:
- Abdomen.
- Outer aspect of the thigh and buttocks.
- The upper outer aspect of the top of the arm.

Drugs are delivered subcutaneously because they would be significantly altered by the oral route or need a greater 'steady state' in the sense of slow and sustained release. Examples of therapies administered via the subcutaneous route include:
- Insulin.
- Vaccines.
- Sustained pain relief (e.g. using a Graseby pump).
- MTX.
- Monoclonal antibodies (e.g. anti-TNFα therapies).

Therapies that are administered via the subcutaneous route for MSC include:
- Monoclonal antibodies (e.g. anti-TNFα therapies):
  - Anti-TNFα therapies (adalimumab, and etanercept).
  - Interleukin 1 receptor agonist (anakinra).
- PTH—an anabolic treatment for osteoporosis: Preotact®.
- MTX—a cytotoxic immunosuppressant therapy that is also co-prescribed with monoclonal antibodies such as adalimumab, etanercept (also delivered subcutaneously), and infliximab.
  - Metoject® a prefilled syringe of MTX—different dosing regimens.
- ▶ Subcutaneous MTX is an important therapeutic option for patients who have:
  - Intolerance due to GI symptoms.
  - Require greater bioavailability.
  - If nurses are administering subcutaneous therapies (rather than patient self-administered) this may be used to resolve some issues in relation to concerns related to compliance of oral therapies.

Note: where possible it is usual to encourage and support patients (or a carer) to be trained to self-administer subcutaneous injections to optimize efficiency of service /resources and cost effectiveness of nurse time.

Community support for patients receiving subcutaneous therapies

There are a number of organizations that can provide community support for patients requiring subcutaneous therapies. These organizations can provide:

- A package of care as part of the purchase of the treatment. For some therapies this service is integral to the prescribing and offers a service that can train the patient to self-administer or check their technique and deliver subcutaneous therapies to the patient's home on a regular basis.
- Regular pre-arranged deliveries that ensure the treatment is managed and stored at the correct temperature whilst in transit for those therapies that require specific temperature control.
- Provide continuity of service.

Patient self-administration of subcutaneous therapies

Patient can self-administer subcutaneous injections providing they:
- Consent to being trained and take responsibility for the treatment and equipment in their own home. In some cases a patient unable to inject themselves may nominate a close relative or partner to be trained to inject.
- Have the ability to recall and sustain the steps involved in self-administration including:
  - Apply appropriate hygiene techniques in preparing to inject.
  - Maintain trained techniques in administering treatment, ensuring aseptic technique.
  - Have the functional ability to administer the treatment (or have a nominated carer who can be trained).
  - Will be able to maintain concordance with monitoring and treatment regimens.
  - Can recognize the risks related to home administration and storage of drugs and equipment (including responsible disposal of equipment and spillage).

A detailed guidance on patient self-administration for biologic therapies and MTX has been developed.[1,2]

Benefits of patient self-administration
- Independence for the patient—flexibility for work and social activities.
- Can encourage the patient to perceive themselves as having an enhanced ability to self-management and reduce perceptions of reliance on healthcare support.
- ↓ nursing activity costs/resources.

Risks related to patient self-administration
- ↓ patient contact and times to carry out opportunistic review/education/support.
- ↓ vigilance by team with regard to disease activity/infections or side effects.
- Risks related to poor concordance to monitoring /failure to adhere to standards of self-administration/drug storages and management

Training patients to self-administer subcutaneous therapies

Training patients to self-administer subcutaneous injections has been undertaken for a number of years and much of the expertise in this field has been developed from the field of diabetes and patient-administered subcutaneous injections of insulin.

A step-wise approach to training patients to self-administers subcutaneous therapies have been specifically developed for patients with MSC. Documentation and frameworks for nursing practice, patient training tools and check lists are available. They include:
- MTX—a cytotoxic drug administered at doses <25mg.[1]
- Biologic therapies—monoclonal antibodies (anti-TNFα).[2]

Key issues in patient-administered subcutaneous therapies

- Patients must express an interest in participating in the training and consent to treatment.
- Select patients who fulfil the criteria for treatment.
- Provide a comprehensive training programme for patients (and partner/carer). Review patient's confidence and technique before home administration.
- Must be able to adhere to aseptic techniques and recommended storage of treatments in home environment.
- Encourage rotation of injection sites.
- Ensure monitoring and co-prescriptions of drug therapies are considered, e.g.:
  - Patient may be self-administering 2 different subcutaneous therapies e.g. adalimumab (biologic) and MTX (cytotoxic therapy). Disposal for MTX requires cytotoxic storage and disposal policy.
- Provide written and verbal information on key point of contact (e.g. telephone advice line).
- If receiving anti-TNFα ensure patient 'alert card' issued—advising patient of when to receive prompt medical advice.[3]
- Review patients on at least an annual basis to check subcutaneous injection technique.
- Training must be provided by competent nurses who can:
  - Provide evidence based drug information, including risks and benefits of treatment.
  - Demonstrate the procedure with clarity and tailor education according to the individual patient's learning needs.
  - Ensure adequate documentation of processes.
  - Recognize limitations of their practice.

References

1. Royal College of Nursing (2004). *Administering subcutaneous methotrexate for inflammatory arthritis.* RCN, London.

2. Royal College of Nursing (2003). *Assessing, managing and monitoring biologic therapies for inflammatory arthritis.* RCN, London.

3. 'Alert card' produced by Arthritis Research Campaign: ⌨ www.arc.org.uk

Frequently asked questions: subcutaneous therapies

Should subcutaneous injections be injected at 45° or 90°?

Evidence supports a 90° angle. You should use a 26-gauge needle, with a 8mm length and then pinch the skin so you can then insert the needle at a 90° angle. The decision to pinch or not to pinch relies upon the needle length (shorter needle will not require a pinch technique) and angle of injection (45° will require a pinch technique).

Are there any specific issues I need to consider for patients who are obese or thin when administering subcutaneous injections?

Studies demonstrate that patients who are obese or thin still receive the drug into the subcutaneous tissues if injected as recommended.

Do patients self-administering MTX need to wear masks, goggles, and aprons?

It is important that routine cytotoxic management and disposal of used equipment are adhered to according to local trust or organizational policy. Patients do not need to wear masks or goggles. Aprons may be appropriate to protect clothing or accidental spillage depending upon the site they are injecting (e.g. an apron will not be appropriate when injecting into the abdomen).

Why are patients giving subcutaneous MTX (an unlicensed indication) when it can be taken orally?

MTX is an inexpensive therapy and research has not been commissioned by the pharmaceutical companies to demonstrate the benefits of the subcutaneous route of administration for IJDs. However, the pharmacokinetics show that MTX is more readily absorbed and reduces some of the unacceptable side effects some patients experience taking MTX orally. A licensed pre-filled subcutaneous MTX is available at different dosing regimens although more costly than the oral route.

Is it common for patients to get reactions following subcutaneous administration of biologic therapies such as adalimumab and etanercept?

Biologic therapies are foreign proteins and have the potential to cause a reaction to treatment in the same way that a blood transfusion can. However, the most commonly reported problem for subcutaneous therapies is that of injection site reactions (>10%) although only ~7% of patients discontinue treatment due to injection site reactions.

Why are patients treated with biologic DMARDs advised to carry an 'alert card'?

The 'alert card' is to remind patients to tell all HCPs that they are receiving a biologic DMARD and highlights the need to treat all infections seriously and to seek specialist guidance on biologic DMARDs.

Intravenous therapies: overview

Issues related to infusions and good practice

Nurses are responsible for the correct administration of prescribed medicines to patients in their care at all times, being guided by the Nursing and Midwifery Council standards. The nurse should have knowledge of the use, action, dosing regimens, side effects, and interactions of any medicines being administered and be competent to prepare and administer the infusion.

Local policies and procedures should be in place to assist the nurse in safe preparation and administration of IV medicines and should be adhered to at all times. Pharmacists should provide appropriate information and advice to all staff and in some cases will have responsibility for preparing medicines to be administered by the parenteral route.

Checklist for preparation and administration of IV medicines[1]

- Pre-plan before drawing up doses.
- Be sure of local protocols.
- Check medicine against prescription—check that the dose, time, and route are correct.
- Check patient identification.
- Check IV site.
- Check that any equipment required is working.
- Know how to administer each medicine, e.g.:
  - Calculation of concentration and rate.
  - Reconstitution.
  - Addition of medicines to recommended diluents.
  - Check package insert, SPC, local medicines information pharmacist.
- Use aseptic technique during reconstitution steps, addition of medicine to diluents, and care of the line.
- Maintain a sterile, particle-free solution.
- Thoroughly mix any additions, checking for precipitation or particles.
- Complete infusion additive label and attach to infusion.
- Understand how the medicine works and explain this to the patient if appropriate.
- Continue to monitor for precipitation, patient response, or adverse effects, where appropriate.

Reference

1. UCL Hospitals (2007). *Injectable Medicines Administration Guide*. Blackwell Publishing, Oxford.

Further reading

Dougherty L, Lister S (eds) (2006). *The Royal Marsden Hospital Manual of Clinical Nursing Procedures*, 6th edn. Blackwell Publishing. Oxford.

Royal College of Nursing (2003). *Standards for Infusion Therapy*. RCN, London.

Summary of Product Characteristics for individual medicines.

Abatacept

Abatacept selectively modulates the activation of T cells involved in the immune system's inflammatory response which can lead to joint pain, swelling, and ultimately damage in RA. It is licensed for the treatment of RA in combination with MTX in patients who have had an inadequate response or intolerance to DMARDs and at least 1 anti-TNF treatment. It is currently being reviewed by NICE.

Pre-treatment screening
- Detailed history and physical examination.
- Chest x-ray.
- TB screening.
- Viral hepatitis screening.
- Routine blood tests.
- Baseline DAS28 measurements.

Contraindications
- Hypersensitivity to abatacept or to any of the excipients.
- Active acute or chronic infection.
- Concomitant use of other biologic agents.
- Demyelinating disease.
- Pregnancy.
- Use in children (safety not yet established).
- Live vaccines at time of treatment or within 3 months of use.

Cautions
- COPD.
- Any underlying condition that predisposes to infection.
- History of recurrent or persistent infection.

Treatment regimen
- Infusion given at weeks 0, 2, 4, and then every 4 weeks thereafter (Table 18.1) (☐ see Administration/nursing care, p.507).
- MTX weekly.

Table 18.1 Abatacept infusion

Body weight	Dose	Number of 250mg vials
<60kg	500mg	2
≥60kg to ≤100kg	750mg	3
>100kg	1000mg	4

Drugs which may be needed at time of infusion
- Chlorpheniramine: 10mg IV tds.
- Hydrocortisone: 100mg IV tds.
- Metoclopramide: 10mg IV tds.
- Paracetamol: 1g orally qds (max 4g in 24 hours).

Practical considerations

- **_Equipment:_** full resuscitation facilities and infusion pump are required. A sterile non-pyrogenic, low-protein-binding filter (pore size 0.2μm to <1.2μm) is essential. A silicone-free disposable syringe is provided and this must be used to reconstitute each vial.
- **_Time and nursing resources:_** infusions take 30min. Close monitoring required.
- **_Handling:_** abatacept does not require any special handling precautions.

Administration/nursing care

Prior to treatment

- Check there are no contraindications to treatment (📖 see Contrindications, p.508).
- Check any recent blood tests are within satisfactory parameters.
- Record baseline observations of: temperature, pulse, blood pressure.
- Urinalysis if symptoms of infection are reported.

Preparation

Prepare the infusion according to manufacturer's guidelines. Abatacept is supplied in 250mg vials as a dry powder. Each vial is reconstituted with 10mL of sterile water for injections using the silicone-free disposable syringe provided with each vial and an 18–21-gauge needle.

The reconstituted solution must be immediately diluted to 100mL with sodium chloride 0.9% solution i.e. withdraw the equivalent volume of fluid from a 100mL bag (20mL for 2 vials; 30mL for 3 vials; 40mL for 4 vials) and replace with the abatacept solution.

Administering the infusion

- Abatacept is infused through a filter into a peripheral cannula using an IV pump with a primed line.
- Abatacept should be administered over 30min.

Clinical observations during infusions

No routine observations during the infusion are required; however, in the event that the patient reports feeling unwell, observations should be monitored and recorded. Observe for any signs of respiratory deterioration in those with COPD.

Repeat baseline observations 1 hour after the infusion starts (see 📖 Post infusion care, p.510).

Observe for side effects throughout—take appropriate action as listed next and record any adverse events in the patient's notes:

- ⚠ Anaphylactic reactions have been reported. In this event:
  - Stop infusion.
  - Call physician.
  - Administer IV hydrocortisone, IV chlorpheniramine and/or any emergency treatment as indicated.
- Acute infusion–related events (i.e. those that occur within 1 hour of the infusion) are most commonly dizziness, headaches, and hypertension.
- Headache and nausea are the most common side effects occurring in ≥1/10 patients following the infusion.
- For full list of adverse effects please see SPC.

Post-infusion care and advice to patients

- Discharge patient post-infusion providing observations taken 1 hour after the infusion start time are satisfactory.
- Advise patient to:
  - Seek medical advice if any symptoms develop suggestive of an infection, e.g. fever in the hours or days after the infusion (provide contact numbers for the Rheumatology Department or first contact point e.g. GP and/or attend A&E).
  - Maintain regular MTX monitoring according to BSR and local guidelines.
  - If diabetic, patients need to be aware that abatacept interferes with blood glucose monitoring strips (GDH-PHQ) resulting in falsely elevated blood glucose readings on the day of the infusion.
- Ensure follow-up for assessment or next infusion has been arranged.
- Ensure patient has a Biologics Alert Card.

Patient information

Patient information leaflets are available from:
- Arthritis Research Campaign: ᐀ www.arc.co.uk
- National Rheumatoid Arthritis Society: ᐀ www.rheumatoid.org.uk

Further reading

BSR website: ᐀ www.rheumatology.org.uk

Joint Formulary Committee (2008). *British National Formulary*, 56th edn. British Medical Association and Royal Pharmaceutical Society of Great Britain, London.

NICE website: ᐀ www.nice.org

Summary of Product Characteristics, see: ᐀ www.medicines.org.uk

Ibandronate

Ibandronate is a bisphosphonate licensed in 2005 to treat osteoporosis in postmenopausal ♀. It selectively inhibits osteoclast activity without affecting bone formation, leading to an ↑ in bone mass. There is evidence for reduction in vertebral fractures; however, efficacy in femoral fracture reduction is yet to be established.

Contraindications (*BNF*)
- Clinically significant hypersensitivity to ibandronate.
- Hypocalcaemia (see 'Cautions').

Cautions
- Renal impairment
- Uncorrected hypocalcaemia—this should be treated before starting Ibandronate therapy.
- Rarely, osteonecrosis of the jaw has been reported in patients receiving IV bisphosphonates for the treatment of cancer and also in some patients taking oral bisphosphonates with concomitant corticosteroids. Most cases are linked with invasive dental procedures. Patients with risk factors (e.g. corticosteroids, cancer, chemotherapy, poor oral hygiene etc.) should have dental examination prior to treatment and avoid invasive procedures during treatment.

See *BNF* or SPC for full list.

Treatment regimen
- Ibandronate IV injection 3mg every 3 months
- Calcium and vitamin D supplementation

Practical considerations
- *Equipment:* access to resuscitation facilities.
- *Time and nursing resources:* given over 15–30 seconds as bolus IV injection.
- *Handling:* no special precautions required.

Administration/nursing care
- *Preparation of ibandronate:* ibandronate is supplied as pre-filled syringe.
- *Administering the infusion:* given over 15–30sec as bolus IV injection.
- *Observations:* not required unless the patient reports feeling unwell.

Post infusion care and advice
- Advise patient to take any calcium and vitamin D supplements at least 60min after the infusion.
- The patient should remain in the department for 20min after the 1st injection in case of allergic response. They may then be discharged if there are no reported side effects. Subsequently they may be discharged as soon as the infusion is completed in the absence of side effects.
- Advise the patient that they may have transient flu-like symptoms particularly after the 1st injection. Paracetamol can be taken to relieve these symptoms. Occasionally there is temporary pain in bones and muscles and rarely, nausea and/or abdominal pain.

Patient information

Patient information leaflets are available from:
- Arthritis Research Campaign: www.arc.co.uk
- National Osteoposoris Society: www.nos.org.uk
- Paget's society: www.paget.org.uk

Further reading

Joint Formulary Committee (2008). *British National Formulary*, 56th edn. British Medical Association and Royal Pharmaceutical Society of Great Britain, London.

Summary of Product Characteristics, see: www.medicines.org.uk

Iloprost

Iloprost is licensed for the treatment of some types of pulmonary hypertension and recently a nebulized version has been introduced for the treatment of pulmonary hypertension (Ventavis®). However, it may only be used under specialist supervision. The use of iloprost infusions for the treatment of Raynaud's and scleroderma remain unlicensed indications.

Contraindications (*BNF*)

- Unstable angina.
- Within 6 months of MI or 3 months of cardiovascular events.
- Pulmonary occlusive disease.
- Cardiac failure.
- Severe arrhythmias.
- Heart valve defects.
- Conditions which ↑ risk of bleeding.
- Pregnancy or breastfeeding.

Interactions/cautions

↑ risk of bleeding if given with NSAIDS, aspirin, phenindione, clopigrel, eptifibatide, tirofiban, and anticoagulants. Caution with antihypertesives. See *BNF* or SPC for full list.

Treatment regimen for Raynaud's syndrome and scleroderma

- IV iloprost 100mcg in 500mL sodium chloride or glucose 5% (0.2mcg/mL).
- To be infused continuously for up to a maximum of 6 hours daily (as tolerated) on 3–5 consecutive days (see Fig. 18.1).

Drugs which may be needed at time of infusion: paracetamol (or other analgesic) and anti-emetics as required.

Practical considerations

- *Equipment:* full resuscitation facilities and infusion pump required. Bed or fully reclining chair.
- *Time and nursing resources:* each infusion lasts for 6 hours and therefore may be given on an outpatient basis. Close monitoring is required.
- *Handling:* iloprost must be correctly diluted before being administered. If the solution comes in contact with skin or eyes, wash off immediately with large amount of water and rinse thoroughly. Contact with skin may cause a long lasting but painless erythema.

Administration/nursing care

Preparation of iloprost solution for use with infusion pump

Add 1mL (100mcg) iloprost to 500mL infusion fluid (sodium chloride 0.9% or glucose 5%) and mix well. The resulting solution of iloprost is at a concentration of 0.2mcg per mL. In units where the staff are using a syringe driver, make up according to manufacturer's guidelines.

Administering the infusion/observations

Take baseline observations of temperature, pulse, blood pressure.
- Days 1–3 (dosage titration): see Fig. 18.1

- Day 4 to the end of treatment (infusion of optimal dose): start the infusion at the optimal rate[b] and infuse at this rate for 6 hours.

Start the infusion at 10mL/hour
Check heart rate and blood pressure after 30min

↓

| **If previous dose has been tolerated, ↑ to 20mL/hour** Check heart rate and blood pressure after 30min | → | If unacceptable adverse effects[a] reduce rate by 10mL/hour |

↓

| **If previous dose has been tolerated, ↑ to 30mL/hour** Check heart rate and blood pressure after 30min | → | If unacceptable adverse effects[a] reduce rate by 10mL/hour |

↓

| **If previous dose has been tolerated, ↑ to 40mL/hour** Check heart rate and blood pressure after 30min | → | If unacceptable adverse effects[a] reduce rate by 10mL/hour |

↓

| Continue as above, ↑ **the rate by 10ml/hour** every 30min (providing the previous dose has been tolerated) until the optimal rate is established[b] Continue observations every 30min | → | If unacceptable adverse effects,[a] reduce rate by 10mL/hour |

↓

Stop the infusion after 6 hours[c]

Fig. 18.1 Iloprost infusion

Figure 18.1 notes: iloprost infusion treatment issues

[a]*Adverse effects*

- Common adverse effects: facial flushing, headache, nausea and vomiting, abdominal cramps.
- If these are considered unacceptable by the patient, reduce the rate as above.
- Give analgesics and/or anti-emetics as required.
- Serious adverse effects: persistent clinically significant drop in BP, persistent clinically significant tachycardia, vagal reaction with bradycardia, nausea and vomiting.
- If these occur, **stop the infusion**. The infusion may be restarted one hour after the symptoms have resolved at HALF the previous rate.

ᵇOptimal rate/dose:
- The infusion rate is ↑ by 10mL/hour every 30min as detailed above until unacceptable adverse effects occur. The infusion rate is then reduced by 10mL/hour. This reduced rate is the optimal infusion rate.
- For the majority of patients the optimal infusion rate will not exceed 50ml/hour. For patients weighing <75kg the optimal infusion rate will rarely exceed 40mL/hour. A small proportion of patients may tolerate higher rates.

ᶜLength of infusion:
- The total maximum length of the infusion, including the rate titration, is 6 hours.

Post-infusion care

The patient may be discharged at the end of the infusion providing they are not experiencing any adverse effects and observations at the end of the infusion are satisfactory.

Patient information

Patient information leaflets are available from:
- Raynaud's and Scleroderma Society: ⁰ www.raynauds.org.uk
- The Scleroderma Society: ⁰ www.schlerodermasociety.co.uk

Further reading

Joint Formulary Committee (2008). *British National Formulary*, 56th edn. British Medical Association and Royal Pharmaceutical Society of Great Britain, London.

Summary of Product Characteristics, see: ⁰ www.medicines.org.uk

Wigley FM *et al.* (1994). Intravenous iloprost infusion in patients with Raynaud phenomenon secondary to systemic sclerosis: a multicenter, placebo-controlled, double-blind study. *Annals of Internal Medicine* **120**(3), 199–206.

Infliximab

Infliximab is a biologically engineered monoclonal antibody. It inhibits activation of TNFα, an important cytokine implicated in activating inflammatory responses.. It is licensed for use in RA, AS, psoriasis, PsA, ulcerative colitis, and Crohn's disease. Criteria for patient selection, use, and response are available from NICE, RCN, and BSR.

⚠ Infliximab should be co-prescribed with MTX once weekly

Pre-treatment screening
- Detailed history and physical examination.
- Chest x-ray and TB screening.
- Routine blood tests.
- Baseline DAS28 measurements.
- ANA.
- DNA binding (dsDNA).
- Hepatitis B screening.

Contraindications
- Hypersensitivity to infliximab or other murine proteins.
- Active acute or chronic infection.
- Previous sepsis in prosthetic joints where replacement remains in situ.
- Severe heart failure NYHA Class III/IV (caution in NYHA I/II).
- Demyelinating disease.
- Pregnancy.
- Use in children <18 years of age (safety not yet established).
- Live vaccines.

Treatment regimen
- RA—initial dose 3mg per kg body weight.
  - Infusions at weeks 0, 2, 6, and then every 8 weeks.
- PsA—initial dose 5mg per kg body weight.
  - Infusions at weeks 0, 2, 6, and then every 8 weeks.
- AS—initial dose 5mg per kg body weight.
  - Infusions at weeks 0, 2, 6, and then every 6–8 weeks.
- All indications—dose ↑ may sometimes be considered for inadequate response (see SPC).

Drugs which may be needed at time of infusion
- Chlorpheniramine: 10 mg IV   tds.
- Hydrocortisone: 100mg IV   tds.
- Metoclopramide: 10mg IV   tds.
- Paracetamol: 1g orally qds (max 4g in 24 hours).

Practical considerations
- *Equipment:* full resuscitation facilities and infusion pump are required. A sterile low protein binding filter (pore size <1.2μm) is essential.
- *Time and nursing resources:* infusions take between 1–2 hours. Close monitoring required. Patient must be observed for 2 hours following first 4 infusions, and then for 1 hour following subsequent infusions.
- *Handling:* infliximab does not require any special handling precautions.

Administration/nursing care

Prior to treatment

- Check that there are no contraindications to treatment.
- Check recent blood tests are within satisfactory parameters.
- Urinalysis.
- Record baseline observations of:
  - Temperature, pulse, and blood pressure.
- Prepare the infusion according to manufacturer's guidelines. It is supplied in vials as a dry powder. One vial mixed with 10mL sterile water equates to 100mg infliximab. The prescribed dose is added to 250mL 0.9% sodium chloride. Vials should not be shared between patients as this can ↑ the risk of contamination. .

Administering the infusion: infliximab is infused through a filter (see 'Equipment') into a peripheral cannula using an IV pump with a primed line.

Clinical observations during infusions

- Every 30min—temperature, pulse, and blood pressure.
- Observe for side effects throughout: take appropriate action as shown below and record any adverse events in the patient's notes.

Infusion reactions and adverse events (Table 18.2)

Table 18.2 Infliximab infusion reactions and adverse events

Infusion reaction	Action
Mild fever, chills, pruritus	• Slow down rate of infusion
Chest pain, hypertension, hypotension and/or dyspnoea	• Stop infusion • Alert physician—consider use of IV hydrocortisone and /or IV chlorpheniramine • Review with physician—consider restarting infusion after 20min at a slower rate
Anaphylactic reaction	• Stop infusion • Call physician—administer IV hydrocortisone IV chlorpheniramine and any emergency treatment as indicated

Post infusion care and advice to patients

Discharge patient post-infusion providing all observations are satisfactory. Monitor blood pressure, temperature, and pulse every 30min for 2 hours following first 4 infusions, and then for 1 hour following subsequent infusions. Advise patient to seek medical advice for symptoms of infection and to maintain their regular monitoring and clinical attendances. Ensure next infusion date booked and patient has a Biologics Alert Card. Provide first contact point telephone numbers to the patient

Patient information

Patient information leaflets are available from:
- Arthritis Research Campaign: ⌐ www.arc.co.uk

Further reading

Additional information can be accessed from BSR website: ⌐ www.rheumatology.org.uk.

Methylprednisolone

Intravenous methylprednisolone is given to patients in a number of rheumatological conditions to suppress inflammation.

Contraindications
- Active infection.

Cautions
- Unstable diabetes mellitus.
- Unstable cardiac conditions.
- Avoid concomitant use of live vaccines.
- Recent contact with shingles/chicken pox.

Refer to BNF for complete listings

Treatment regimen
- Methylprednisolone 500mg or 1g in 250mL 0.9% sodium chloride.
- 3 infusions may be prescribed to be given over a 3-day period.

Practical considerations
- *Equipment:* full resuscitation facilities and infusion pump required.
- *Time and nursing resources:* infusions usually last for 60min. Close monitoring required.
- *Handling:* no special precautions required.

Administration/nursing care
- Prepare the infusion according to manufacturer's guidelines.

Administering the infusion
As prescribed on the drug chart. Commonly the infusion will be given over a period of 60min.

Clinical observations during infusions
Pre infusion: record pulse and blood pressure as a baseline. Further observations are not required unless the patient reports feeling unwell.

Infusion reactions and adverse events
- Rare cases of anaphylaxis have been reported.
- Rarely, cardiac arrhythmias and/or circulatory collapse and/or cardiac arrest can occur. Usually associated with rapid administration of large doses (>500mg in <10min).
- Refer to *BNF*/SPC for complete list.

Post infusion care
The patient should remain in the day unit for 1 hour after the 1st infusion for observation. If further infusions are given, the patient may be discharged as soon as the infusion is completed, providing there are no reported side effects.

Patient information

Patient information leaflets are available from:
• Arthritis Research Campaign: www.arc.co.uk

Further reading

Joint Formulary Committee (2008). *British National Formulary*, 56th edn. British Medical Association and Royal Pharmaceutical Society of Great Britain, London.

Summary of Product Characteristics, see: www.medicines.org.uk

Pamidronate

Pamidronate is a bisphosphonate used to treat the over-production of bone and relieve pain associated with Paget's disease. It is given to treat osteoporosis when oral preparations are not deemed appropriate or cannot be tolerated. Other licensed uses include tumour induced hypercalcaemia and metastatic bone pain.

Contraindications

- Clinically significant hypersensitivity to Pamidronate disodium or other bisphosphonates

Cautions

- Should not be given with other bisphophonates.
- Rarely, osteonecrosis of the jaw has been reported in patients receiving IV bisphosphonates for the treatment of cancer and also in some patients taking oral bisphosphonates with concomitant corticosteroids. Most cases are linked with invasive dental procedures. Patients with risk factors (e.g. corticosteroids, cancer, chemotherapy, poor oral hygiene etc.) should have dental examination prior to treatment and avoid invasive procedures during treatment.
- In patients with Paget's who may be at risk of calcium or vitamin D deficiency, oral supplementation should be considered.

See *BNF* or SPC for full list.

Treatment regimen for Paget's

Pamidronate 60mg in 250mL sodium chloride 0.9% is often prescribed but other regimens may be used. See *BNF* and SPC for complete listings.

Practical considerations

- ***Equipment:*** full resuscitation facilities and infusion pump required.
- ***Time and nursing resources:*** infusions may last for 1–3 hours.
- ***Handling:*** no special precautions required.

Administration/nursing care

Preparation of pamidronate

Pamidronate is supplied as a dry powder and should be prepared according to the instructions given by the manufacturer. It should never be given as a bolus injection.

Administering the infusion/observations

- In order to minimize local reaction a large vein should be selected for cannula insertion.
- Infusion rate should not exceed 60mg per hour and in renal impairment, the rate should not exceed 20mg hour.
- Pre infusion: record pulse and blood pressure as a baseline.
- These observations do not need to be repeated unless the patient reports feeling unwell.

Post-infusion care and advice

- The patient should remain in the department for 1 hour after the 1st infusion in case of allergic response. They may then be discharged if there are no reported side effects. Subsequently they may be discharged as soon as the infusion is completed in the absence of side effects.
- Serum electrolytes, calcium, and phosphate should be monitored as levels may fall 24–48 hours post infusion, normalization is achieved between 3–7 days. It is therefore suggested that blood levels are checked prior to the infusion and after 1 week.
- Advise the patient that they may have a rise in body temperature in the next 24–48 hours and/or flu-like symptoms. Paracetamol can be taken to relieve these symptoms. Occasionally there is temporary pain in bones and muscles and rarely, nausea and/or abdominal pain.
- There are rare cases of somnolence and /or dizziness after the infusion therefore the patient should be advised not to drive home.

Patient information

Patient information leaflets are available from:
- Arthritis Research Campaign: www.arc.co.uk
- National Osteoposoris Society: www.nos.org.uk
- Paget's society: www.paget.org.uk

Further reading

Joint Formulary Committee (2008). *British National Formulary*, 56th edn. British Medical Association and Royal Pharmaceutical Society of Great Britain, London.

Summary of Product Characteristics, see: www.medicines.org.uk

Rituximab

Rituximab is a genetically engineered chimeric mouse/human antibody designed to deplete pre-cursor B cells. It is indicated for use in severe active RA in combination with MTX in adult patients who have had an inadequate response or intolerance to other DMARDs, including 1 or more TNFα inhibitor therapies. NICE approval was granted in 2007.

Pre-treatment screening

- Detailed history and physical examination.
- Chest x-ray.
- Routine blood tests.
- Hepatitis B screen.
- Immunoglobulin levels.
- Baseline DAS28.
- CD19 may be considered.
- Any inactivated vaccinations should be given 1 month prior or at least 7 months after treatment (no live vaccines).

Contraindications

- Hypersensitivity to rituximab or other murine proteins.
- Active acute or chronic infection.
- Severe heart failure NYHA Class IV.
- Pregnancy.
- Use in children (safety not yet established).

Treatment regimen

- IV 1000mg rituximab on day 1 and day 15.
- MTX weekly.

Further courses of may be considered 6–12 months after initial course.

Drugs prior to infusion

All given 60min prior to infusion:
- Methylprednisolone: 100mg IV (100mg in 100mL normal saline infused over 30min)
- Paracetamol: 1g orally
- Chlorpheniramine: 10mg IV

Drugs which may be needed at time of infusion

- Chlorpheniramine: 10mg IV tds
- Hydrocortisone: 100mg IV tds
- Metoclopramide: 10mg IV tds
- Paracetamol: 1g orally qds (max 4g in 24 hours)

Practical considerations

- *Equipment:* full resuscitation facilities and infusion pump required.
- *Time and nursing resources:* 1st infusion may take between 6–7 hours, the 2nd can be completed more quickly if no adverse effects during first one. Close monitoring required.
- *Handling:* as rituximab is not an irritant there are no special handling precautions in the case of extravasation.

Administration/nursing care

- Check no analgesics containing paracetamol have been taken within last 4 hours and that any morning dose of anti-hypertensives have been omitted.
- Take baseline observations of temperature, pulse, blood pressure and SaO_2.
- Administer pre-infusion medications as per drug chart 60min before rituximab.
- In units where the staff prepare the infusion, make up rituximab according to manufacturer's guidelines.

Administering the infusion

- Rituximab is infused through a peripheral cannula using an IV pump with a primed line.
- The following regimen is based on a concentration of 2mg/mL i.e. 1000mg in 500mL.
- The rate of the infusion will depend on the concentration of the rituximab and whether it is the 1st or 2nd infusion. In the event of a reaction to the 1st infusion, the 2nd infusion should be administered as per instructions for the 1st infusion (Tables 18.3, 18.4, 18.5).

Table 18.3 Rituximab infusion rate for day 1

Time	mg/hour	mL/hour
1st 30min	50mg/hour	25mL/hour
2nd 30min	100mg/hour	50mL/hour

Then the rate can be ↑ by 50mg/hour (25mL/hour) every 30min to a maximum rate of 400mg/hour (200mL/hour) providing no adverse reactions occur

Table 18.4 Rituximab infusion rate for day 15—if the patient had no reaction to the 1st infusion

Time	mg/hour	mL/hour
1st 30min	100mg/hour	50mL/hour
2nd 30min	200mg/hour	100mL/hour

Then the rate can be ↑ by 100mg/hour (50mL/hour) every 30min to a maximum rate of 400mg/hour (200mL/hour) providing no adverse reactions occur

Table 18.5 Rituximab can be diluted to a concentration of between 1–4mg/mL normal saline

Concentration	1mg/mL	2mg/mL	4mg/mL
Volume of fluid	1000mL	500mL	250mL

Clinical observations during infusions

- Blood pressure.
- Pulse.
- Temperature.
- Oxygen saturation levels.

1st hour every 15min then every 30min (prior to ↑ the rate of infusion and until infusion completed).

NB: most reactions have been noted during the first few minutes of the infusion so observe the patient carefully during this time and following each ↑ in infusion rate

Infusion reactions and adverse events

Acute infusion reactions may occur within 1–2 hours of the 1st rituximab infusion (Table 18.6). These may include:
- Fever.
- Headache.
- Rigors.
- Flushing.
- Nausea.
- Rash.
- URTI symptoms.

Transient hypotension and bronchospasm are usually related to the infusion rate. A small ↑ in serious infections has been noted (not opportunistic infections such as TB).

Table 18.6 Rituximab infusion reactions

Reaction	Action to take
Mild-to-moderate reactions (30–35% at 1st infusion; less with the 2nd)—e.g. low grade fever; hypotension <30mmHg from baseline	• Halve the infusion rate • Consider giving prn medication
Moderate-to-severe reactions (uncommon: frequency is reduced by the concomitant use of IV steroids)— e.g. fever >38.5°C; chills; mucosal swelling; SOB; hypotension by >30mmHg from baseline	• STOP the infusion and treat the symptoms. • Contact the doctor. • The infusion should be restarted at half the previous rate only when the symptoms have resolved

Post infusion care advice for the patient

- Can leave the department once infusion is complete and observations satisfactory.
- Seek medical advice if any symptoms suggestive of an infection e.g. fever in the hours or days after the infusion (provide contact numbers for the Rheumatology Department or 1st contact point e.g. GP and/or attend A&E).
- Restart any anti-hypertensive drugs on next day.
- Maintain regular MTX monitoring according to BSR and local guidelines.

• Ensure follow-up assessment at 16 weeks to assess response.

Patient information

Patient information leaflets are available from:
• Arthritis Research Campaign: ✍ www.arc.co.uk
• National Rheumatoid Arthritis Society: ✍ www.rheumatoid.org.uk

Further reading

NICE (2007). *Rheumatoid arthritis (refractory)–rituximab. Rituximab for the treatment of rheumatoid arthritis.* NICE, London. Available at: ✍ www.nice.org.uk/TA126

Smolen JS, Keystone EC, Emery P *et al.* (2007). Consensus statement on the use of Rituximab in patients with rheumatoid arthritis. *Annals of the Rheumatic Diseases,* **66**, 143–50.

Non-pharmacological therapies

Joint protection

What is joint protection? Why use it?

The pain, strain, and frustration of undertaking daily activities are common features in many types of arthritis, back pain, and soft tissue conditions (e.g. CTS, de Quervains, repetitive strain injury (RSI)). Joint protection is used to:

- Protect joints that are vulnerable as a result of pain, swelling, or weakness of the ligaments and muscles.
- Provide improved movement patterns and activities to conserve energy and protect the joints.
- Ensure correct posture and positioning when undertaking activities.
- Restructuring activities to improve function, reduce pain, swelling, risk of deformities, and maximize independence.

▶ For people with inflammatory arthritis or hand OA refer to OT for detailed advice and training to preserve joint function long term. If they have lower limb OA refer to PT.

Joint protection, pacing, and exercise

People can be confused why they are recommended to protect joints and pace activities and yet to exercise. It can seem contradictory. Joint protection is not about stopping activity but doing it differently. Pacing reduces fatigue so they can exercise. Exercise builds muscle and endurance to protect joints and reduce fatigue. Present these strategies as working together (see Table 19.1).

Making changes

Research supports the value of joint protection. Finding easier ways of carrying out tasks makes common sense and over time people will naturally find ways to ease pain and avoid activities that produce pain. There are benefits in enabling patients to be convinced of the benefits of such strategies early on during the course of their problems.

Adjusting to change

Many people find change difficult, experience frustrations, and find the 'need' to change as feeling as if they have 'given in'. Patients may need time and support to adapt to these changes. They should be encouraged to recognize that they are taking control, not giving in. Start by:

- Asking about everyday problems they experience and how their arthritis limits them doing things they really want to do (e.g. at work, hobbies, socially, in the home). Encourage them to review the way they use their affected joints and note which activities and movements cause them aches, pain, and/or fatigue.
- Ask them how they see being able to do these things in 5 years' time?
- Discuss the pros and cons of making changes to help them achieve what they want to. Remind them adapting is not giving in.
- When they have accepted the principles of change and benefits, reiterate the value of joint protection, how it works, and key principles (Table 19.1). Provide some practical ideas and help them set goals to practise using the solutions outlined.

- Then progress to ask about activities they have difficulty with and/or find painful. Encourage them to problem-solve alternative solutions by: listing on paper the different stages in the activity; analyse how they do each stage—discuss movements and equipment used and which aspects cause difficulty, aches, or pain. Focus on changing the elements of a problem; use the principles in Table 19.1 to jointly brainstorm different ways of doing these stages. Note these on paper and give the person a copy to help them remember.
- At the next follow-up appointment, review their progress and encourage them to try problem-solving again for another problem— and repeat if you have time.

Table 19.1 Key joint protection principles

Principle	Example
1. Reduce force and effort	Use levers, labour-saving devices, slide, or use wheels to move objects, use assistive technology (📖 see Chapter 11, Care in the community)
2. Spread load over several joints	Use palms of 2 hands to carry, not fingertips (use a cloth for hot items)
3. Use larger, stronger joints	Hold bags over forearm/shoulder or use backpack not hands; use hip/shoulder to open/close doors and drawers
4. Use joints in stable positions; avoid positions of potential deformity (e.g. bent sideways or down)	Avoid twisting at knee: stand up with knees facing forward, not to side; push up with palms of hands, not knuckles. Avoid lifting heavy objects with wrists bent down. Avoid pushing fingers towards little finger
5. Avoid strong pinch and grip	Enlarge and pad handles, pens, and tools; use gadgets for easy grip, e.g. jar openers (📖 see Chapter 11, Care in the community). Don't press hard on thumb
6. Correct posture	Avoid poking head and leaning forward when active or sitting. Use supportive seating and beds

Further reading

Adams J, Hammond A, Burridge J, et al (2005). Static orthoses in the prevention of hand dysfunction in rheumatoid arthritis. *Musculoskeletal Care*, **3**, 85–101.

Arthritis Research Campaign leaflet: *Looking After Your Joints When You Have Arthritis*. Available at: ⚓ http://www.arc.org.uk/arthinfo/patpubs/6055/6055.asp

Cordery J, Rocchi M (1998). Joint protection and fatigue management. In: Melvin J, Jensen G (eds), *Rheumatologic Rehabilitation Volume 1: Assessment and Management*. American Occupational Therapy Association, Bethesda, MD.

Hammond A, Freeman K (2001). One year outcomes of a randomised controlled trial of an educational-behavioural joint protection programme for people with rheumatoid arthritis. *Rheumatology*, **40**, 1044–51.

Why splint joints?

Hand/wrist splints are commonly provided for RA, thumb OA, and RSIs such as CTS and other types of tenosynovitis. They are provided to:
- Reduce pain.
- Improve function.
- Reduce inflammation.
- Re-align or correct deformity.

When to splint?

Indications for splint referral are given in Table 19.2 Referral to OT is recommended as splints are best combined with joint protection and hand exercise training. An individual assessment is often needed as many designs are available. The provision of splints must meet Medical Devices Agency regulations. Splint adherence is significantly improved by effective patient education.

Wrist working splints (Fig. 19.1)

There are many commercial, working splint designs and they are made out of a range of products including elasticated fabric, neoprene, or lycra with aluminum or plastic support inserts. It is essential that the splint is the correct size and fit. If one design does not suit, try another. The insert must be moulded to the person: They should be moulded according to need:
- 20–30° extension for a functional splint.
- Or neutral–10° extension in CTS for symptom relief.

The splint straps should be firm enough to control wrist movement. The splint should not impede hand movement at the transverse palmar or thenar creases as this may cause stiffness. Patients should be informed that these splints initially will reduce grip strength as they take 1 or 2 weeks to get used to. After this, most benefits are gained in moderate-to-heavy activities (e.g. vacuuming, ironing, gardening, and lifting) as grip improves and pain reduces. They should not be worn for long periods or a stiff wrist may develop. Splints need replacing every 6 months or so as they wear out.[1]

Hand resting splints (Fig. 19.2)

These are usually custom-made in thermoplastic, placing the hand in a comfortable rest position. They are most beneficial in RA, other inflammatory diseases and RSIs if the person is being kept awake at night by pain. If 2 splints are necessary it might be more appropriate to recommend alternate use or a modified design with finger/thumb ends free to enable some hand function, e.g. pulling covers or flipping light switches.

Thumb splints (Fig. 19.3)

The thumb contributes 60% of hand function. Thumb pain and instability can significantly affect daily activities and work. OA carpometacarpal (CMC) joint affects >30% of postmenopausal ♀. Many do not realize that a splint and therapy would help. There are many designs:
- Hand-based C bar.
- Elasticated thumb wrap.
- Thumb/wrist splints.

The choice will be dependent on the extent of the problem—to effectively reduce pain. Early splint provision may avoid the need for later surgery.

MCP and finger deformity splints

Custom-made splints can correct early finger deformities and realign MCPJs for improved hand function in RA. These may avoid need for later surgery.

Table 19.2 Indications for hand splints

Splint type	Indication
Wrist working	RA: wrist pain limiting hand function; weak grip.
	CTS: wrist pain (day or night); pins and needles; weak grip
Hand resting	RA: night-time hand/wrist pain; acute inflammation wrist/ MCP joints.
Thumb	RA or OA: CMC joint or 1ˢᵗ MCP joint pain reducing function
Figure of 8/ silver ring	RA: correctable swan neck/ boutonnière deformity
MCP ulnar deviation	RA: correctable MCPJ deformity (to realign fingers for improved function).

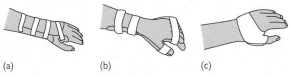

(a)   (b)   (c)

Fig. 19.1 Joint protection splints. a) Elastic wrist working splint; b) hand resting splint; c) thumb splint. Reproduced with kind permission from the Arthritis Research Campaign.

Reference

1. Adams J et al (2005). *Musculoskeletal Care*, **3**, 85–101.

Fatigue and stress

Fatigue in arthritis

Fatigue is common in inflammatory forms of arthritis and OA and is increasingly recognized as an important factor affecting quality of life of those with long-term MSC. Pacing uses the principle that regular short rests help 'recharge batteries' when fatigue, pain, and stress are factors in disease. However, there are many contributing factors and possible solutions to pacing. See Table 19.3 for ideas.

Activity pacing

Adjusting to limitations of a condition such as arthritis can frustrate people. As they attempt to maintain activities they used to be able to achieve easily, they may state that they do not wish to be 'beaten' by their condition and may result in a tendency to overdo things on 'good days' and suffer for it later: the 'boom and bust' cycle. People may fail to accept the condition and restrictions (e.g. the over-doers) or become fearful of damaging joints or pain and become 'deconditioned' by a cycle of muscle weakness and loss of vitality (insufficient activity).

Research shows that pacing achieves effective outcomes for those who learn to adapt to these frustrating limitations. Activity pacing works on the links between activity levels, fatigue, and pain and the use of simple principles such as pacing techniques (Table 19.3) and an activity diary.

Table 19.3 Pacing techniques

Use of pacing to take:	Activity: advise patients to use an alarm or timer to remind them of when to take breaks. Encourage adhering to time allocation.
Micro breaks	Stretch and relax: 30–60 second breaks every 5–10min
Short breaks	Every 1–2 hours take a 5–10min break
Measure	How long an activity can be carried out before pain/fatigue starts (reduce 25% off the set quota) and review ability with 25% reduction in task
Measure	If under active; gradually ↑ activity quote through goal setting
Plan ahead	Break activities into smaller components to enable rest breaks; plan the same amount of activity and rest each day; balance heavier and lighter activities out through the day and week
Prioritize	Carry out activities which are essential. Ensure time and energy left for hobbies, and social and family activities. Are there any activities which can be done less often or omitted/ delegated?
Problem solve	Identify ways to make activities easier by using joint protection and correct positioning

Rest

Research shows 'overdoers' who pace are *more* active—and do not get exhausted so rapidly. 30–60min daily rest is effective but many find this difficult, with short breaks feeling more acceptable than longer periods. Ideally they should progress to longer rests which are *relaxing*—in a comfortable chair, head and shoulders supported or lying; relaxing music or deep breathing to mentally and physically slow down (they should not keep busy watching TV/reading). They should also aim for at least 8 hours sleep a day (see Table 19.4).

Relaxation

Some people find relaxation CDs helpful. This can be combined with the use of deep breathing (as a quick stress buster): advise patients to sit with arms and head relaxed, eyes closed, listen to the sound of their breath. They should breathe in slowly through the nose (count of 4), breathe out slowly through slightly parted lips (count of 6), whilst thinking 'relax' (or other phrase that would help visualization of something pleasant, e.g. favourite place). Repeat breaths 6–10 times.

Table 19.4 Possible causes and solutions for fatigue

Possible cause	Possible solutions
The disease itself	Fatigue and pain are common in RA, SLE, and OA. Ensure prescribed appropriate drug therapy
Overdoing activities	Activity pacing. Refer to: OT for joint protection, Activity Pacing and Relaxation training and education programme and support groups (📖 see Expert patient programme, p.330) Encourage positive approach to condition
Underactvity/over resting	Activity pacing. Refer to: OT and refer to PT Pacing training; arthritis education or EPP Encourage more activity; explain consequences of resting too much; dispel myth that activity will cause damage
Deconditioning/lack of fitness	Support to enable ↑ activity/fitness programme. Refer to OT for pacing and/or PT for exercise training Arthritis education or EPP .
Stress/depression	Assess the person's mood state. Provide support and self-help references for managing stress and low mood, e.g. Arthritis Care booklet *Coping with Emotions* www.arthritiscare.org. If clinically anxious/depressed, refer to mental health practitioner.
Poor sleep	Assess cause. If nocturnal pain—review analgesia prescribed prior to bedtime. For insomnia and sleep management advice: • www.helpguide.org/Life/insomnia_treatment.htm • www.sleepfoundation.org • www.rcpsych.ac.uk—search for 'sleep problems'

Thermotherapy and transcutaneous electrical nerve stimulation

Thermotherapy

Thermotherapy is the application of heat or cold to alter cutaneous, IA temperature and core temperature. It has been self-administered for millennia and is widely recommended for many MSC because it is a safe, effective, popular, easy way to apply treatment that does not require complex, expensive equipment. It also enhances the individual's perceptions of control and adds a simple approach to self-management strategies (Table 19.5).

Table 19.5 Effects of thermotherapy

	Heating	Cooling
'Shutting the pain gate'	Yes	Yes
Muscle relaxation	↑	↓
Tissue temperature	↑	↓
Blood flow	↑ (vasodilaition)	↓ (vasoconstriction), followed by ↑ to prevent hypoxic damage
Metabolic rate	↑	↓
Neuronal excitability	↑	↓
Neuronal conduction rate	↑	↓
Tissue extensibility	↑	↓

There are a number of ways thermotherapy can be applied. Warmth can be achieved using commercially available hot packs, a hot water bottle wrapped in a towel, taking a hot bath, wearing thermal clothing or bandages can reduce pain considerably. Cooling can be achieved using commercially available cool packs or coolant sprays or a homemade ice pack (a bag of frozen peas wrapped in a towel). Since heating and cooling can relieve pain, patient preference can be taken into consideration when deciding which to use.

Simple forms of thermotherapy (heat/ice packs) are safe for people with normal vasculature and neurological sensation. Care should be taken with patients who have diabetes, peripheral vascular disease, or peripheral neuropathies. It is appropriate to use for patients who can adhere to simple guidelines. The patient can be advised to:
- Wrap a hot water bottle/bag of frozen peas or ices cubes in a towel.
- Lie or sit down and relax.
- Place the hot/cold pack on the painful, inflamed joint for 10min.
- Remove the pack and gently move their joint.
- Replace the hot/cold pack on the joint for another 5–10min.

Whether heat or cold packs are used it should never become uncomfortably hot or cold.

TENS

TENS is a form of electrotherapy usually administered by PTs in the first instance. Laboratory studies suggest that TENS works by blocking pain pathways by inhibiting nociceptive at the presynaptic level, inhibiting the central transmission of pain sensations. It is often used to relieve pain, reduce inflammation, and improve muscle function. Indications for TENS include:

- Neurogenic or post-herpetic pain.
- Mild-to-moderate musculoskeletal pain (e.g. low back pain).

TENS is an easily applied, non-invasive modality; the only adverse effect is occasional, mild skin irritation. A small, inexpensive battery-operated TENS machine delivers a low frequency electrical impulse via surface skin electrodes. Patients can be easily advised on how to place electrodes to self-administer treatment.

There are 5 TENS protocols—the selection used is based upon the underlying condition and which pain relief mechanism is required (Table 19.6). The waveform, pulse duration, pulse frequency, intensity, and electrode position can be adjusted to achieve optimal pain relief. High frequency, 'strong burst' TENS for >4 weeks has been shown to be most effective.

Table 19.6 The treatment plans for TENS—rationale for pain relief

Indication	Definition	Treatment parameters
Conventional: • Rationale: via pain gate • Indication: less severe pain	• High frequency 90–130Hz • Pulse width <100μsec	• *Time*: 30 min periods applied regularly as needed • *Intensity*: feel comfortable buzz
Acupuncture: • Rationale: via opiod • Indication: chronic conditions	• Low frequency 2–5Hz • Pulse width >200μsec	• *Time*: 30min • *Intensity*: strong but comfortable buzz
Burst: • Rationale: via all pain • Indication: long-term use	• Low frequency 10Hz • Burst impulses, 2–3 per sec	• *Intensity*: strong but comfortable buzz
Brief intense: • Rationale: via pain gate • Indication: short term for severe pain	• High frequency >80Hz • Pulse width >150 μsec	• *Time*: 15–30min • *Intensity*: close to maximum tolerance
Modulation: • Rationale: all pain relief • Indication: long-term use	• All characteristics are varied throughout application	• *Intensity*: strong but comfortable buzz

Further reading

Brosseau L, Wells G A, Tugwell P (2004). Ottawa panel evidence based clinical practice guidelines for electrotherapy and thermotherapy interventions in the management of rheumatoid arthritis. *Physical Therapy*, **8**, 1016–43.

Assessment tools and outcome measures

Assessment and outcome tools: overview

Most aspects of care start with some form of consultation/discussion with the patient to explore the patient's problem, clinical history taking and assessments (health/disease assessment), followed by a treatment or management plan (process), and finally reviewing the outcome of the treatment or management plan (outcome measures). For those who have little experience in the use of assessment tools and wish to identify an appropriate instrument to use as assessment or outcome measure a strong suggestion would be to use a well validated tool until experienced in the use of tools development. In a simple form consider:

Individual in a health or disease state: assessment → process → outcome

All tools are set out in a standardized way, usually in the form of a questionnaire style measuring either a single or multiple concepts. Multidimensional tools will provide either a global score (all the scores are combined to give one number) or be analyzed using subscales. In some cases, a mixture of both scoring systems will be used. The relative advantages and disadvantages of these methods need to be considered when selecting a tool.

Validated objective measures are vital in identifying baseline and essential changes in health or disease status; increasingly tools are used for diagnostic or treatment criteria and are frequently incorporated into ICPs. Future evaluations may include measures to assess outcomes at specific points in the patient pathway of care. Many tools are internationally validated.

Tools can be used as part of an assessment prior to treatment to demonstrate disease or health states (at baseline and following treatment or intervention). They could also be used to identify benefits of services/interventions (e.g. benefits of a nurse clinic on symptom control for those with joint pain), looking at pre- and post-treatment effects. The data collected may need to include a combination of clinical indicators and outcome measures (such as Visual Analogue for Pain, Quality of Life Tool, and the Health Assessment Questionnaire for functional ability).

Also see Selecting the right tool for the job, p.542.

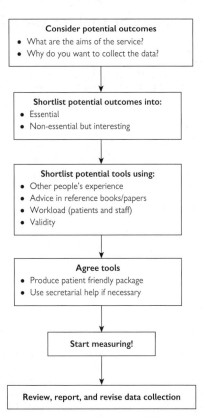

Fig. 20.1 The process of selecting the right tools. Adapted with permission from Oliver S (ed.) (2004). *Chronic Disease Nursing. A Rheumatology Example.* John Wiley & Sons Ltd: Chichester.

Selecting the right tool for the job

Tools can be used as:
- A validated method of evaluation using clearly defined parameters—assessment tools.
- A validated methods of measuring changes as a result of a specific intervention/ treatment/time fram—outcome measure.

The decision about what type of tool to use (assessment or outcome) will rely on:
- What is the aim of the data being collected.
- What is being measured.
- If there a potential treatment or effect/change over time.
- What will be the best way to measure these changes.

In addition, consideration should be given to whether there is a need to use a:
- Generic tool—relevant to the general population and could be used to compare activities across disease areas such as diabetes, cardiovascular disease and arthritis.
- Disease-specific tool—e.g. relevant to just 1 disease, such as RA
- Dimension-specific tools—measuring specific aspect of health status e.g. social well-being or physical function.

Then consider:
- Single topic tools—e.g. a VAS for pain.
- Multi-dimensional tool—global score for the full assessment or broken down into subscales.

Additional factors to consider include:
- Individual *self-reported* (subjective tools) such as the Pain or Fatigue Scale.
- *Clinical indicators* (objective measures) such as an investigation e.g. an x-ray result.

The data may also be used to demonstrate the effective use of specific resources (e.g. the benefit of a nurse-led clinic) to improve patient outcomes. This can present very real challenges because the essence of nursing is:
- Holistic and responsive to patient need.
- Multi-dimensional.
- Crosses numerous aspects of healthcare delivery.
- Difficult to define and evaluate.

In many cases these limitations have to be worked with and flaws identified in the interpretation of the data (e.g. what the tool has failed to measure). The patient's perspective on their condition, care received, and outcomes of care are increasingly of interest and important to capture.

Consider:
- Subjective assessments, e.g. patient-reported outcome measures (PROMs):
  - patient perspective on treatment.
  - psychological factors (e.g. self-efficacy).
  - Expectations/needs (quality of life issues).
  - Measures to explore specific symptoms (e.g. VAS of pain).

- Objective measures such as:
  - Functionally important measures (ADLs, ROMs).
  - Measures required to assess disease process (e.g. x-rays).
  - Measures to assess treatment efficacy (reduction in CRP).

It is common for a set of tools to be used (e.g. 1 or 2 PROMs with an objective clinical assessment tool). When selecting an assessment tool it is imperative to clarify whether the tool has a copyright There are useful websites that can provide this information or your local audit department will be able to provide information.[1]

Reference

1. ⌐ www.gl-assessment.co.uk

Further reading

Bowling A (1997). *Measuring Health*, 2nd edn. Open University Press, Buckingham.

Bowling A (2001). *Measuring Disease*, 2nd edn. Open University Press, Maidenhead.

Hewlett S (2004). Nurse clinics, using the right tools for the job. In Oliver S (ed) (2004). *Chronic Disease Nursing: A Rheumatology Example*. Whurr Publishers, West Sussex, UK.

Assessment tools: are they valid?

Is it a valid tool?

All assessment/outcome measures must be valid, reliable, and sensitive to change:
- Covers the relevant aspects of the concept.
- Is consistent and accurate.
- Sensitive to change.
- Makes sense to the concept being studied.

In essence they must be reliable and have credibility in the context of evidence-based care. This means that measures should demonstrate meaningful criteria to assess outcomes (from patient, clinician, and provider perspective).

For those inexperienced in the use of assessment tools it is strongly recommended that a well validated tool is used until expertise in the use of tools is developed. Designing assessment tools requires a sound knowledge of strength and weakness of tools as well as considering key aspects that must be considered to ensure an effective and valuable tool (Table 20.1).

A combination of tools can provide a holistic view of meaningful aspects of care—provided the correct tools are selected and there is clarity about what the purpose of the measure is:
- To demonstrate improvements in quality of life indicators.
- Specific disease state outcomes such as scleroderma skin score.
- Changes in psychological factors following an intervention (e.g. ↑ in self-efficacy following a patient education programme) (Fig. 20.1).

Data collection without well-validated tools can be labour intensive and lack validity in a wider clinical or research based settings. Audit tools may be a useful adjunct to evidence required for example specific aspects of care can be evaluated using audit tools against recognized standards or guidelines (benchmarking) or care delivered before changes in treatment criteria were applied.

📖 Also see Selecting the right tool for the job, p.542.

Further reading

Bowling A (2005). *Measuring Health: a review of quality of life measurement scales.*, 3rd edn. Open University Press, Buckingham.

Bowling A (2001). *Measuring Disease*, 2nd edn. Open University Press, Buckingham.

Hewlett S (2004). Nurse clinics, using the right tools for the job. In Oliver S (ed) (2004). *Chronic Disease Nursing: A Rheumatology Example*. Whurr Publishers, West Sussex, UK.

Table 20.1 What to consider in selecting a tool

Choosing tools	Consider
Disease specific (face validity)	• Is it credible from a clinician/ patient perspective • Has the tool been validated in the disease area?
Disease specific (construct validity)	• Does the measure reflect the true biological aspects of the condition?
Disease (content validity)	• Does it cover all the relevant aspects needed to evaluate? • Is it measuring the aspect of the disease you need to measure?
Consistent and accurate (discriminant and criterion validity)	• Is it *responsive*—ability to measure a significant change in the condition over time (sensitive to change) • Is it stable and consistent and accurate when repeated (consistency)
Language	• Has the tool been used and researched in the same patient population (language, community, cultural issues)
Ease of use	• Is it easy to use? • If a patient-completed tool, pilot for ease of completion and relevance of questions. Is the tool relevant/too long? • Is it easy to score/analyse?
Is it the best tool for job?	• Are there better tools that will cover the topic more succinctly or reduce the overall number of tools to be used?
Strengths and weaknesses	• All tools have strengths and weaknesses—it helps to know what they are when using and analysing the results
Finally	• Does the tool (or tools) give a truthful and accurate representation of all the clinical aspects necessary to consider for the condition and changes/activity in relation to outcomes?

Examples of assessment tools

The selection of tools outlined is not by any means exhaustive but aims to outline some examples of the types of tools that are available and may be useful to consider for MSC.

Some diagnoses are mild, self-limiting, and of short duration whilst others are incurable and will require continuing care and treatment. It might be useful to consider some key health issues that are common to all conditions (in varying degrees) and which might be considered 'core' data sets to measure because of their common presentation in many MSC:

- Pain.
- Functional issues.
- Quality of life factors including; social participation, independence, well being.
- Psychological factors that affect the individual in coming to terms or managing their conditions (e.g. self-efficacy, self-esteem, helplessness).

Health state measures

Health is considered an essential and valued concept that affects quality of life (social, emotional, and physical well being not just the absence of disease). There is a plethora of tools to explore different components of quality of life in relation to changes in perceived or actual health or disease states. Many of these are generic and have a value in identifying differences in health status across a number of diseases.

Examples includes the patient-reported outcome of:

Short form 36 (SF36 © (Ware and Sherbourne 1992)[1]
There are 9 health concepts (physical function, physical role, emotional role, social function, pain, mental health, vitality, general health, health transition). This is not a simple tool to score yourself but a good tool to use if you want to compare changes against other LTCs. A computer scoring package is available with the questionnaire.[2]

Health Perceptions Questionnaire and General Health Rating Index © Algorithmic Medicine (Ware 1976)[3]
A tool that consists of 32 questions divided into 8 subscales related to a patient's perception of health. A subset of 22 questions making up the General Health Rating Index, with subsets used for faster evaluations. The questionnaire is simple and fast to administer, and has been widely studied.

Quality of life measures

European Quality of Life Questionnaire. (EuroQoL EQ-5D) EuroQoL Group (1990)[4]
A generic, patient self-completed, state of health tool that can be for clinical, economic, and population health state assessments. Contains 5 domains; anxiety and depression, mobility, pain and discomfort, self-care, and usual activities. It also uses a vertical 20cm VAS to ask the patient to rate from worst imaginable state to best imaginable state of their perception of their health state. The weighting of the tool and each health state were determined by exploring view of the general population (societal preference weights) and the weighting given may not be the same if explored with a patient who has a LTC. Designed to complement other quality of life and disease-specific tools.

References

1. Ware JE, Sherbourne CD (1992). The MOS 36-Item Short-Form Health Survey (SF-36®): I. conceptual framework and item selection. *Med Care*, **30**, 473–83.

2. ⤷ www.sf-36.org

3. Ware JE (1976). Scales for measuring general health perceptions. *Health Serv Res*, **11**, 396–415.

4. ⤷ www.EuroQoL.org

Assessment tools: clinical indicators and disease-specific tools

The decision to review patient outcomes must consider the appropriate tools to use. Assessment tools are often combined with clinical indicators.

The clinical indicators that could support patient-reported outcome measures could include:

- Individual's health status over time (with or without an underlying disease state), e.g. monitoring blood pressure, body weight.
- Monitoring disease states (e.g. monitoring of diabetic control) as a result of treatment. The monitoring may be to assess changes to the individual (from baseline) or part of a treatment criteria for stopping or starting treatment (e.g. in RA a DAS >5.1 indicates eligibility for new therapies).
- Evaluation of patient outcomes against recognized standards of care /guidelines in management (e.g. comparing patient populations against the national average expected outcomes). Includes aspects of benchmarking or audit.

An example of a tool measuring clinical indicators

SLE

The British Isles Lupus Assessment Group index (Hay et al. 1993)

This tool assesses 86 clinical signs, symptoms, and laboratory measures across 8 areas (mucocutaneous, neurological, musculoskeletal, cardiovascular and respiratory, vasculitis, renal, haematological, and general aspects). Shown to be valid, reliable, and sensitive to change. Scoring is based upon the physicians' intention to treat with each system or organ being scored separately—the scoring is based upon changes seen and whether they are new, worse, better, the same, or improving from the previous assessment. Basic haematology and renal function determine scores of the different systems. It categorizes disease states into 5 different levels from A to E. With A level being the highest level of disease activity. A computer-scoring package is available as it is complex to score.

Examples of disease specific tools

Arthritis (general tool covering 'arthritis')

The Arthritis Impact Measurement Scales (AIMS-2) © (Meenan et al. 1980)

The AIMS contains 57 items with 12 subscales measuring function, social life, pain, work, tension and mood, satisfaction, and prioritization questions.

OA

The Western Ontario McMaster Universities Arthritis Index (WOMAC) (Bellamy et al. 1988)

A popular tool that has undergone several revisions and changes during its development. It is valid, reliable and sensitive to change and uses three subscales with 24 items to assess pain, function and stiffness in knee and Hip OA. This can be scored using either a 5-point Likert scoring system (none, mild, moderate, severe, extreme) or 100mm VAS. (www.womac.org).

The AIMS and WOMAC could be supported by measures specifically for the condition or joint affected, e.g. Oxford Hip Score (OHS) or the Hip Disability and Osteoarthritis Outcome Score (HOOS).

The Knee and Hip Assessment Tools

The Oxford Knee Score (Dawson *et al.* 1998) and The Oxford Hip Score (Dawson *et al.* 1996). These tools have 12 questions. The OHS covers pain and disability experienced over the past 4 weeks. Each item has 5 response categories. The response was formatted as a Likert scales.

AS

In arthritis the 3 commonly used and validated tools are:

- *The Bath Ankylosing Spondylitis Functional Index (BASFI)*. A patient-completed form on patient perceived functional ability. It uses 10 questions to measure aspects of functional ability which are scored using a VAS measuring 10 aspects of functional ability.
- *The Bath Ankylosing Spondylitis Disease Activity Index (BASDI)*. Patient-completed form. 6 components of perceived disease activity are scored as a patient self-assessment (fatigue, spinal pain, joint pain and enthesis, together with morning stiffness and severity of stiffness). Range of scores are 0–10 (none to very severe) although duration of morning stiffness is scored on length of time from 0 to >2 hours.
  - The scores are added for questions 1–4; this is then combined with the mean scores of questions 5 and 6 (duration of morning stiffness and severity of stiffness) to give a score out of 50. Then multiply by 2 and divide by 10 to get the BASDAI score.
- *The Bath Ankylosing Spondylitis Metrology Index (BASMI)*. A clinical assessment tool measuring spinal mobility. Aggragate score is 0–10 using the variables in Table 20.2 (see ⌁ www.nass.co.uk/bath_indices.htm).

Table 20.2 BASMI assessment tool[1,2]

Measurement	Score 0	Score 1	Score 2
Tragus to wall	<15cm	15–30	>30
Lumbar flexion (mod schobert test)	>4cm	2–4cm	<4cm
Cervical rotation	>70°	20–70°	<20°
Lumbar side flexion	>10cm	5–10cm	<5cm
Intermalleolar distance	>100cm	70–100cm	<70cm

Low back pain

The Roland and Morris Disability Questionnaire (RDQ) (Roland and Morris 1983). A self-report, self-complete questionnaire to assess degree of functional ability. 24 items were modified from the Sickness Impact Profile (SIP). Quick and easy to understand, complete and score. (www.csp.org.uk)

References

1. Calin A et al. (1994). A new approach to defining functional ability in Ankylosing Spondylitis: the development of the Bath Ankylosing Spondylitis Functional Index (BASFI). *Journal of Rheumatology*, **21**, 2281–5.

2. Jenkinson TR et al. (1994). Defining Spinal Mobility in Ankylosing Spondylitis (AS): the Bath AS Metrology Index. *Journal of Rheumatology*. **21**, 1694–8.

Examples of domain- and disease-specific measures

Domain specific

Fatigue

The Functional Assessment of Chronic Illness Therapy (FACIT) (Cella 1997)
The FACIT contains a collection of health-related quality of life (HRQOL) questionnaires targeted to the management of chronic illness. 27 items compiled and divided into 4 primary QOL domains: physical well-being, social/family well-being, emotional well-being, and functional well-being. Initially developed for cancer but has been validated in a number of areas including RA. Can be administered or patient-completed. FACIT enables a tailored assessment using the most relevant questions. Completion usually takes about 10–15min.

Pain

VAS Single Item tool
A VAS uses a horizontal or vertical line measuring 10cm in length. The VAS scale uses verbal descriptors of 'no pain' at one end and 'pain as bad as it could be' at the other end (🔲 see Fig. 9.1, p.293).

Functional

Health Assessment Questionnaire (HAQ) (Fries 1980;[1] Bruce and Fries 2003)
Probably the most widely used tool in rheumatology clinics. Arthritis-specific tool to measure function. There are 2 domains: disability and discomfort.

There are 9 patient self-completed topics which include dressing and grooming, rising, eating, walking, hygiene, reach, grip, activities. The patient completes the form on a 4-point scale from: without any difficulty (score 0), with some difficulty (score 1), much difficulty (score 2), and unable to do (score 3). In addition they are asked to tick in sections at the end of the 2 domains whether they use additional help or, in the case of function domain, if additional aids are used (e.g. special utensils).

For each of the bottom sections (see Fig. 20.2) ticked related to additional help or aids the score is adjusted to maximum score of 3 for the area, e.g. if the question on hygiene was ticked as 'with some difficulty' yet the additional box at the end of the section is also ticked as using a bath seat, the new score for hygiene would be a maximum score of 3. A simple scoring system attributes the scores. Scores of 0 = 0 to a maximum score of 24 points = 3.0 HAQ score for maximum disability. Quick to complete and score and frequently used as part of a battery of tools in research trials (🖰 www.aramis.standard.edu). Validated for use in UK population by Kirwan and Reeback.[2]

References

1. Fries JF, Spitz P, Kraines RG, *et al.* (1980). Measurement of patient outcome in arthritis. *Arthritis and Rheumatism*, **23**, 137–45.

2. Kirwan JR, Reeback JS (1986) Stanford Health Assessment Questionnaire modified to assess disability in British patients with rheumatoid arthritis. *British Journal of Rheumatology*, **23**, 210–13.

HEALTH ASSESSMENT QUESTIONNAIRE (HAQ)

Date: [   ]   Patient Name: [   ]

Please tick the one response which best describes your usual abilities over the past week

	Without ANY difficulty	With SOME difficulty	With MUCH difficulty	UNABLE to do

1. DRESSING and GROOMING
Are you able to:

a. Dress yourself, including tying shoelaces and doing buttons? ☐ ☐ ☐ ☐

b. Shampoo your hair? ☐ ☐ ☐ ☐   [----------]

2. RISING ⭐
Are you able to:

a. Stand up from an armless straight chair? ☐ ☐ ☐ ☐

b. Get in and out of bed? ☐ ☐ ☐ ☐   [----------]

3. EATING
Are you able to:

a. Cut your meat? ☐ ☐ ☐ ☐

b. Lift a full cup or glass to your mouth? ☐ ☐ ☐ ☐   [----------]

c. Open a new carton of milk (or soap powder)? ☐ ☐ ☐ ☐

4. WALKING
Are you able to:

a. Walk outdoors on flat ground? ☐ ☐ ☐ ☐

b. Climb up five steps? ☐ ☐ ☐ ☐   [----------]

PLEASE TICK ANY AIDS OR DEVICES THAT YOU USUALLY USE FOR ANY OF THESE ACTIVITIES:

Cane (W) ☐   Walking frame (W) ☐   Built-up or special utensils (E) ☐

Crutches (W) ☐   Wheelchair (W) ☐   Special or built-up chair (A) ☐

Devices used for dressing (button hooks, zipper pull, shoe horn) ☐

Other (specify)..

PLEASE TICK ANY CATEGORIES FOR WHICH YOU USUALLY NEED HELP FROM ANOTHER PERSON:

Dressing and Grooming ☐   Eating ☐

Rising ☐   Walking ☐

⭐ Subscale – example of an
Activities subscale

ID [   ]
For office use only

Fig. 20.2 Health Assessment Questionnaire.

Assessment tools measuring psychological aspects

Anxiety and depression

Hospital Anxiety and Depression (HAD) (Zigmond and Snaith 1983) ©
A quick and easy tool to complete. 1-page self-report questionnaire. Measures depression and generalized anxiety. Comprises of 14-item scale, has 7 questions each for anxiety and depression. Outlines cut off points to indicate 'within the normal range', or in a 'mildly', 'moderately', or 'severely' disordered state A useful tool in hospital, outpatient, and the community setting. Easy to score (🖰 www.gl-assessment.co.uk).

Helplessness

Arthritis Helplessness Index (Stein et al. 1988)
This questionnaire uses 6 categories for scoring (strongly agree to strongly disagree). This is a 15-item questionnaire. Scores range from 5–30. The higher the score the higher the helplessness.

Self-efficacy

The Arthritis Self-Efficacy Scale (ASES) (Lorig et al. 1989)
This tool has subscales for pain, function, and other symptoms. 20 items and 3 subscales; self-efficacy pain, self-efficacy function, and self-efficacy other symptoms. The tool uses a number of VAS which are totalled and averaged to give a score. The higher scores indicate high levels of SE.

The Rheumatoid Arthritis Self-Efficacy scale (RASE) (Hewlett et al. 2001)[1]
A relatively new, disease specific tool developed for use in UK. Self-administered; easy to use. Measures perceived stress and methods of coping. Measures task specific self-efficacy for the initiation of self-management and related behaviours. 28 items, no subscales.. High scores indicate higher self-efficacy (Table 20.3).

Attitude

The Rheumatoid Attitude Index (RAI) (Nicassio et al. 1985)© Algorithmic Medicine
This tool explores beliefs related to helplessness (e.g. actions do not affect outcomes). A self-reporting questionnaire focusing on learned helplessness and was originally developed from the Arthritis Helplessness Index (AHI).

Changes in knowledge following educational intervention

Patient Knowledge Questionnaire for OA (PKQ-OA) (Hill and Bird 2007)
Patient-completed questionnaire to identify level of knowledge and use of self-management techniques. Studies have also demonstrated the validity of this tool for measuring knowledge in early RA. Comprises 16 multiple choice questions with 30 correct answers. A tool that is easy to read, complete and interpret.

Table 20.3 Example of the RA self-efficacy tool[1]. Adapted with permission from Tugwell P, Shea B, Boers M, et al. (eds) (2003). *Evidence Based Rheumatology.* Copyright John Wiley & Sons Limited, Chichester, UK.

We are interested in finding out what things you believe you could do to help you with your arthritis.

We want to know what you think you *could* do, even if you are not actually doing it at the moment. Please tick one column for each question.

Do you believe you *could* do these things to help you with your arthritis?

	Strongly disagree	Disagree	Neither disagree nor agree	Agree	Strongly agree
I believe I *could* use relaxation techniques to help with pain					
I believe I *could* think about something else to help with pain					
I believe I *could* use my joints carefully (joint protection) to help with pain					
I believe I *could* think positively to help with pain					
I believe I *could* avoid doing things that cause pain					

Reference

1. Hewlett S, Cockshott Z, Kirwan J, *et al.* (2001). Development and validation of a self-efficacy scale for use in British patients with rheumatoid arthritis. *Rheumatology*, **40**, 1221–30.

Specialist nursing support: the role and nurse prescribing

The nurse specialist role

The role of the rheumatology nurse specialist (RNS) initially developed from research nurse roles. Today many nurses working in rheumatology have developed their roles through an interest in the specialty. As with other specialist roles many have gained qualifications at diploma, degree, or Masters degree level. The RNS role involves the following components:

Advanced nursing practice

Patient assessment and delivery of care

Acts as an advocate and provides nurse-led review of patients using a holistic approach to assess ADL, pain, disease activity, psychological status, coping styles, social circumstances, and employment issues.

- Advanced level of knowledge/competencies and autonomous clinical decision making and negotiating a plan of care and disease management with the patient.
- Extended roles such as prescribing and administering joint injections.
- Coordinates referrals to the MDT.

Educator

Uses a patient-centred approach to ascertain the patients' knowledge, beliefs and perceptions of their condition and treatment options as an advocate. Provide a nurse-led review of patients using a holistic approach to assess ADL, pain, disease activity, psychological status, social circumstances, and employment issues:

- Signposts the patient to voluntary and support agencies.
- Provides relevant written information to support education given.
- Provides patient (and carer) education and facilitates development of patient self-management. This may be delivered either as formal (group) or informal (individual) sessions and may be in collaboration with MDT.
- Engages in teaching all HCPs in the clinical setting and in universities.
- Develops the role of junior nurses and works with them to enhance their learning opportunities.
- Acts as an expert resource in the clinical setting with opportunistic teaching of clinical care aspects of specialism.

Leadership and management role

- Day-to-day management of the rheumatology department.
- Considers succession planning and sustainability of services.
- Line management, clinical supervision, and assessment of competency for a team of nurses.
- Acts as role model for nurses and supports nursing development.
- Responsibility for clinical governance.
- Providing strategic direction for the Trust and incorporating user patient involvement in rheumatology service development.

Research and audit role

Research studies are increasingly being undertaken and published by RNSs and along with audit both are important to demonstrate:

- Quality and safety of care given.
- Access to treatment and adherence to specific guidance (e.g. organizations such as NICE).

- Introduction of service change.
- Health outcome and cost effectiveness.

Nurse specialist (NSs)—extended roles

Many NSs have extended their roles with formal training, achieving practice base competencies and practice development. The rationale for role expansion is to provide a complete package of care for patients and this has taken place in the following areas of practice:

- A full and thorough physical assessment of patients to include examination of joints, heart, abdomen, and lungs, and performing disease activity scores.
- Assessment and management of comorbid conditions such as hypertension, coronary heart disease, hypercholesterolemia, osteoporosis, and diabetes.
- Consulting with patients, taking a history, and determining a management plan.
- Prescribing drug treatment and titration of therapy.
- Provision of IA and soft tissue injections.
- Referral and communicating with medical and surgical colleagues regarding the patient's management.
- Ordering and interpreting a range of imaging and blood investigations.

In addition a key component of the NS role is that of ensuring that a proactive patient-centred approach is applied to management:

- Patients get rapid access to care and treatments to optimize patient outcomes.
- Proactive review and assessment to review efficacy of treatment.
- Empowering the patient to ensure that they have the ability to make informed decisions about their care and adhere to treatment.
- Adherence to guidelines particularly of new therapies to ensure open and transparent access to treatments.
- Ensure that symptom control is achieved to the satisfaction of the patient.
- Enable patients to access opportunities to participate in research trials.

Nurse prescribing

Prescribing legislation has resulted in amendments to the original Medicines Act 1968 and following the Crown Report in 1989 which recommended that the development of nurse prescribing would improve patient care. The details of the development of nurse prescribing has been outlined by Beckwith and Franklin.[1]

The principles of nurse prescribing are:
- Improved patient access to medicines and subsequent improvements in health outcome.
- Better use of the doctors, nurses, and the patient's time.
- Clarification of professional responsibilities.
- Improved patient safety by fewer drug interactions and serious adverse events
    - This includes ensuring that all HCPs involved in the patient's care are aware of any prescribed medications and treatment plans made, including patient review.
- Framework of regular audit of prescribing practice, continued professional development, and prescribing updates.
- Reduction in costs as nurses can only prescribe generically.

Since May 2006 nurses with an ENB V300 qualification can act as Independent and or as Supplementary prescribers:

Methods of nurse prescribing

Independent nurse prescribing
The nurse prescriber takes legal responsibility for the clinical assessment of the patient, arriving at a diagnosis for the condition to be treated, the management of that condition, the decision to prescribe, and the suitability of the prescription

Supplementary prescribing
Is a voluntary partnership between a nurse prescriber and a doctor or dentist facilitated by drawing up an agreed clinical management plan (CMP) in conjunction with the patient. There is no identified formulary or restrictions on the type of medical conditions that can be treated within supplementary prescribing.

Nurse prescribers are entitled to prescribe drugs independently from the entire *BNF* but many NHS Trusts ask for an approval to practice form that outlines what will be prescribed, thus limiting the range of drugs prescribed to the specialist area of practice. Other exceptions apply; see The nurse prescriber: managing drug interactions, p.560.

The CMP

A variety of CMPs exist. The Department for Health or National Prescribing Centre recommends using CMPs they have developed as a tool to generate the prescription. The CMP must provide detail on:
- Guidelines, protocols, publications, and best evidence supporting the prescribing practice.
- Patient review schedule by the supplementary and independent prescribers.
- The process for reporting adverse drug reactions.

- The date from which the CMP became effective.
- The CMP, if not lapsed, should be reviewed at 1 year; this is an ideal opportunity for nurses working with patients who have a LTC to review them and their medication.
- The condition(s) to be treated and a single aim of treatment. A term to cover a wide patient group may be preferable, e.g. using the term 'Inflammatory Arthritis' thus enabling the nurse to prescribe for a variety of conditions e.g. AS, RA, CTD, etc. Likewise, the aim of treatment could be 'To control inflammation and limit the progression of the disease'.
- A list of medications that are to be prescribed—defined by class, e.g. NSAID or by named drug, e.g. diclofenac.

Examples of CMPs can be found at the Department of Health website: www.dh.gov.uk/—select 'Medicines' and type in 'clinical management plans' for templates and examples

Reference

1. Beckwith S, Franklin P (2006). *Oxford Handbook of Nurse Prescribing*. Oxford University Press, Oxford.

The nurse prescriber: managing drug interactions

Patients with arthritis often have other comorbid conditions, may be elderly, and are usually taking several drugs at any one time which makes drug interactions more likely. It is therefore essential that nurse prescribers identify and avoid use of concomitant drugs that are likely to cause the patient harm. Nurses must be aware of the pharmacokinetics and pharmacodynamics of the drugs and check the SPC and *BNF*.

Adverse event reporting

A nurse prescriber must complete a full nursing assessment on the patient and should be aware of potential drug interactions and the risks specifically related to the patient's current medications and individual comorbidities or other risk factors. In the event of an adverse event the nurse should:
- Report it via yellow card reporting scheme found in the *BNF* to the CSM or report to the Medicines Healthcare products Regulatory Agency at 🖰 www.mhra.gov.uk
- Report the details in the patient's medical records.
- Notify the Medicines Management Committee within their organization.
- Make colleagues in your department and hospital Trust aware.
- Report it to pharmacovigilance department of the drug company whose product is alleged to have caused the adverse event.

Therapies unlicensed—exceptions that apply

- Controlled drugs—only by independent midwife prescribers and nurse prescribers working in palliative care.
- A clinical trials certificate—enables unlicensed and off-label drugs to be prescribed independently.

A supplementary prescribing arrangement needs to be in place to support nurse prescribing of:
- Controlled drugs.
- Unlicensed drugs.
- Off-label drugs, such as using a licensed drug for an unlicensed indication, e.g. amitriptyline prescribed for neuropathic pain instead of at higher doses for depression.

Further reading

Beckwith S, Franklin P (2006). *Oxford Handbook of Nurse Prescribing*. Oxford University Press, Oxford.

Ryan S (2007). *Drug therapy in rheumatology nursing*. John Wiley and Sons Ltd., Chichester.

Nurse specialists: rapid access and early arthritis clinics

Rapid access to specific services (such as early arthritis clinics) has developed to ensure patients benefit from prompt early diagnosis and rapid aggressive treatment. In addition, improved access for patients with severe side effects, e.g. breathing difficulties with suspicion of suspected pneumonitis or gross knee effusion and suspicion of septic arthritis, can access rapid referral.

Principles of monitoring

Monitoring does not just refer to the blood testing schedule for DMARDS but should incorporate a holistic assessment of the patient. A typical monitoring visit should involve the following actions:

- Review of medical records, treatment plans, and current health status of patient. Considers joint assessment and expected treatment response.
- The DMARD treatment and monitoring plans. Dose escalation/cessation of treatment in accordance with local, regional, or national guidelines.
- Monitoring of overall disease status taking into consideration drug therapies and patient issues/ diagnosis.
- Inflammatory markers (ESR/CRP) to assess disease activity.
- Review of other systems evaluating weight, blood, urine, and physical examination function, e.g. renal and liver profiles, blood pressure. Consider results in the context of treatment plan, health status, and issues indicating referral or review of treatment.
- Identify side effects such as rash, nausea, diarrhoea, mouth ulcers, headache, dyspnoea, cough, hair loss, signs of infection, and bruising or bleeding.
- Adhere to Monitoring time frames and identify appropriate steps in treatment pathway, e.g. reduction in monitoring frequency.
- Support and advise patients on symptom control e.g. short-term use of NSAIDs and analgesics whilst waiting for DMARDs to become effective.
- Document information on blood monitoring and educate the patient about the values and results.
- Joint changes or damage that may indicate prompt referral, e.g. presence of nodules, rashes, wasted muscles, or flexion deformities requiring referral or review of treatment.
- Identify any educational opportunities or gaps in the patient's knowledge and provide education tailored to the patient's needs.
- Provide 1st point of contact for patients, e.g. access to telephone advice line and reasons to contact the nursing service.
- Document fully all decisions made, actions taken, and information given, and convey this information in writing to the GP and patient.

Index